MAGNETIC RESONANCE IN CHEMISTRY AND MEDICINE

D0221787

St. Louis Community College
at Meramec
Library

Magnetic Resonance in Chemistry and Medicine

RAY FREEMAN

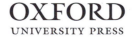
OXFORD

UNIVERSITY PRESS

OXFORD

UNIVERSITY PRESS

Great Clarendon Street, Oxford OX2 6DP

Oxford University Press is a department of the University of Oxford.
It furthers the University's objective of excellence in research, scholarship,
and education by publishing worldwide in

Oxford New York

Auckland Bangkok Buenos Aires Cape Town Chennai
Dar es Salaam Delhi Hong Kong Istanbul Karachi Kolkata
Kuala Lumpur Madrid Melbourne Mexico City Mumbai Nairobi
São Paulo Shanghai Taipei Tokyo Toronto

Oxford is a registered trade mark of Oxford University Press
in the UK and in certain other countries

Published in the United States
by Oxford University Press Inc., New York

© Ray Freeman, 2003

The moral rights of the author have been asserted
Database right Oxford University Press (maker)

First published 2003

All rights reserved. No part of this publication may be reproduced,
stored in a retrieval system, or transmitted, in any form or by any means,
without the prior permission in writing of Oxford University Press,
or as expressly permitted by law, or under terms agreed with the appropriate
reprographics rights organization. Enquiries concerning reproduction
outside the scope of the above should be sent to the Rights Department,
Oxford University Press, at the address above

You must not circulate this book in any other binding or cover
and you must impose this same condition on any acquirer

A Catalogue record for this title is available from the British Library

Library of Congress Cataloging in Publication Data

Freeman, Ray, 1932-
Magnetic resonance in chemistry and medicine / Ray Freeman.
Includes bibliographical references and index.
1. Nuclear magnetic resonance spectroscopy 2. Magnetic resonance imaging   I. Title.
QD96.N8F75 2003   543′.0877–dc21   2002193109

ISBN 0 19 926061 3 (hbk. : acid-free paper)
ISBN 0 19 926225 X (pbk. : acid-free paper)

1 3 5 7 9 10 8 6 4 2

Typeset by Kolam Information Services
Printed in Great Britain on acid-free paper by Biddles Ltd, Guildford & King's Lynn

To our grandsons, Tristan and Philip

Preface

One of the most impressive examples of high-technology health care is the magnetic resonance imaging (MRI) scanner, a device for viewing the internal structure of the human body without surgery of any kind. It exploits the magnetic properties of the nucleus of the atom to obtain these images. The same fundamental principles govern the science of high-resolution nuclear magnetic resonance (NMR) spectroscopy, which allows the chemist to picture the architecture of molecules too small to be seen under the most powerful microscope. This book draws together these quite different applications and emphasizes their common origins. The atomic nucleus obeys the laws of quantum mechanics, but it is nevertheless possible to understand MRI and NMR without delving into mathematics or heavy physics. All the complex manipulations of the tiny magnetic nuclei can be described in a largely pictorial fashion. The aim of this book is to explain magnetic resonance in the simplest possible terms and to show that the chemical and medical applications are based on the same fundamental concepts. The differences are largely in the practical details.

The basic principles underlying magnetic resonance are set out in the first nine chapters of this book, making few assumptions about prior knowledge. This sets the stage for the treatment of chemical and medical applications in the remaining chapters, with extensive cross-referencing. Every effort has been made to keep the descriptions as simple as possible, so citations of the scientific literature have been kept to a minimum. However, there are suggestions for further general reading at the end of each chapter. Because the various practitioners of chemistry, magnetic resonance and clinical medicine have their own particular brands of scientific jargon, care has been taken to avoid the use of abbreviations and acronyms as far as possible.

The aim is to make this text accessible to a wide spectrum of readers—from busy medical practitioners at one extreme to undergraduate students of chemistry at the other. A broad general understanding of magnetic resonance should prove of interest to doctors who make use of the MRI scanner, and to those of their patients who wish to learn more about these daunting machines, even if it is only the question of their own personal safety. Many in the medical fraternity will benefit from a general appreciation of how high-resolution NMR has advanced our understanding of human biochemistry, diagnostic medicine, and the search for new drugs. Chapters on *in vivo* NMR spectroscopy and the analysis of body fluids examine the way human body reacts to drugs, toxic substances, or disease.

Chemists and biochemists who use NMR spectroscopy in their everyday investigations have much to gain by extending their horizons to cover the exciting new developments in imaging and *in vivo* spectroscopy, as one justification for their research is the eventual benefit to health care. Insights and cross-fertilization from the less-familiar realms of the subject can be very valuable. Anyone interested in how the human mind works (cognitive neuroscience) will find a chapter devoted to the fascinating new developments in functional magnetic resonance imaging of the brain. Each disparate group has something useful to learn from the others.

In a book that covers such a wide range of different applications, it has been very helpful to have established experts look over specific sections on the alert for 'howlers'. So I would like to thank Peter Barker, Jim Feeney, Gareth Morris, Jeremy Nicholson, Toshiaki Nishida, Brian Ross, and Kamil Ugurbil for kindly reading and correcting parts of the text. Several colleagues have been kind enough to provide illustrations of typical spectra or images, notably Peter Barker, William Edelstein, Laurie Hall, Eriks Kupče, Gareth Morris, Jeremy Nicholson, Toshiaki Nishida, Brian Ross, and Michael Woodley. Finally, I owe a huge debt of gratitude to my editor, Michael Rodgers, for his long-standing patience and unwavering support for a project that, at times, seemed to have no end.

Jesus College, Cambridge
R. F. *May 2002*

Contents

1

Introduction

1.1 Imaging and spectroscopy

If the man in the street has heard about magnetic resonance at all it is probably in the context of the 'MRI scanner', a large and expensive piece of equipment used to diagnose medical problems associated with the vital internal organs—the heart, brain, liver, kidney, etc. In his mind, he might well associate this machine with the earlier X-ray device, sometimes called the CT (computer-aided tomography) scanner. If ever he needs medical examination with a magnetic resonance scanner, he will be relieved to learn that it is a 'non-invasive' technique, in the sense that it does not involve the more usual exploratory surgery with a sharp knife. He should also feel reassured, because no ionizing radiation is involved, in contrast to X-ray procedures. To the medical fraternity X-ray scanning and magnetic resonance imaging are usually grouped under radiology, and they occupy the high-technology end of medical practice, reminiscent of the wizardry visualized in certain science fiction films.

Anyone acquainted with chemistry would have a more intimate relationship with magnetic resonance, for this subject has been turned on its head by the introduction of nuclear magnetic resonance (NMR) spectroscopy. Soon after the first observations of NMR in bulk matter at Harvard[1] and Stanford[2] it was discovered that the observed NMR frequencies were sensitive to the chemical environment of the nucleus[3–6] although the effect is quite small. Within a year a group at Stanford[7] demonstrated that the three chemically distinct protons in the ethanol molecule gave a spectrum with three corresponding NMR responses and it became clear that high-resolution NMR offered a powerful new technique for chemical studies.

The structures of all relatively simple chemical molecules were established many years ago by painstaking experiments in 'wet chemistry', followed by deductions made from the way chemicals react. Many of these structures are based on the principle that the carbon atom has four valence bonds, usually pointing in a tetrahedral arrangement in space. High resolution NMR has confirmed these simple structures and goes much further, allowing us to probe the detailed architecture of macromolecules such as proteins. These days, no serious structural research in chemistry or biochemistry can be carried out without access to a high resolution NMR spectrometer.

Magnetic resonance is a technique that allows us to meet two very important challenges—the investigation of the internal organs of the human body without surgery, and the study of the structure of molecules too small to be observed under the most powerful microscope. These two fields of science may seem far removed, but it turns out that the underlying basic principles of magnetic resonance are common to both; they exploit the magnetic properties of the nucleus of the atom. The clinician and the chemist rely on identical physical laws. Furthermore, the clinician has much to gain by familiarity with the chemical aspects of the subject, and every chemist should be aware of the amazing new developments in medicine. The two disciplines begin to overlap in an application called magnetic resonance spectroscopy (MRS), where a high resolution NMR spectrum is recorded from a localized region of the body, for example the heart, or a particular muscle. Perhaps the most exciting new area is functional magnetic resonance imaging (fMRI), in which a particular region of the brain 'lights up' according to a specific stimulus. Even the layman should be aware of this development, if ever it proves to be a viable technique for monitoring what a person is actually thinking.

The chemical and medical aspects of magnetic resonance have hitherto been treated as separate disciplines, for both have become vast subjects in their own right. But if we draw a schematic diagram of the applications of magnetic resonance in chemistry and medicine it is clear that the tentacles of NMR are inextricably entwined with those of MRI (Figure 1.1). To take just one simple example, the study of human body tissues and fluids relies heavily on high resolution NMR spectroscopy to identify and quantify trace amounts of important chemicals, but the thrust of this research is undoubtedly medical (§ 15.1). It therefore makes sense to consider the entire edifice of magnetic resonance as a single entity, not least because the underlying science is the same for both MRI and NMR.

Any rigorous treatment of magnetic resonance must be grounded on quantum mechanics, but this monograph takes the view that all the essential concepts can be described in a pictorial fashion, with a minimum of mathematical formalism. Quantum effects can be explained in terms of the existence of a set of energy levels of the nuclear spin system. The images we see (or the spectra we record) involve radiation at just the right frequency to cause a 'transition' from one such level to another. That is why we speak of 'quanta' of radiation. These frequencies fall in the radiofrequency range, similar to those used to transmit television pictures.

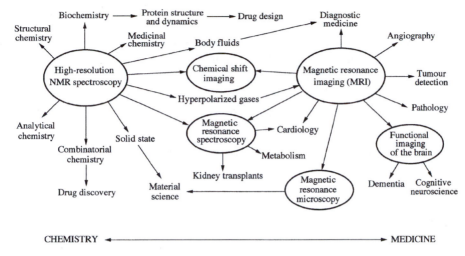

Figure 1.1 The chemical and medical applications of magnetic resonance are inextricably linked, although the technique of high-resolution NMR was established two decades before magnetic resonance imaging. Applications like magnetic resonance spectroscopy and chemical shift imaging borrow from both disciplines.

1.2 Nuclear magnetism

The medical profession has quietly dropped the term 'nuclear' from the vocabulary of magnetic resonance, on the grounds that it could be unnecessarily alarming to a patient—the nuclei we deal with are not radioactive, they are simply an integral part of the atoms and molecules that make up human tissue or everyday chemical substances. They are far removed from the dangerously radioactive nuclei (uranium or plutonium) used to create nuclear fission. It is the innocuous magnetic properties of the nucleus that are of interest here.

We are taught that an atom is made up of a small central nucleus surrounded by a diffuse cloud of electrons. The nucleus accounts for most of the mass of the atom, and it also carries a positive electric charge. If we disregard the 'atom smashing' experiments of the physicists, that is about all we need to know about the nucleus, except for one very important property—many nuclei are continually spinning about an axis. This is such a fundamental property that we often speak of a 'spin' as if this were a noun synonymous with 'nucleus'. Now a spinning charge creates an electric current. Since the work of Faraday we know that a circulating electric current generates a magnetic field, so these nuclei behave like tiny bar magnets.

If these tiny nuclear magnets are immersed in a magnetic field they line up with one another, creating *macroscopic* magnetism, but the resultant is extremely weak, for reasons set out below.

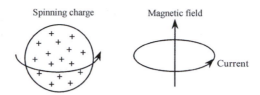

For our purposes, the most important types of nuclei that possess 'spin' are hydrogen (the proton), carbon-13, nitrogen-15, fluorine-19 and phosphorus-31. Their characteristic properties are set out in Table 1.1. Of these, the proton will turn out to be the most important because it gives a strong signal and is widely distributed. Hereafter we shall use the terms 'nucleus' and 'spin' essentially interchangeably. According to the context, 'spin' may mean a single nucleus or a particular spin species, for example, protons.

There are also two very important *non-magnetic* nuclei—carbon-12 and oxygen-16; these are both almost 100 % abundant in nature. For the purposes of magnetic resonance we may disregard their presence in a given molecule. For example, in ethanol (CH_3CH_2OH) we are concerned only with the protons; the carbon-12 and oxygen-16 atoms give no magnetic resonance response at all. (However, in some special applications we might deliberately set out to look for some very weak NMR signals from one of the low-abundance isotopes, carbon-13 or oxygen-17.)

There is also an entire class of nuclei (including nitrogen-14, chlorine-35 and chlorine-37) that are also magnetic but the macroscopic effect is quickly dissipated and is consequently difficult to detect. This is because the nuclear charge is distorted from the spherical shape, rendering them very susceptible to interaction with local electric fields (§ 4.1). These so-called 'quadrupolar' nuclei can be disregarded for many NMR purposes—we can therefore concentrate on the class of nuclei that have a spherical distribution of electric charge, like those listed in Table 1.1.

Much of our interest will be focused on the proton because it possesses very strong nuclear magnetism, is widely distributed in chemical compounds, and, in

Table 1.1 Properties of some common magnetic nuclei

Nucleus	Abundance	Frequency[a]	Frequency[b]
Proton	100 %	900.0 MHz	63.9 MHz
Carbon-13	1.1 %	226.3 MHz	16.1 MHz
Nitrogen-15	0.4 %	91.2 MHz	6.5 MHz
Fluorine-19	100 %	846.7 MHz	60.1 MHz
Phosphorus-31	100 %	364.3 MHz	25.9 MHz

[a] At a magnetic field of 21.14 tesla (NMR); [b] At 1.5 tesla (MRI)

the form of water, makes up a large proportion of the human body. When we obtain a routine magnetic resonance image of a patient we are in fact observing the spatial distribution of water protons. Chemical applications of magnetic resonance tend to explore a wider range of magnetic nuclei than do imaging experiments, depending on the composition of the sample under investigation.

As mentioned above, the magnetic properties of the nucleus may not be evident under normal everyday circumstances. First of all the patient or the sample of material must be placed in a strong magnetic field. Even then, there is very little overall magnetism because the individual nuclear magnets tend to cancel one another. Think of the nuclei as tiny compass needles that have the special property that they can only align themselves along the applied field direction (parallel) or opposed to it (antiparallel). This is because quantum mechanics permits only two states, not a continuum of states. We often represent these two possible orientations as little arrows (vectors) pointing 'up' or 'down' with respect to the direction of the applied magnetic field.

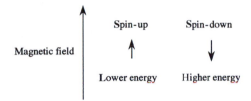

The 'spin-up' case is slightly favoured over the 'spin-down' case, although the difference in energy is very small. Later we shall see that the tiny excess population of 'spin-up' nuclei turns out to have a very important influence on the ability to detect magnetic resonance.

1.3 Resonance

A platoon of soldiers marching across a bridge would be ordered to 'break step' for fear that the regular tramp, tramp, tramp in unison might force the bridge into a dangerous vibration at its natural 'resonance' frequency, possibly collapsing the structure. This would only be a real problem if the cadence of the march closely matched the mechanical vibration frequency of the bridge. Resonance effects are quite widespread in the mechanical world—the tuning fork is a good example.

Resonance is a key feature of MRI and NMR phenomena. We can only make nuclear spins jump between their two energy states by applying radiation at precisely the right frequency—any other frequency is quite ineffective. Hence the term 'magnetic resonance'. So what is so special about this particular frequency? Well, the picture of nuclear magnets aligned parallel or antiparallel to the external magnetic field is something of an oversimplification. We should rather say that the vectors representing nuclear spins *precess* about the direction of the field, moving on the surface of a cone, but there are still only two possibilities, which we can continue to call 'spin-up' and 'spin-down':

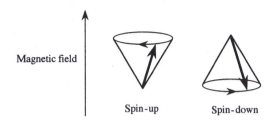

The frequency of this precession (ω) is in fact the resonance frequency. It is called the *Larmor frequency*[8] and it is directly proportional to the strength of the applied magnetic field (B_0) according to the expression

$$\omega = \gamma B_0$$

1.1

where γ is a characteristic constant for the nucleus in question—called the *gyromagnetic ratio*. This proportionality pervades all of magnetic resonance; whenever there is some effect that changes the magnetic field, there is always a corresponding proportional shift of the Larmor precession frequency.

Early NMR experiments were performed by slowly sweeping the radiofrequency until it reached this resonance condition, then measuring the tiny absorption of energy as nuclei were 'flipped' from the lower energy level to the upper level. Present-day experiments operate in a distinctly different mode where an intense pulse of radiofrequency energy 'shocks' the nuclei into emitting their characteristic resonance frequency, rather like a sharply-struck tuning fork. Just as the tuning fork continues to 'sing' for a few seconds, the note slowly dying away, the nuclear spin response persists for a few seconds, becoming weaker and weaker with time. This decay is caused by a process known as 'relaxation' which we shall examine in detail later (§ 4.5). The magnetic resonance response to the radiofrequency pulse is known as the *free precession signal* or the *free induction decay* and it is this tiny transient signal that is amplified electronically, detected, and then converted into either a spectrum (for high-resolution NMR) or an image (for MRI).

1.4 Spies at work

How do these arcane properties help us study human disease (or indeed the structure of molecules)? Consider this everyday analogy. Someone strikes a sequence of certain keys on a piano. Without observing this action directly, a musician with the gift of absolute pitch could identify the notes and deduce the locations of the keys on the keyboard. He has translated *frequency* information into *position*. Magnetic resonance imaging employs the same principle—a frequency is detected and used to deduce the location of the spins that generated that frequency.

Think of the nucleus as a spy, present in all living, and indeed, all inanimate matter. For the moment we can focus our attention on the hydrogen nucleus (the proton). The human body is made up of a high proportion of water and fat, both of which contain protons. The proton acts as a spy, reporting back a radiofrequency (its natural Larmor precession frequency) corresponding to the exact value of the magnetic field at his location. If we deliberately vary the intensity of the magnetic field applied across a human patient, let us say a high field at the head, falling off to a lower field at the toes, then the spy 'knows' where he is located with respect to the main axis of the body. The field *gradient* defines a specific direction, and the spy uses the local value of the field as a reference to establish his position in that dimension. He 'broadcasts' this information to the outside world as the Larmor precession frequency, always exactly proportional to the local magnetic field strength. If the measurement is twice repeated with field gradients in the other two dimensions, the spy can then report all three spatial coordinates. We often speak of 'encoding' the spatial information in the form of a frequency; once again implicitly employing the vocabulary of espionage.

In this manner the MRI technique generates a three-dimensional picture of the density of protons within the patient. In practice such a three-dimensional array is awkward to handle and we normally work with a two-dimensional display from a selected 'slice' through the subject. (Note that this 'slice' is defined by magnetic resonance conditions and in no sense involves physically *sectioning* the patient.) The relative intensities in the MRI scan may be represented on a grey-scale or they may be colour-coded. The radiologist is trained to interpret any abnormalities in this image. For example, if a tumour has developed within a particular organ, its presence may show up as an enhanced proton signal from that region, a bright area on the MRI scan.

The MRI information is thus loosely related to that obtained from an X-ray scanner, but we shall see that it is far more detailed and specific. The magnetic resonance technique is said to be non-invasive, in the sense that it does not involve the use of a scalpel, although we should remember that the subject is bathed in an intense magnetic field, with rapidly-switched applied field gradients, and penetrated by electromagnetic fields in the radiofrequency region, which in certain circumstances could cause undesirable heating effects (§ 13.4). However, unlike X-ray tomography, ionizing radiation is not involved, and tissues are not damaged. Our only intervention has been to change some nuclei from the 'spin-up' state to the 'spin-down' state, and vice versa. After a few seconds to allow the spins to return to their equilibrium condition ('relaxation'), there is no evidence to show that a magnetic resonance experiment has been performed. Nothing has been permanently altered by the MRI scan.

The CT scanner differentiates very clearly between bone and soft tissue, in effect giving a clear picture of the skeletal structure, but is less effective than MRI in distinguishing between various types of soft tissue. Indeed, MRI contrast can be improved by any one of an entire armoury of special techniques, based on relaxation, diffusion, flow effects, oxygenation level, or the deliberate injection of chemical reagents (although here the 'non-invasive' claim is infringed to some extent). This very flexibility is characteristic of magnetic resonance in general—the image (or the spectrum) is susceptible to complex manipulations that can improve the quality and provide more detailed information.

Our spy has a quite different role in chemistry. He still reports on the local magnetic field, broadcasting this information as a radiofrequency signal, but normally no field gradients are applied, indeed the magnetic field is made as uniform as possible, so the resonance frequency is no longer a function of the coordinates in space. Each individual nucleus is surrounded by a cloud of electrons. If we represent the applied magnetic field by a set of parallel 'lines of force' then the closer the lines of force, the stronger the field. The extranuclear electrons tend to bend these lines away from the nucleus, which then experiences a magnetic field that is lower than the external field. This very slight reduction in magnetic field manifests itself as a corresponding lowering of the Larmor precession frequency of the nucleus. In effect the electrons act to 'shield' the nucleus from the external magnetic field to a very small degree (§ 7.1).

The structural chemist has to deal with molecules that contain many spies, in different electronic environments. So each spy has a different frequency to transmit—he reports on the local density of electrons, which in turn determines the chemical properties of that particular atom. Only the outermost electrons are affected by the formation of chemical bonds—they are referred to as *valence* electrons. Chemical bonding modifies the shape and density of this outer electron cloud, slightly changing the magnetic field at the nucleus. The corresponding change in the nuclear precession frequency is called the *chemical shift*. Instead of a single Larmor frequency there is a characteristic *spectrum* of discrete frequencies. For example, the ethanol molecule mentioned above contains three different types of hydrogen atom, situated in the CH_3, CH_2, and OH groups, with three different chemical shifts, leading to three resonance lines in the NMR spectrum.[7] Our spy reports three different frequencies (with intensities in the ratio 3:2:1). To the chemist this is an invaluable 'fingerprint' that identifies the molecule and determines its structure. Martin Packard, the physicist who first observed the three resonance lines of ethanol, claims that he never really believed the molecular structures written by chemists until he saw this spectrum.

The chemical shift is a parameter of enormous interest to an analytical or structural chemist for it allows him to identify the chemical environment of any given atom. For example, a nitro group is known to withdraw electrons from neighbouring atoms, so a proton close to a nitro group has a weakened electron cloud which has a smaller shielding effect on the applied magnetic field. The resonance frequency is thus slightly increased. Protons on aromatic rings are affected by the π electrons which circulate around the ring, generating a current that induces a slightly increased magnetic field at the proton sites, so they have a slightly higher resonance frequency.

Of course a molecule of any complexity harbours several nuclear spies, and they provide further useful information by informing on their near neighbours. Since each nucleus behaves like a tiny bar magnet, it creates a weak additional magnetic field at the site of its neighbour, positive or negative depending on whether the nucleus is aligned 'spin-up' or 'spin-down'. This rather weak effect, called *spin–spin coupling*, is carried through the electrons that form the chemical bonds and consequently only operates over relatively short distances.[9]

Spin–spin coupling (represented by the symbol J) imposes a characteristic pattern on each chemically-shifted resonance response. The form of this 'spin multiplet' pattern depends on the number of close nuclear neighbours. Common patterns are the 1:1 doublet, the 1:2:1 triplet and the 1:3:3:1 quartet. These are analysed in detail in Chapter 8. They serve as an additional aid to the assignment of the NMR response to a particular site in the molecule. Ethanol has three such responses, a 1:2:1 triplet from the CH_3 group and a 1:3:3:1 quartet from the CH_2 group. The OH group is a special case (§ 7.8). It generates a single resonance line, as if it were not coupled to any of its neighbours in the molecule. We might think of it as a 'sleeper', a spy without any contact with his colleagues.

Owing to this wealth of information, spectrometers for structural chemistry are designed to have high resolving power in order to reveal all the interesting fine structure. This entails the use of an applied magnetic field that is extremely uniform in space and highly stable in time; otherwise the fine details of the spectrum would be blurred. We are talking about a resolving power of the order of one part in a thousand million; if an astronomical telescope could achieve a comparable resolving power it would be able to pick out an individual 40 cm rock on the surface of the Moon, at a distance of about 400,000 km. The technique is therefore known as *high-resolution* nuclear magnetic resonance. (In this chemistry context the term 'nuclear' has no negative connotations.)

Most clinical applications of magnetic resonance are principally concerned with the distribution of proton density, irrespective of chemical shift effects, so it is usual to apply magnetic field gradients so intense that they swamp any small differences in chemical shifts, coding only the spatial information. Nevertheless, it can sometimes be useful to exploit the chemical shift to distinguish different tissues, for example, water and fat. Indeed, two different images can be obtained, one reflecting the distribution of fatty tissue and the other the spatial distribution of water (§ 14.9). Even the spin–spin splitting can be put to good use, for example, to distinguish the important lactate moiety (which has a detectable spin–spin splitting) from other molecules that lack spin–spin interactions.

Chemical applications employ the highest possible applied magnetic field and the highest attainable field uniformity. The sample is usually a pure liquid or, more commonly, a solution in a deuterated solvent (so that there are no protons in the solvent to interfere with the spectrum of interest). It is contained in a cylindrical glass tube (usually 5 mm in diameter) which is often rotated about its long axis by an air turbine in order to increase the effective uniformity of the applied field. Field gradients are only applied to disperse unwanted signal components or to distinguish between different types of signal.

Medical applications employ much weaker magnetic fields; indeed there are regulations that limit the magnetic field that can be used for routine clinical examination of human patients to an intensity about fourteen times weaker than the highest field employed in high-resolution NMR spectroscopy. However, the magnets used for MRI are physically much larger since the enclosed volume has to be big enough to accept the entire human body.

We see that the two main applications of magnetic resonance—imaging and high resolution NMR—are related by the fact that they both use the nucleus as a probe of the local magnetic field. Both rely implicitly on the Larmor relationship between magnetic field and the resonance frequency. Magnetic resonance imaging uses the Larmor relationship to convert a position in space into a characteristic frequency; high resolution NMR uses it to measure chemical influences on the electron cloud that surrounds the nucleus.

It is easy to fall into the trap of assuming that the medical applications of magnetic resonance are more important than the chemical ones, they certainly touch many more people directly and entail a considerably higher expenditure on the equipment. But that would be to underestimate the pivotal role that high resolution NMR has had on chemistry in general, particularly the life-saving developments in pharmaceutical chemistry (Chapter 16) and biochemistry (Chapters 14 and 15). We must always bear in mind that MRI is only a diagnostic technique; it does not *cure* disease. Any subsequent therapy must rely on drugs.

The clinical and chemical fields are combined in magnetic resonance spectrosopy (MRS), where a high-resolution NMR spectrum is obtained from a particular organ, for example, the kidney, heart, or brain. This involves localization of the excitation, using methods related to imaging, yet detecting the response under high-resolution conditions (Chapter 14). This technique, sometimes known as *in vivo* spectroscopy, offers the possibility of studying metabolic processes within a living animal or patient. Another hybrid technique is chemical shift imaging, which produces different images according to the chemical species under investigation (§ 14.9). These applications strengthen the argument for treating MRI and NMR under the same head.

1.5 A word about jargon

To the layman reading about magnetic resonance for the first time, there is a disagreeable surprise in store—practitioners of this art have constructed a defensive barrier of abbreviations and acronyms that make it very hard to follow their scientific presentations, be they written or oral. Although these terms are well-known within the magnetic resonance 'family', they can be bewildering to the outsider. Some are very common, while others are quite specialized and appear to have been invented to satisfy a very narrow clique of investigators. They fall into four main categories.

The first group comprises the terms for the various branches of magnetic resonance, NMR (nuclear magnetic resonance), MRI (magnetic resonance imaging) and MRS (magnetic resonance spectroscopy). Their use is perhaps justified by the fact that they are required so often, and abbreviations save time and space. In this book these will be the only abbreviations used without further explanation. There are also a few related terms such as CT (computer-aided tomography), and PET (positron emission tomography) that also seem to have entered the common lexicon.

The second type of abbreviation is widespread among magnetic resonance scientists—the use of *acronyms* to describe popular radiofrequency pulse sequences, for example, STEAM, an abbreviation for stimulated echo acquisition mode (§ 14.8). Fortunately the total number of these sequences in common usage is relatively small and they can sometimes add a certain humour to the proceedings. Without a specific name, it would be very tedious to define a pulse sequence in detail every time it is mentioned, and an acronym is easy to remember. Except for the situation where experts are addressing experts, these acronyms should always be defined, and the appropriate references cited. In the present text, acronyms will be kept to the absolute minimum; a list of those used is set out in Table 1.2.

The third category comprises abbreviations for the names of biochemical molecules commonly encountered in these magnetic resonance studies. These three- or four-letter codes are not acronyms and are very difficult to decipher unless the speaker or writer defines them once and for all at the beginning of the presentation. Common examples are NAA (N-acetyl aspartate) and GABA (γ-aminobutyric acid) but the list of less obvious names is endless. The root of the problem lies in the *specialized* nature of biochemical research; the scientist has to deal every day with the same, very limited, number of chemical substances and soon slips into the habit of using jargon. However, in presentations or scientific papers he risks losing his audience if just one such abbreviation remains obscure. It is encouraging to see that some journals now require that the authors provide a list of chemical abbreviations used in their text. In diagrams or slides, where space is at a premium, it may well be necessary to annotate the individual resonances of a high resolution NMR spectrum with the abbreviated forms, but the figure legend should nevertheless spell out the full name of these compounds.

The fourth category, which seems to have even less merit than the others, represents abbreviations of pathology terms such as NHL (non-Hodgkin's lymphoma) and TLE (temporal lobe epilepsy). While a husband and wife may well use pet names for each other, they are obliged to employ their given names for communication with the rest of the world. There seems to be no good reason why clinicians should not spell out their terminology in talks and in the scientific

Table 1.2 Acronyms and abbreviations

BEST	Blipped echo-planar single-pulse technique
BOLD	Blood oxygen level dependent contrast
BURP	Band-selective, uniform response, pure-phase pulse
COSY	Correlation spectroscopy
CP-MAS	Cross-polarization with magic angle spinning
CPMG	Carr–Purcell–Meiboom–Gill
CSF	Cerebrospinal fluid
DOSY	Diffusion-ordered spectroscopy
EXSY	Exchange spectroscopy
fMRI	Functional magnetic resonance imaging of the brain
HMQC	Heteronuclear multiple-quantum correlation
HOHAHA	Homonuclear Hartmann–Hahn technique
HPLC	High-performance liquid chromatography
HSQC	Heteronuclear single-quantum correlation
INADEQUATE	Incredible natural abundance double-quantum transfer experiment
INEPT	Insensitive nuclei enhanced by polarization transfer
ISIS	Image-selected *in vivo* spectroscopy
MLEV	Malcolm Levitt's phase cycle
MRI	Magnetic resonance imaging
MRS	Magnetic resonance spectroscopy
NOESY	Nuclear Overhauser enhancement spectroscopy
NMR	Nuclear magnetic resonance
PRESS	Point-resolved spectroscopy
ROESY	Rotating-frame Overhauser enhancement spectroscopy
STEAM	Stimulated echo acquisition mode
TOCSY	Total correlation spectroscopy
WAHUHA	Magic pulse cycle of Waugh, Huber and Haeberlen
WALTZ	Wideband alternating-phase technique for zero splitting
WURST	Adiabatic soft radiofrequency pulse shaped like a sausage

literature; the modest savings in space offered by abbreviations will never be matched by the confusion that they create. Does HI signify hydrogen iodide or hypoxic-ischaemic?

Put together all four types of abbreviation in the same article and we have a classic problem of impenetrable cryptography, similar to that which has made computer jargon such a problem. For this reason the present text avoids abbreviations as far as possible.

2

Excitation of magnetic resonance

2.1 Equipment

Before we consider the instrumental equipment needed for magnetic resonance experiments it is perhaps helpful to take a look at a more familiar subject—television. A television transmitter sends out intense radiation at a precise frequency which is picked up by an aerial on the roof of the house. The greater the distance between the transmitter and this antenna, the weaker the signal that is detected. This tiny signal is amplified in a tuned receiver and processed to form a picture. If the house is too far from the television station, or the antenna misaligned, or the receiver poorly tuned, the detected signal is so weak that it is lost in a sea of random noise arising from the electronics. The television screen shows only 'snow', a chaotic pattern of bright spots on a dark background, containing no useful information. Magnetic resonance has many features in common with this familiar scenario—there is a powerful transmitter operating at a fixed frequency, but the signals from the nuclear spins, picked up by the receiver, are very weak indeed, so some degree of noise is always present in NMR spectra or MRI scans. This is probably the most serious limitation of the magnetic resonance method.

In all magnetic resonance experiments (NMR or MRI) there are certain instrumental requirements common to all applications First, the sample must be immersed in a strong magnetic field (for convenience we shall take the word 'sample' to include not only a chemical substance in a glass tube but also that part of the human anatomy under investigation—the head, the chest, a limb, or an internal organ). Then radiofrequency radiation is fed from a transmitter to a coil surrounding or very close to the chosen sample. This induces a weak radio-frequency response from the nuclear spins, picked up on the coil and fed to a sensitive tuned receiver which amplifies this tiny signal and converts it to a form suitable for processing and display. This implies conversion of the signal into digital form followed by manipulation in a computer. A schematic diagram of these basic units is set out in Figure 2.1.

2.2 The magnet

The first requirement for NMR or MRI is to provide a strong magnetic field. In childhood, our initial experience of magnetism was probably with a toy 'horse-shoe' magnet that has the apparently magical property that iron or steel objects are attracted to the vicinity of the two 'poles' (one labelled north and the other south). Although there is nothing to see or touch there, this particular region of space between the poles clearly possesses some special property—physicists call this a 'field'. The magnetic field has a 'shape' which can be made evident by sprinkling iron filings onto a piece of card placed just over the horseshoe magnet. The filings line up along the 'lines of force' that run from one pole to the other. The magnetic field is strongest where these lines of force are packed close to-gether.

There are also bar magnets with the north and south poles at their extremities. Two such magnets may attract or repel each other according to their relative configuration. For example, two north poles repel, whereas a north and a south pole attract. A magnetic compass, long used as an aid to navigation, consists of a bar magnet in the form of a needle mounted on a pivot so that the needle aligns itself along the direction of the earth's magnetic field. This is how we define the north and south poles of a magnet.

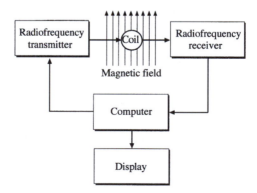

Figure 2.1 Schematic diagram showing the essential elements of a magnetic resonance device. The axis of the radiofrequency coil is at right angles to the direction of the main magnetic field.

Magnetic fields can also be created by passing a current through a coil of wire or 'solenoid'. This is the basis of the electric motor. The stronger the current and the more turns on the coil, the stronger the magnetic field. On the other hand, if a coil of wire is moved through an existing magnetic field, a current is induced in the wire—this is the basis of all electrical power generation. We shall see later (§ 3.1) that the same phenomenon is used to detect magnetic resonance signals—a tiny 'nuclear magnet' rotating inside a small coil of wire induces a high-frequency alternating current. This is the magnetic resonance signal.

Iron and steel have exceptionally strong magnetism because the individual magnetic atoms act in a cooperative manner, many atomic magnets lining up together in 'domains' where the magnetism is magnified by a large factor. These metals are said to be *ferromagnetic*. Most other materials are much more weakly magnetic. When placed near an existing magnetic field, some are drawn into the field (these are said to be *paramagnetic* materials) and others tend to be forced out of the field (these are called *diamagnetic* materials). Paramagnetic and dia-magnetic effects are so weak that we need a strong magnetic field and a rather sensitive measuring device to detect the resulting force. Fortunately, living systems fall into the diamagnetic category; we can normally disregard magnetic forces for most purposes, and even quite intense magnetic fields seem to have no detectable physiological effect (§ 13.1). So the MRI patient can be immersed in a strong magnetic field without any real danger; indeed he has no means of sensing the presence of the field. (However, we may need to qualify this statement for magnetic fields that change rapidly with time.)

The unit of magnetic field is the tesla, named after the scientist who invented the world's first alternating-current power station at Niagara Falls. One tesla is quite a strong field, as can be appreciated from the fact that the earth's magnetic field is only approximately 50 millionths of a tesla yet it is strong enough to move a compass needle. For the purposes of magnetic resonance we shall need fields somewhere in the range of 1–20 tesla. To generate such intense fields by passing electric current through a coil of copper wire requires enormously high currents with attendant heating effects that are usually prohibitive. This problem can be alleviated by winding the coil on a core of soft iron. For a given current and number of turns on the coil, the magnetic field is enormously increased. Unfortunately such *electromagnets* have an upper limit to the magnetic field (near 2.3 tesla), caused by magnetic 'saturation' of the soft iron. Increasing the current does not then increase the strength of the field.

Certain ferromagnetic materials (for example, an alloy containing alumi-nium, nickel and cobalt) can be permanently magnetized. Once energized by an electrical current, they retain their magnetism when the current is switched off. However, these permanent magnets use expensive materials and are limited to even lower maximum field strengths (around 1.4 tesla). They are only used for small-scale magnetic resonance experiments where low cost is the main consider-ation.

Most magnets used for magnetic resonance take a third route. When certain materials (special alloys involving metals such as niobium, tin, titanium or zirconium) are cooled to very low temperatures (typically only a few degrees above absolute zero) they lose all electrical resistance, and a current can be passed through them without any heating effect at all. They are said to be *superconducting*. This remarkable property means that a coil of wire can be initially energized with an electrical power supply, but when the power is cut off and the circuit closed, the current continues to flow 'forever'. There is absolutely no energy lost and the magnetic field is remarkably stable. This is one of the few physical phenomena that could be said to constitute perpetual motion. The associated technology is difficult and expensive, and it is probably true to say that most of the costs of state-of-the-art high-resolution NMR spectrometers and MRI systems stem from the superconducting magnet.[1] Future systems may employ new materials that retain their superconductivity at much higher temperatures, perhaps eventually at room temperature.

The most common form for a superconducting magnet for MRI is a solenoid with its axis horizontal. The patient is then eased into the core of the solenoid on a sliding support, either the whole body, or one limb, or just the head, depending on the site chosen to be imaged. An alternative magnet design employs a 'Helmholtz pair' of superconducting coils. This is a pair of parallel coils separated by a distance equal to the coil radius, a configuration that generates a particularly uniform magnetic field. The physical dimensions are large enough to allow a surgeon and technician to enter the enclosed space between the coils and perform surgery in the strong applied magnetic field, being guided by the MRI images (Figure 2.2).

Cooling is achieved by immersing the superconducting coil in a liquid helium bath, usually surrounded by a dewar vessel of liquid nitrogen (which is far cheaper to replenish, being, pint for pint, about as expensive as beer). There is an inherent danger associated with this scheme. If the magnet suffers a mechanical shock (for example, by impact with a large iron or steel object attracted by the strong field) or if the level of the helium cryogenic liquid is allowed to fall low enough to expose the coil to higher temperatures, there could be a catastrophic 'quench' of the magnetic field as the coil material makes a sudden transition from superconducting to resistive wire. The very high magnetic energy previously stored in the coil is rapidly transformed into heat, boiling away all the liquid helium in a very short time and possibly damaging the coil itself. Any large tool made of iron or steel should be rigorously excluded from a magnetic resonance laboratory because of the danger that it could be suddenly pulled up against the superconducting magnet and thus provoke a catastrophic quench. In order to avoid the danger of asphyxiation for personnel in the room as the oxygen in the air is displaced by helium and nitrogen gases, large high-field superconducting magnets must have a very efficient gas venting system. Fortunately, a quench is a relatively rare phenomenon and most superconducting solenoids used for magnetic resonance remain energized for years without any loss of magnetic field.

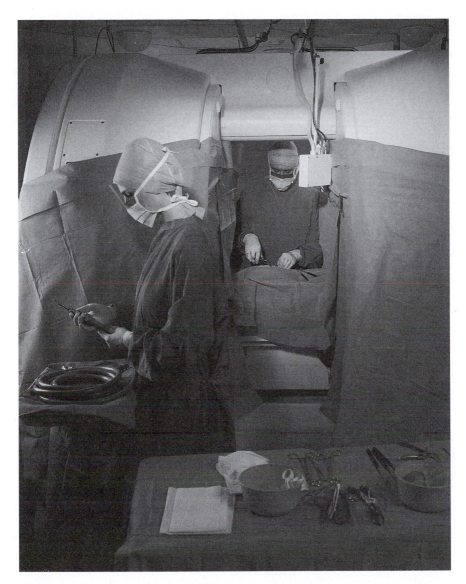

Figure 2.2 A 0.5 tesla superconducting magnet used for imaging, made up of a pair of super-conducting coils with a separation large enough to permit the surgeon to operate inside the main magnetic field, guided by magnetic resonance images. (© 1998 General Electric Company; photo-graph by courtesy of G. E. Medical Systems.)

The field strength of a superconducting magnet is inherently quite stable, and the solenoid also has a shielding effect, minimizing any fluctuating external magnetic fields generated in the laboratory. For high-resolution studies, further stabilization is provided by a servo-loop that monitors the dispersion-mode signal from the deuterium resonance of the solvent (often deuterochloroform), pulling the magnetic field back when it tends to drift away from the correct value. Another version of this deuterium signal (the absorption-mode) is employed as an aid to adjustment of the spatial uniformity of the magnetic field.

Scientists working in NMR and MRI often refer to the strength of their magnets in terms of MHz rather than tesla, which can be confusing to the outsider. They are merely using the Larmor condition, Equation 1.1, to relate the magnetic field intensity to the characteristic precession frequency of protons in that field. Frequency is directly proportional to field strength with a proportionality constant set by the magnetogyric ratio (γ) of the proton. Thus, a field strength of 21.14 tesla corresponds to a 900 MHz proton spectrometer, while a magnetic field of 1.5 tesla (common for MRI measurements) represents a proton resonance frequency of 63.9 MHz.

As a general rule we aim for a high magnetic field intensity because this favours a strong NMR response and improves the presentation of spectra. But the requirements for high-resolution NMR and MRI are rather different. Other things being equal, the magnetic field inside a solenoid is stronger the smaller the radius of the coil. A superconducting magnet for high-resolution NMR needs only a rather narrow bore, typically a diameter of about 50 mm, which makes it possible to generate fields as high as 21 tesla. A clinical MRI magnet must have a much larger enclosed volume in order to accept a human patient, and this limits the field that can be easily achieved. Because of this, and because of concerns about the possible physiological effects of very high fields, many MRI systems are operated at 1.5 tesla. Whole-body research systems at 4 tesla and even 7 tesla are in use, but the magnets are large and heavy. More seriously, the 'stray' field outside these higher-field magnets can extend a considerable distance, posing a potential hazard for passers-by with cardiac pacemakers (§ 13.1). Large (and costly) installations have to be built to house such high-field whole-body MRI systems.

Stray fields are also a nuisance in high-resolution NMR research. Scientists in nearby rooms often complain about this invisible 'magnetic pollution'. The fringe field of a high-resolution solenoid extends to considerable distances (particularly above and below the magnet), interfering with computer monitors and making heavy demands on precious laboratory space. There is a growing tendency to use actively shielded superconducting solenoids that limit the extent of these stray magnetic fields.

2.3 The radiofrequency

The detailed characteristics of the radiofrequency transmitter need not concern us too much here. Typically the source is a crystal-controlled oscillator at a frequency chosen to match the Larmor frequency of the nuclei under investigation. This is followed by a power amplifier designed to generate intense pulses of radiofrequency radiation. These pulses are under computer control because many experiments involve complex sequences of pulses and delays, where duration, intensity and phase of the various pulses are set according to some predetermined strategy for manipulating the nuclear spins.

The radiofrequency transmitter coil determines which region of the sample is excited. It must generate a radiofrequency field (B_1) that is at right angles to the external magnetic field (B_0). The intensity of the radiofrequency field is high inside the coil and much weaker outside, so in high-resolution NMR we may define an 'effective volume' of the sample—the region actually enclosed by the coil windings—which may be significantly smaller than the actual volume because the liquid is enclosed in a long cylindrical tube.

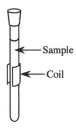

We can also define a 'filling factor' representing the proportion of the enclosed coil volume actually occupied by the sample; this directly influences the attainable sensitivity. Usually, but not always, the coil used to excite the nuclear spins (the transmitter coil) and the coil used to pick up the NMR response (the receiver coil) are one and the same. The properties of the receiver coil have an important influence on the quality of the magnetic resonance response; they are examined in detail in Chapter 3.

After radiofrequency amplification, the magnetic resonance response is converted to an audiofrequency signal and then put into digital form. From this point on, a computer takes over, processing the signal by an entire armoury of special techniques, the most important being Fourier transformation (§ 3.7).

2.4 Polarization

When a chemical sample is first placed in the magnet we are not quite ready to observe a signal; the nuclear spins need a certain time (usually measured in seconds) to become 'polarized'. A similar restriction applies when a human patient is eased into an imaging magnet, although the polarization delay would then be masked by the hiatus involved in positioning the patient. So what exactly do we mean by polarization and why is it not established immediately?

As we saw in Chapter 1, a nuclear spin may be 'up' or 'down' with respect to the applied magnetic field. These two states have slightly different energies and are called the ground state ('spin-up') and the excited state ('spin-down'). The separation ΔE of the two energy levels is directly proportional to the strength of the applied magnetic field. We might have imagined that all the nuclear spins would congregate in the ground state, but this is only the case at the absolute zero of temperature, some 300°C below room temperature. At ambient temperatures, where magnetic resonance experiments are normally performed, the energy associated with thermal agitation is very much greater than the separation between magnetic energy levels. Under these conditions the Boltzmann law states that, if the system is at equilibrium, the number of spins in the lower level N_{lower} is related to the number in the upper level, N_{upper} by the expression

$$(N_{lower} - N_{upper})/N_{lower} = \Delta E/kT \qquad \textbf{2.1}$$

where k is the Boltzmann constant and T is the absolute temperature. Equation 2.1 is a simplification of a slightly more complicated expression and is an excellent approximation provided that the energy gap ΔE is very much smaller than the thermal energy kT, which is the case in all present-day magnetic resonance applications. Consequently, the right-hand side of the equation is very small compared with unity, and the two energy levels are almost equally populated; there is only a very small excess of nuclei in the lower level. In a typical situation, if there are a 10,000 spins in the upper energy level, there would be 10,001 in the lower level. As the applied magnetic field is increased, ΔE increases in proportion, boosting the excess population in the ground state. This is the main reason for working at high magnetic fields.

Now Einstein showed that when a system is stimulated by radiation the intrinsic probabilities of upward and downward transitions between energy levels are the same, so the effect of most upward 'flips' is cancelled by an equal number of 'flops' in the opposite direction. If the two energy levels are equally populated, the effect of upward transitions is exactly matched by that of downward transitions; the energy absorbed by the nuclear spins is exactly equal to the energy emitted, so we can detect no signal at all. The spin system is said to be 'saturated'.

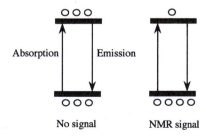

We rely entirely on the tiny excess population in the lower level if we wish to measure an absorption of energy by the nuclei. The rest of the spins, although they are in the vast majority, have no observable influence at all. This is the fundamental reason why magnetic resonance signals are rather weak.

When the sample (or the patient) is outside the magnet, both energy levels are equally populated to all intents and purposes, because ΔE is essentially negligible, being determined by any stray field from the magnet and the very weak magnetic field of the Earth. So we can write the initial condition as $N_{upper} = N_{lower}$, and the nuclear spin system is saturated. If it were possible to apply the external magnetic field very suddenly, the populations would remain equal, and initially we would see no magnetic resonance response. An excess population in the lower level builds up only quite slowly, by a mechanism called 'spin–lattice relaxation' which is treated in detail in § 4.1. Relaxation is an exponential process with a time constant of a few seconds; only when it is complete can we observe the full magnetic resonance response.

The most common mode of operation in MRI and NMR is to apply radio-frequency pulses repetitively, acquiring the magnetic resonance response after each pulse. The radiofrequency pulse equalizes the spin populations on the upper and lower levels and the system is temporarily saturated, but some spins then begin to drop down to the lower level by the process of spin–lattice relaxation and they can then be excited again by the next pulse. Very often, sensitivity considerations force us to repeat the pulse-acquire cycle quite quickly, with the result that the spin populations do not have time to reach equilibrium before the next excitation pulse. This partial saturation regime means that the signals have less than opti-mum intensity. A reasonable compromise has to be reached between saturation and relaxation, maintaining a sufficiently long 'recycle time' between successive excitations but nevertheless achieving a profitable rate of signal acquisition. It is rather like asking one's bank manager for an overdraft, it works better if the requests are judiciously spaced out in time.

2.5 The rotating reference frame

So far we have tacitly assumed that if we supply the correct radiofrequency, it will excite a magnetic resonance response. But we need to examine this mechanism more closely to see what happens if the transmitter frequency is not quite at reso-nance. When a pulse of radiofrequency energy is supplied from the transmitter, this radiofrequency (ω_0) must somehow interact with spins precessing at their characteristic Larmor frequencies (ω_L). In the general case there are many such Larmor frequencies—in high resolution NMR there is an entire *spectrum* of dis-crete resonances from the different chemical sites, while in MRI there is a con-tinuum of precession frequencies because the magnetic field varies with position (§ 12.2). To understand how the applied radiofrequency pulse excites all these different nuclear frequencies in a reasonably uniform manner we employ the concept of a rotating reference frame to simplify the analysis of the various motions.

Imagine you are riding a wooden horse on a merry-go-round. To an observer actually aboard the merry-go-round you would seem to be executing a simple up-and-down motion, but to another observer on *terra firma* the movement would appear to be far more complicated. It is all a question of choosing the most appropriate frame of reference. It turns out that there is a considerable simplification of magnetic resonance problems if we make a transformation into a new coordinate system, called the *rotating reference frame*.

The radiofrequency current supplied by the transmitter generates a linearly oscillating field. We decompose this into two equal rotating components, one turning clockwise and the other anticlockwise, and then use the component (B_1) that rotates in the same sense as the nuclear precession, disregarding the other component.

A new Cartesian coordinate frame (X, Y, Z) is now defined. It rotates about the Z axis at just the right rate to make B_1 stationary in the XY plane. Furthermore, it greatly reduces all the nuclear Larmor precession frequencies viewed in this frame. Frequencies that were expressed in hundreds of MHz (hundreds of millions of rotations per second) in the real world become frequencies of the order of kHz (thousands of rotations per second) in the rotating frame. It is now a much simpler matter to calculate the interaction of B_1 with the various nuclear spins. We have essentially stepped onto the nuclear merry-go-round. The general result is that all spins are excited essentially uniformly if B_1 is sufficiently intense. Virtually all treatments of magnetic resonance phenomena consider motion in this rotating frame of reference; often this transformation is assumed implicitly. To see what happens in detail we need the vector picture of nuclear magnetism.

2.6 The vector representation

Nuclear spins obey quantum mechanics, but because we are dealing with a collection of literally billions of billions of spins in a given sample, for many purposes we can conveniently forget about the quantum laws, and deal only with the overall (macroscopic) response which obeys much more 'user-friendly' laws of motion.[2] We can simplify the treatment of nuclear spin dynamics enormously by considering only the resultant magnetization summed over all the spins within the effective volume of the sample. By effective volume we mean that part of the sample (or patient) situated inside the radiofrequency receiver coil. In MRI this might be the entire head of a human patient or, in high-resolution NMR, a short length of liquid in a cylindrical sample tube.

Consider first of all an ensemble of (polarized) nuclear spins at equilibrium. As outlined in Chapter 1, each individual magnetic nucleus can be thought of as a tiny bar magnet and represented by a small vector ↑ or ↓ depending on whether it is aligned along the magnetic field (↑) or in opposition to the field (↓). The former has a slightly lower energy and we focus attention on this slight excess of spins in this ground state, disregarding all the rest. The resultant of all these individual nuclear spin vectors is a macroscopic magnetization vector M_0 aligned along the $+Z$ axis of the rotating reference frame. Almost all NMR or MRI measurements start with this initial condition.

As we saw in Chapter 1 the representation of spins as vectors aligned parallel (↑) or antiparallel (↓) to the magnetic field is really a shorthand notation for two states of nuclear precession:

There are almost equal numbers of spins in these two states, so any resultant is always very small. Even when we single out only the tiny excess population in the ground state, the resultant precessing signal is zero for a system at equilibrium. This is because the precession phases of individual spins are quite random so the resultants in the X and Y directions, summed over the effective volume, are zero.

Now a radiofrequency pulse causes the nuclear spins to precess in step with another; it induces *phase coherence*.

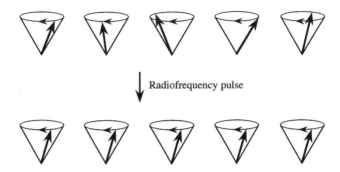

Radiofrequency pulse

The resultant is a precessing macroscopic magnetization vector in the XY plane. As this vector precesses, it interacts with the receiver coil to induce a small radiofrequency current that is then amplified and recorded. This is what we detect when we perform a magnetic resonance experiment. Note that the receiver coil is necessarily in the 'laboratory frame', so the frequency of the detected signal is the sum of the nuclear precession frequency in the rotating frame (measured in kHz) plus the rotation frequency of the reference frame (measured in hundreds of MHz).

These manipulations allow us to represent the process of excitation and detection in simple pictorial terms. By convention B_1 is assumed to be aligned along the $+X$ axis of the rotating frame. When the radiofrequency pulse is applied, the macroscopic magnetization vector (M) rotates about the radiofrequency field B_1 in the rotating reference frame. We choose the intensity and length of the radiofrequency pulse so that M rotates through $90°$, being carried from the $+Z$ axis (the equilibrium state) to the $+Y$ axis of the rotating frame. In this position M induces a maximum absorption-mode signal in the receiver coil.

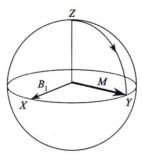

The axis of the receiver coil is at right angles to the direction of the magnetic field. If the radiofrequency pulse is not tuned exactly to the Larmor frequency but is offset by an amount that can be written as a small magnetic field ΔB (along the $+Z$ axis), the rotation occurs about a tilted effective field B_{eff}, the resultant of B_1 and ΔB.

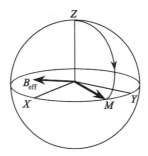

Nevertheless, if the radiofrequency pulse is intense enough that B_1 is very much larger than ΔB, the effective field is essentially along the $+X$ axis, and small variations of the offset ΔB have very little effect. Once again the result is to rotate M from $+Z$ to $+Y$. This is why there is no need to tune an intense radiofrequency pulse to the exact Larmor frequency, and it explains why we can achieve essentially uniform excitation in high resolution NMR or MRI even when many of the nuclear spins are not at exact resonance. The stronger the radiofrequency pulse, the wider the range of action (the *effective bandwidth*) of the excitation and the shorter the duration required to achieve 90° rotation. Typically an excitation pulse would be sufficiently strong that its duration would be of the order of 10 microseconds, giving it an effective bandwidth of the order of tens of kHz.

In this manner the nuclear spin behaviour has been converted from one defined by quantum mechanics to a much more familiar 'classical' problem. We focus attention on a particular spin species and represent the effect of the ensemble of individual nuclear magnets as a simple resultant vector M in the rotating frame, obeying rules which are simple to visualize. The radiofrequency pulse rotates this vector into the XY plane, where it rotates freely, that is to say, in the absence of any driving radiofrequency field. This is called the *free precession signal* or *free induction signal*. As the magnetic vector M precesses it intersects the turns of the receiver coil, inducing a tiny current which is amplified, detected and passed on to the display device.

2.7 The free precession signal

We now need to examine the nature of the free precession signal in more detail. Imagine for a moment that you are listening to the rehearsal of an orchestra made up of neophyte musicians who, although competent to play their own instruments, have not yet learned to pay much attention to what their colleagues are doing. The conductor starts them off in time, but is then called away and leaves them to their own devices. We can readily imagine the 'symphony' gradually degenerating into a 'cacophony' as all sense of relative timing is lost.

In both magnetic resonance spectroscopy and in high-resolution NMR, there are many different resonance frequencies, either from parts of the sample in

different regions of an applied magnetic field or from different chemical components precessing at their characteristic chemical shift frequencies. When excited by
a radiofrequency pulse, all these components start with the same phase, but owing
to their different precession frequencies, they gradually get out of synchronism
with one another. The overall signal is called an *interferogram*; it consists of a
complex sequence of 'beats' between the different frequency components. What
concerns us here is that the beat pattern is difficult to decipher—the information
about the various frequencies is there, but in a very inconvenient form. Later we
shall show that the desired separation into individual frequencies is achieved by a
process called Fourier transformation (§ 3.7).

   This complex free precession signal does not last forever but is gradually
attenuated and eventually disappears. But what causes this decay? There are
two distinct mechanisms, one fundamental and the other imposed by instrumental shortcomings. The first is spin–spin relaxation (§ 4.5). We saw above
how a radiofrequency pulse brings individual precessing spin vectors into phase,
so that they all move in step. Spin–spin relaxation is a process that gradually
interferes with this orderly precession. It is characterized by a time constant
called the spin–spin relaxation time T_2. Left to themselves the nuclear spins
always relax to a chaotic state where there is no relationship between individual
phases.

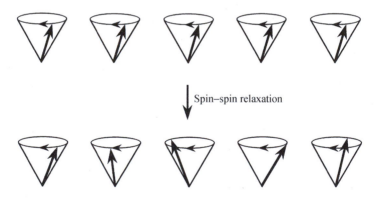

Spins continue to precess but leave no evidence of their precession on a macroscopic scale. Physical chemists would use the term *entropy* to describe this tendency to progress towards a disordered state.

2.8 Field inhomogeneity

In practical situations the free precession signal decays by another, quite distinct,
mechanism that often dominates the effect of spin–spin relaxation described
above. We must accept that the applied magnetic field B_0 can never be perfectly

uniform in space. Only if the lines of force are all exactly parallel and equally spaced can the field be said to be completely 'homogeneous'. When the magnetic field is generated by a superconducting solenoid, its strength necessarily falls off at the ends of the coil where the lines of force begin to diverge. Naturally the solenoid windings are carefully designed to give a highly uniform field at the 'isocentre' where the magnetic resonance measurements are made, but there is a practical limit to the uniformity that can be achieved, even after careful corrections are made to the residual gradients.

The magnetic field uniformity is optimized by adjusting tiny currents in room-temperature correction coils, usually by hand, but increasingly with automated computer programs. These are commonly called 'shim' coils, a historical reference to the early years of high resolution NMR, when the uniformity of an iron magnet was optimized by adjusting the pole caps to be parallel by introducing very thin strips of metal known as shims.

In the case of high-resolution NMR spectroscopy, the effective uniformity can be improved by spinning the sample by means of a small air turbine, using spinning speeds of the order of ten revolutions per second (10 Hz). Each nuclear spin traverses a circular path in a short time and 'sees' essentially the average value of the magnetic field around the circle. The effective homogeneity is thereby improved as far as transverse gradients are concerned, although the effect of variations in the field along the spinning axis are unchanged. Linewidths are typically a fraction of 1 Hz, which corresponds to an effective field homogeneity of the order of one part in a billion for very high-field NMR spectrometers. Since the magnetic field is modulated by this spinning motion of the sample, weak 'spinning sidebands' are inevitably introduced into the spectrum; they flank all the main resonance lines at separations equal to the spinner frequency and its harmonics. With the simpler and more efficient shimming procedures available in the more recent high-resolution NMR spectrometers, and the growing emphasis on biological samples with broader resonance lines, the present-day tendency is to employ non-spinning samples. This not only eliminates spinning sidebands but also some other artefacts attributable to mechanical vibration.

In MRI, the samples are much larger but polarizing field intensities are considerably weaker (typically 1.5 tesla). The *absolute* homogeneity is poorer than in high-resolution NMR, but not catastrophically so. It is usual to specify a field uniformity of better than 2 parts per million over a 25 cm diameter spherical volume at the isocentre of the magnet. This corresponds to an inhomogeneity of approximately 120 Hz in a 1.5 tesla magnet (about 1 part in 500,000). For clinical purposes we are less concerned with the overall inhomogeneity over the organ under investigation (which would merely lead to some distortion) than with the spatial *resolution* of the image, that is, the fineness of the detail that can be achieved. This is influenced by the intensity of the applied field gradients, and typically can be better than 1 mm.

Even if the applied field were perfect, there would always be some distortion caused by the materials used to construct the radiofrequency coil and its supports, and any additional decoupling coil (§ 8.5) and its supports. The magnetic field penetrates some materials slightly more easily than others (they are said to have different *magnetic susceptibilities*), inducing field distortions at the interface between two materials. These effects are more serious the closer these materials are to the sample and the stronger the applied magnetic field. To counter such distortions of the field the radiofrequency coil may be constructed of a composite of two metals having magnetic susceptibilities of opposite sign so that overall susceptibility matches that of air.

In MRI studies, the patient also distorts the magnetic field because of unavoidable variations in magnetic susceptibility in the body. Magnetic resonance imaging relies on an applied magnetic field gradient to encode spatial information, so any residual field inhomogeneity necessarily distorts the image. (An artist prefers to start with a completely blank canvas, not one already splashed with colour.) Because oxygen in the air is slightly paramagnetic, cavities such as the sinuses, the mouth, or the lungs are more easily penetrated by the applied field than normal tissue, creating undesirable local inhomogeneities. As metabolic processes use up oxygen carried by the blood, the latter becomes slightly paramagnetic and distorts the local magnetic field; this is exploited to monitor brain activity in functional MRI (§ 17.2).

Because of field inhomogeneity, nuclear spins in different regions of the sample precess at slightly different frequencies and the initial phase coherence is gradually lost. We must carefully distinguish this macroscopic effect from the atomic-scale loss of coherence caused by interactions between individual nuclear spins. By convention, the decay of the free precession signal caused by field inhomogeneities is represented by another time constant T_2^* on the (debatable) assumption that the decay is exponential.

$$M = M_0 \exp(-t/T_2^*)$$ **2.2**

The parameter T_2^* is generally used to represent the signal decay rate arising from all possible instrumental imperfections or instabilities. It is quite unrelated to the spin–spin relaxation time T_2 (§ 4.5) which determines the natural linewidth. Not only is the decay due to field inhomogeneity a different physical phenomenon, but also it can be reversed, whereas the decay due to spin–spin relaxation cannot. This will be evident when we discuss spin echoes in Chapter 9.

The rate of decay of the free precession signal determines the observed linewidth. This is an inverse relationship—a slow decay corresponds to a narrow resonance response, whereas a fast decay implies a broad resonance line. When the linewidth of a resonance response is determined by instrumental shortcomings it is said to be 'inhomogeneously broadened'. There is a practical test for this situation; it is possible to burn a hole in the line profile (through localized saturation) by irradiation with a suitably monochromatic radiofrequency. When the linewidth is determined by T_2 it is said to be 'homogeneously broadened' and monochromatic irradiation saturates the entire line profile in a uniform manner.

2.9 Hard and soft radiofrequency pulses

So far we have assumed that all the nuclear spins are excited uniformly by a radiofrequency pulse. This is called a 'hard' pulse. On the other hand there are quite a few magnetic resonance techniques where the 'frequency profile' of the excitation needs to be non-uniform, for example in the 'slice selection' experiments widely employed in magnetic resonance imaging (§ 12.3). The idea is to pick out a group of nuclear spins that precess in a chosen narrow frequency range and excite their magnetic resonance response, leaving the remaining spins essentially unchanged. Such a selective radiofrequency pulse is usually called a 'soft' pulse to distinguish it from a non-selective hard pulse. Magnetic resonance aficionados would say that a soft pulse has a 'narrow excitation bandwidth in the frequency domain'. Analogous soft pulses can be used to invert spin populations in a selective manner (§ 4.1).

The vector model of magnetic resonance (§ 2.6) provides insight into this selectivity. As explained above, the problem is transformed into a reference frame that rotates in synchronism with the transmitter frequency, so that the radiofrequency field B_1 is stationary rather than oscillatory (§ 2.5). By convention we place B_1 along the $+X$ axis of this rotating frame. We always measure the magnetic field at a some chosen position by reference to the magnetic field where the spins are at exact resonance with the transmitter frequency, and we call this field offset ΔB. Nuclear spins at an offset ΔB experience an effective field B_{eff} which is the resultant of B_1 and ΔB, tilted in the XZ plane through an angle θ. The nuclear magnetization is rotated about this effective field, and the angle of rotation (called the 'flip angle') is determined by the product of B_{eff} and the pulse duration.

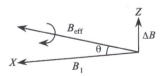

A hard radiofrequency pulse is defined as one where B_1 is very much stronger than ΔB for all practical offsets ΔB. Then B_{eff} has almost the same amplitude as B_1, θ is vanishingly small, and all nuclear magnetization vectors are rotated essentially about the X axis, providing virtually uniform excitation as a function of frequency. The flip angle is determined by the product of B_1 and the pulse duration, and is now set to 90° so that magnetization initially along the $+Z$ axis is rotated to the $+Y$ axis, where it induces a maximum magnetic resonance response in the receiver coil.

By contrast, a 'soft' radiofrequency pulse has a relatively weak radiofrequency field B_1 so that for most nuclear spins the offset ΔB is very much larger than B_1 and the effective field B_{eff} is tilted through an angle θ close to 90°. Rotation takes place about an axis very close to $+Z$ and, although the rotation angle may now be very large, the resultant excitation is negligible.

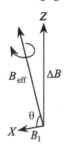

There is significant excitation only very close to exact resonance, at offsets ΔB so small that B_1 is again very much stronger than ΔB.

Frequency selectivity is achieved because a soft pulse only excites spins relatively close to the transmitter frequency. The weaker B_1, the narrower the effective bandwidth of the pulse. Because we still need a 90° flip angle at resonance, the duration of the soft pulse must be correspondingly increased in comparison with a hard pulse, typically from several microseconds (millionths of a second) to several milliseconds (thousandths of a second). High selectivity always implies a long pulse duration.

With soft radiofrequency pulses it is not a good idea to switch the radiation on and off abruptly. In other words, a rectangular pulse envelope is unsuitable, although that would be perfectly acceptable for a hard radiofrequency pulse. The best results are achieved by shaping the pulse envelope, and in particular, making the rise and fall sections very gradual. Sharp leading and trailing edges excite undesirable frequency components. One simple and robust time-domain pulse shape is the Gaussian[3] which excites a frequency region which is approximately Gaussian in shape. Figure 2.3(a) illustrates how the amplitude and phase of the radiation evolve in the time domain during a Gaussian pulse offset by 40 Hz from the frequency of the rotating reference frame. It is customary to truncate the tails of the Gaussian function at about the 2 % level; this has little effect on the shape of the excitation band.

Sometimes a 'band-selective' pulse is required. We choose a range of nuclear frequencies that are to be excited essentially uniformly and require that all frequencies outside the chosen band have negligible excitation, apart from narrow transition regions between the 'pass band' and the 'stop band'. In magnetic resonance imaging (§ 12.3) where the radiofrequency pulse must have a short duration,

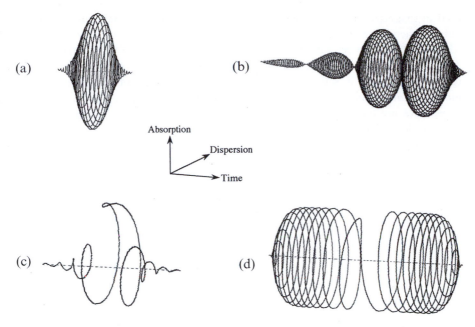

Figure 2.3 Time-domain evolution of the radiofrequency amplitude and phase for a selection of soft radiofrequency pulses: (a) the frequency-selective Gaussian excitation pulse, (b) the band-selective E-BURP excitation pulse, (c) the hyperbolic secant pulse used for wideband spin inversion, (d) the WURST-40 wideband spin inversion pulse. Both (c) and (d) are employed for decoupling, with the radiofrequency being swept during the pulse. (Simulations courtesy of Eriks Kupče.)

slice selection is often implemented with a pulse that has been shaped according to a sinc function, truncated at the third crossing points.

In high-resolution NMR it is more usual to employ a radiofrequency pulse shape that has been optimized for band selection, for example, one of the so-called 'BURP' pulses.[4] They have the practical advantage that the excitation is in pure absorption throughout the excitation band. Figure 2.3(b) shows the time-domain evolution of the radiofrequency during one of the band-selective BURP pulses.

Not all radiofrequency pulses are used for excitation. Sometimes it is necessary to invert the spin populations, flipping nuclear spins from the lower energy level to the upper level and vice versa, with no excitation of transverse magnetization. Inversion requires a 180° pulse rather than a 90° pulse. This is important for the measurement of spin–lattice relaxation times (§ 4.1) and in the ISIS sequence used in magnetic resonance spectroscopy (§ 14.6). A simple hard radiofrequency pulse is ineffective for spin inversion over a wide frequency band, but this is just what is required for broadband decoupling experiments (§ 8.5). Furthermore, the decoupler should use only a low level of radiofrequency power so as to avoid undue heating of the sample or the patient. Schemes that involve sweeping the radiofrequency during the pulse have proved very efficient in this context. The sweep rate normally obeys the 'adiabatic condition' (§ 8.5) so these are some-times called adiabatic pulses. One example is a pulse shaped according to a hyperbolic secant.[5] Figure 2.3(c) illustrates the time evolution of the radiation during this type of decoupling pulse. Even wider decoupling bands can be covered by one of the 'WURST' family of pulses where the pulse amplitude has a sausage shape—constant through most of the pulse, but with carefully shaped rise and fall sections.[6] The time evolution of a WURST-40 pulse is shown in Figure 2.3(d) where it can be seen that the rate of change of phase increases continuously during the pulse.

Further reading

E. Fukushima and S. B. W. Roeder, *Experimental Pulse NMR: A Nuts and Bolts Approach*, Addison-Wesley, Reading, Massachusetts (1981).

A. E. Derome, *Modern NMR Techniques for Chemistry Research*, Pergamon Press, Oxford (1987).

H. Günther, *NMR Spectroscopy*, 2nd ed., Wiley, Chichester, UK (1994).

3

Detection of magnetic resonance

3.1 The magnetic resonance response

We first observe the magnetic resonance response from the nuclei as a tiny voltage induced on a coil surrounding the sample—the receiver coil. How does this arise? In most forms of spectroscopy there are three possible mechanisms to describe the interaction of radiation with matter. *Stimulated absorption* or *stimulated emission* describe the absorption or emission of radiation by the sample provoked by the radiation field itself. *Spontaneous emission* occurs in the absence of any imposed radiation field, for example, the light emitted from a heated metallic filament. Spontaneous emission is far too weak an effect to be relevant to magnetic resonance experiments. The free precession NMR signal occurs after extinction of the radiofrequency pulse used for excitation and subsequently evolves in the absence of any imposed radiation field, so none of these three phenomena can properly account for magnetic resonance signals.

The simplest way to explain the generation of a magnetic resonance response is in terms of a concerted motion of the individual tiny nuclear magnets such that they all move in phase, creating a macroscopic resultant that behaves rather like a small rotating bar magnet. We might liken this to the reaction of a field of sunflowers as they are first exposed to the rising sun. As a consequence of Faraday's law of electromagnetic induction, the concerted motion of the spins generates a small electrical voltage on the receiver coil, just as in a dynamo.

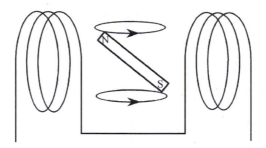

In the vast majority of cases this radiofrequency voltage is very weak, of the order of one-millionth of a volt, and any induced radiofrequency current is correspondingly small. A high degree of amplification is usually needed. However, just occasionally the high-resolution NMR signal from a sample (such as water) is sufficiently strong that the induced current can no longer be neglected, and it generates an appreciable radiofrequency field within the coil. This so-called 'radiation damping' field[1] acts in opposition to the main excitation field, causing a premature decay of the NMR signal.

Even in the absence of radiation damping, the phase coherence between the precessing nuclear magnets is gradually dissipated, causing an irreversible decay of the free precession signal. This is usually known as spin–spin relaxation (§ 4.5) or (occasionally) decoherence. Although individual nuclear spins continue to precess, the tiny magnets point in random directions and no net signal can be observed.

3.2 The radiofrequency coil

The NMR response is picked up on a radiofrequency coil, usually made of copper wire or copper foil, forming part of a resonant tuned circuit.

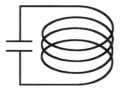

The haphazard motion of electrons in the coil induces small random fluctuations in voltage, called 'noise'. A tuned circuit has the effect of boosting the ratio of true magnetic resonance signal to this background noise. The effectiveness of a tuned circuit for this purpose is measured by its 'quality factor, Q' normally of the order of 500, although Q can be significantly increased if the coil is cooled to a very low temperature. To make the best use of this resonant circuit, it must be carefully tuned to match the precession frequency of the nuclei under investigation, otherwise the signal-to-noise advantage is degraded.

The same coil is usually used as receiver and transmitter, although some spectrometers use two separate coils disposed at right angles—the so-called 'crossed-coil' arrangement.

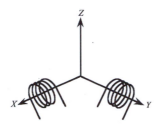

The transmitter coil generates the excitation pulses and the receiver coil picks up the magnetic resonance response. We retain these terms to denote *purpose* even when they may in fact be the same coil. The physical size of the receiver coil is governed by the desire to keep the 'filling factor' (the proportion of the enclosed volume occupied by the sample) as high as possible. Copper is employed for most radiofrequency coils because it is an excellent conductor. We are principally concerned with the 'signal-to-noise ratio', the strength of the desired magnetic resonance response compared with the level of meaningless noise; this increases as the square root of the quality factor Q, and in direct proportion to the filling factor.

At low temperatures the noise level decreases as the random motion of the electrons in the wire becomes less agitated, while the quality factor improves owing to the lower resistive losses in the coil. There are technical developments underway in high-resolution NMR spectroscopy that exploit 'cryogenic' coils[2,3] operating at around 20° to 25° above absolute zero, some with copper coils and others with new 'high-temperature superconducting' materials. Contrary to what one might expect, these superconducting coils do not have zero resistance for radiofrequency current, but the resistive losses are nevertheless very small. At the time of writing, cryogenic coils offer about a fourfold improvement in the signal-to-noise ratio compared with the equivalent room-temperature coils. This is lower than the enhancement expected on the basis of the higher quality factor and the reduced noise, because the filling factor is reduced through the necessity of leaving a suitable gap for thermal insulation between the very cold coil and the warm sample. Cryogenic coils are not yet used in MRI.

Biochemical applications of high-resolution NMR often involve aqueous solutions containing ions, and their random motion introduces additional noise, normally represented as a degradation in the quality factor Q. In imaging applications the presence of a patient inside the receiver coil similarly reduces the quality factor. In this situation these 'dielectric losses' can easily outweigh the inherent noise from the random thermal motion of electrons in the coil. One important factor determining MRI sensitivity is the ratio of the Q factor of the empty coil to that of the same coil occupied by the head or torso of the patient. The degradation in Q factor by the head is about the same as that from a 0.2 % saline solution. MRI performance is also degraded by any motion of the patient, voluntary or involuntary.

Radiofrequency coils may take several possible forms. The solenoid shape is the simplest and most effective of all (Figure 3.1(a)). For high-resolution NMR spectroscopy a 'saddle coil' is normally employed which wraps around a long cylindrical sample tube aligned along the field direction (Figure 3.1(b)). For magnetic resonance spectroscopy, as well as certain localized imaging applications, a 'surface coil' is often used (Figure 3.1(c)). It consists of a flat loop of wire placed directly on the surface of the patient over some interesting region of the body, and it is only sensitive to nuclear spins relatively close to the surface. With surface coil geometry the radiofrequency field has poor uniformity.

In MRI, the radiofrequency coil arrangement may be more complex because we need to enclose a head, a limb or even the entire torso within a suitable coil geometry. The coil should achieve a high filling factor (typically 70 %) and hence may be designed specifically to enclose the head, the chest or a limb. The spatial uniformity of the radiofrequency field is important because a non-uniform driving field distorts the intensities across the image; in contrast, high-resolution NMR can more easily tolerate radiofrequency inhomogeneity because the signal is an integral over the total effective sample volume.

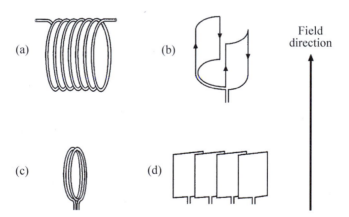

Figure 3.1 Various radiofrequency coil configurations: (a) a simple solenoid has a high filling factor, (b) a saddle coil enclosing a cylindrical sample tube, commonly used for high-resolution NMR, (c) a flat surface coil is the basis of many experiments in magnetic resonance spectroscopy (MRS) and some imaging protocols, (d) an array of overlapping surface coils can be used for imaging an elongated feature such as the spine. In all cases the direction of the radiofrequency field of the coil is at right angles to the direction of the main magnetic field.

Mention has already been made of the surface coil (described in the context of MRS in § 14.3). The problem of imaging the spine can be addressed by using a phased array of several partially overlapping surface coils (Figure 3.1(d)), producing separate responses that can be combined together to give an extended image. The degree of overlap is important in determining the uniformity of the image along the axis of the spine. Figure 3.2 shows a 1.5 tesla sagittal image of the lumbar region of a normal human spine obtained by this technique. The use of a surface coil array accounts for the change in brightness from left to right across the image.

An alternative approach is to design a flexible 'wraparound' coil, shaped to enclose the desired anatomical feature, such as the knee or the ankle. In a sense this is a bilateral surface coil, but it has the great advantage that the radiofrequency field is far more uniform than a simple surface coil and the filling factor is much higher. Figure 3.3 shows the example of magnetic resonance imaging of the knee, using a wraparound radiofrequency coil with the patient sitting inside a large superconducting magnet.

Widespread use has been made of the 'birdcage coil'[4] for MRI of the human head or the whole body.

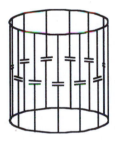

We can imagine the birdcage configuration as evolving from a pair of parallel radiofrequency coils similar to the saddle-coil arrangement. These can be represented schematically as shown in Figure 3.4(a), neglecting the leads in order to simplify the diagrams. Suppose we add a second pair of coils at right angles to create a crossed-coil arrangement (Figure 3.4(b)). If the upper and lower edges of these four coils are now joined (Figure 3.4(c)) the structure begins to resemble the birdcage configuration. An actual birdcage coil with eight vertical conductors incorporates eight tuning capacitors (Figure 3.4(d)) but it is possible to employ any even number of vertical elements. Calculations and experiments indicate that the radiofrequency field inside a birdcage coil is considerably more uniform in space than that of a simple saddle coil, and that the uniformity increases as more elements are introduced; a sixteen-element birdcage is often employed. The radiofrequency uniformity only falls off significantly at the top and bottom of the coil, so a long coil is well adapted to coronal and sagittal images, while axial images

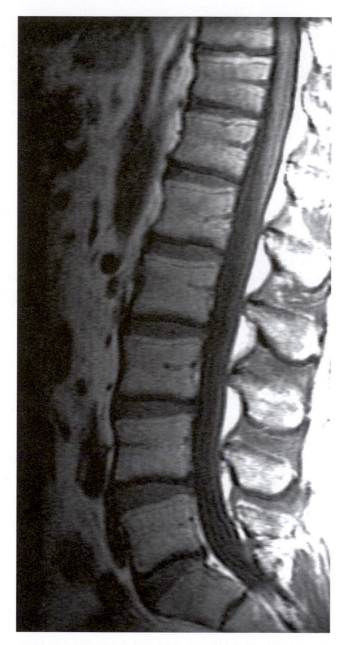

Figure 3.2 A 1.5 tesla sagittal image of the lumbar region of the spine obtained with a phased array of surface coils. The non-uniformity of the radiofrequency field and the spatial variation in the coupling of nuclear spins to the coils causes the change in brightness from left to right across the image. (Photograph courtesy of Peter Barker.)

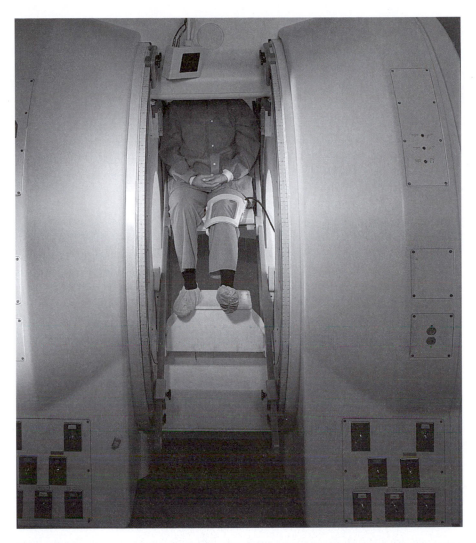

Figure 3.3 A wraparound radiofrequency coil designed specifically for magnetic resonance imaging of the knee. The patient sits inside the field of a 0.5 tesla superconducting magnet. (© 1998 General Electric Company; photograph by courtesy of G. E. Medical Systems.)

favour a shorter coil that gathers less noise from parts of the body beyond the imaging plane. Imaging coils are appreciably larger than coils used for high-resolution NMR, but since they operate at much lower radiofrequencies, the increased inductance of the large coils is not a problem.

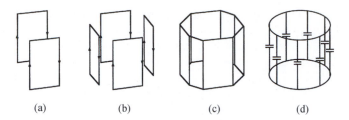

(a)   (b)   (c)   (d)

Figure 3.4 Evolution of the design of the birdcage coil: (a) a pair of parallel radiofrequency coils, (b) the 'crossed-coil' configuration, (c) crossed coils joined together, (d) the birdcage. The introduction of capacitors permits operation at a relatively high radiofrequency.

3.3 Amplification

The magnetic resonance response picked up on the receiver coil is very weak, typically of the order of a millionth of a volt. The random motion of the electrons in the wire of the receiver coil generate 'noise' that is amplified along with the magnetic resonance signal, spoiling the final image or high-resolution spectrum. The same phenomenon causes the 'hiss' in a poorly tuned radio set or the 'snow' on a television screen. In MRI the random motion of charged particles within the body also contributes a fluctuating response and may well be the dominant source of noise. However, in MRI, *contrast* is usually more important than signal-to-noise ratio, so one often speaks of the *contrast-to-noise* ratio.

The task of the receiver is to amplify the magnetic resonance signal by a very large factor without introducing additional noise. All electronic amplifiers contribute a certain amount of intrinsic noise, but once the desired magnetic resonance signal has been raised to a level appreciably above the noise, further amplification does not significantly degrade the signal-to-noise ratio. For this reason the first stage of amplification is critical; this 'preamplifier' is specially designed so that it introduces the least possible noise; the electronic engineer would say that its 'noise figure' is close to unity.

When the radiofrequency voltage has been amplified to a convenient level, it is converted to an audiofrequency signal through what is known as 'heterodyne' action. This low-frequency version of the response is what we normally think of as the 'free precession signal' or 'free induction decay'. It is converted to digital form and processed in a computer, the main program involving Fourier transformation (§ 3.7), to give a magnetic resonance image for clinical applications or a high-resolution spectrum to be used by the chemist.

Computer processing can also improve the presentation of the MRI display or the high-resolution NMR spectrum. Although these data manipulations may enhance certain features, suppress others, and even hide the noise, we must always bear in mind that the information content is fundamentally determined by the initial signal-to-noise ratio of the raw response picked up on the receiver coil. We must be very wary of 'magical' schemes that promise to suppress noise altogether because they also hide signals that are so weak that they lie below the random noise. In particular there are several non-linear procedures that can enhance the signal-to-noise ratio for signals above the noise, but actually degrade signals weaker than the noise. They may make a spectrum or image *look* much 'cleaner' but that is dangerously deceptive. They are of no use at all for enhancing *sensitivity*—the ability to detect very low concentrations of nuclear spins.

3.4 Quadrature detection

A high-resolution NMR spectrum contains several distinct resonances at different frequencies, while MRI involves a continuum of observed frequencies. When these have been converted from radiofrequencies to audiofrequencies by heterodyne action, the transmitter frequency becomes the zero point, and the magnetic resonance frequencies may be positive or negative, depending on whether they fall above or below the frequency of the transmitter. Some of the spins precess clockwise in the rotating frame and other process anticlockwise, depending on where we chose to set the transmitter frequency. So we need to be able to distinguish the *sense* of nuclear precession in the rotating reference frame. Otherwise, in NMR the left-hand section of the spectrum would appear to be 'folded' onto the right-hand part, and in MRI, one region of the image would become superimposed on the remainder. In both cases the resulting confusion is unacceptable. We could of course move the transmitter frequency to one edge of the spectrum or the image, so that the NMR frequencies are all positive or all negative, but that would make poor use of the available transmitter power and would also admit noise contributions from a region where there are no magnetic resonance signals, a recipe for poor sensitivity.

So how do we determine the sense of the nuclear precession? First consider a practical analogy. Suppose we employ a rotary engine to expand or compress gas inside a cylinder.

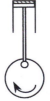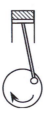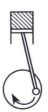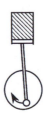

Because the piston is only sensitive to up-and-down movement, it does not matter which way the wheel is turning; exactly the same configurations of piston and cylinder would be achieved for anticlockwise rotation. Now imagine that we employ the same engine to drive two pistons arranged at right angles. When the wheel rotates clockwise it leaves only a small volume of gas in the second cylinder.

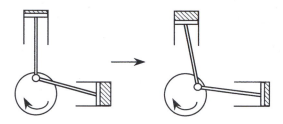

Starting from the same initial condition, we now let the wheel rotate anticlockwise and observe that the final result is different—the piston leaves a large volume of gas in the second cylinder.

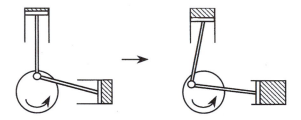

By making two 'measurements' at right angles we have succeeded in determining the sense of rotation of the wheel. More mathematically inclined readers would point out that this is merely a question of representing the two senses of rotation as $(\cos\theta + i\sin\theta)$ and $(\cos\theta - i\sin\theta)$.

The same principle applies to the observation of magnetic resonance signals. If we detect only the component of the free precession signal along one axis (say the $+Y$ axis) it is a linearly oscillating voltage and the sense of precession remains ambiguous. On the other hand, if we detect two components at right angles (say along the $+X$ and $+Y$ axes) then we know whether the precession is clockwise or anticlockwise. This can be achieved by detecting the magnetic resonance signal in two separate receiver coils arranged at right angles. In practice it is usually carried out electronically by extracting two orthogonal components of the signal. This 'quadrature detection' scheme[5] eliminates the problem of folding the spectrum or the image with respect to zero frequency.

It is also possible to achieve quadrature *excitation*. A crossed coil arrangement (or a birdcage coil with fourfold symmetry) can be driven by two equal radio-frequency fields with phases differing by 90°. With the correct choice of the relationship between these phases ($+90°$ or $-90°$) this generates a circularly polarized radiofrequency field that rotates in the same sense as the nuclear precession. Compared with the more usual linearly polarized radiofrequency field (the equivalent of two equal counter-rotating fields), this halves the required transmitter power.

3.5 Sampling the time-domain signal

The early cartographers were well aware that their view of the civilized world was restricted to the geographical region that had been properly explored, so they annotated the outer margins of their maps with comments like '*There be dragons*', thereby hoping to absolve themselves of any responsibility. High resolution NMR spectra and MRI images are similarly confined to a limited frequency 'window'; any signals that would normally fall outside this window are not properly processed. We have to learn to avoid these dragons. The problem arises during the process of sampling the magnetic resonance signal.

The use of Fourier transformation presupposes conversion of the analog signal from the receiver into digital form suitable for processing. A digital representation of a smooth analog function can only be an approximation. The fundamental problem is the rate at which the analog signal is sampled. Clearly, if we only take one sample while the signal completes a hundred oscillations, most of the information will be lost. So we must decide on how fine the sampling should be in the time domain. We cannot be too profligate with sampling points because that would make unreasonable demands on the hardware for analog-to-digital conversion, and slow down the Fourier transformation stage unnecessarily, but if we are too parsimonious, the image (or spectrum) is degraded, and important information may be obscured.

As an illustration of this last point, consider the related problem of recording a motion picture of a stagecoach in a western movie film. The frame speed of the camera corresponds to the sampling rate, and because this is slower than the speed of rotation of the wheels of the stagecoach, it cannot handle this information properly. As a result, on the film, the wheels appear to revolve more slowly than in real life. If the frame speed is exactly synchronized with the rotation rate, there is no evidence on the film that the wheels are turning at all, and they appear to be stationary, giving the ludicrous impression that the stagecoach is skidding. At a slightly faster framing speed the wheels even appear to turn backwards. And they say the camera never lies!

In magnetic resonance the problem reduces to the question of how many sample points are required to define a given nuclear precession frequency without danger of falsification. The answer is given by the Nyquist sampling theorem[6] which states that the highest frequency F that can be properly digitized requires two sample points per period of the oscillation. Suppose that the usual quadrature detection scheme (§ 3.4) is employed where the receiver detects two orthogonal components

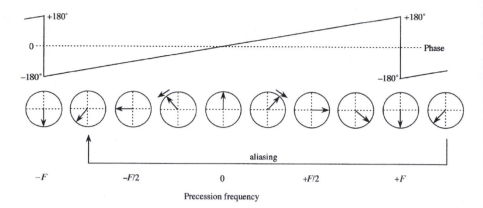

Figure 3.5 The origin of aliasing. As various frequency components in an NMR spectrum evolve between successive sampling operations, they build up phase angles proportional to their precession frequencies. If the sampling rate is $2F$ Hz, all NMR frequencies must be kept within the range $\pm F$ Hz so that all accumulated phase angles are less than $\pm 180°$. Otherwise there is an ambiguity in the phase angle and the corresponding frequency component is reduced by $2F$ Hz.

(say along $+X$ and $+Y$) of the precessing magnetization, in order to discriminate positive and negative frequencies. We can represent a typical nuclear precession signal by a vector rotating clockwise or anticlockwise, depending on whether its NMR frequency is positive or negative. Suppose we take $2F$ samples per second. The key to the problem is the phase change measured in the interval between two consecutive sampling operations—the product of the NMR precession frequency and the sampling interval. There is no problem with low frequencies (positive or negative) because the phase change between successive samples is small. But when the frequency reaches $+F$ Hz or $-F$ Hz, the phase change reaches $+180°$ or $-180°$, and beyond that 'aliasing' occurs (Figure 3.5). For example, the position of the precessing nuclear magnetization vector is the same for a phase change of $+185°$ as for a phase change of $-175°$, owing to the cyclic nature of the motion.

   In other words, if the nuclear precession frequency is $F + \Delta F$ Hz (slightly above the Nyquist frequency), the corresponding vector is in exactly the same position as if the precession frequency had been $-F + \Delta F$. The *apparent* precession frequency has been aliased by subtracting $2F$ Hz from the *actual* frequency.

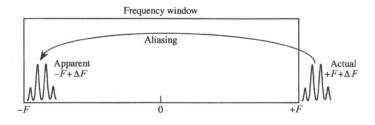

In exactly the same manner, a negative precession frequency $-F - \Delta F$ (just beyond the left-hand edge of the window) would be aliased to $+F - \Delta F$ (just inside the right-hand edge). As in the stagecoach analogy above, we see that an experimental NMR signal actually at $+2F$ or $-2F$ Hz would appear to be perfectly stationary! Because of the intrinsic periodicity of this phase diagram, NMR frequencies may be aliased many times by addition or subtraction of $2nF$ where n is an integer. The process of sampling has created a 'Nyquist window' in the frequency domain, and all experimental frequencies (however high they are in reality) are constrained to appear within this window. The analog-to-digital converter is just not capable of recognizing high frequencies, for the same reason that the movie camera cannot deal properly with speeding stagecoaches.

Aliasing in magnetic resonance is to be avoided at all costs. Unless the entire range of experimental high-resolution NMR frequencies falls naturally inside this Nyquist window, some lines will appear in the wrong part of the spectrum, causing confusion. In two-dimensional NMR spectroscopy, aliasing can occur in both frequency dimensions, further complicating the display. The remedy is to increase the sampling rate, or filter out any NMR responses carried at frequencies outside the permitted window. In MRI, aliasing must similarly be avoided, otherwise part of the proton density map that should properly appear, say, just outside the right-hand edge of the picture, appears instead inside the left-hand edge, or responses just above the top of the map are moved to the bottom (Figure 3.6). In the worst-case scenario, the image of a tumour could be translated to a completely different part of the anatomy.

The moral of the story is that the sampling rate must be twice the frequency of the highest-frequency component of the magnetic resonance response. We must remember that instrumental noise may also be carried at frequencies outside the Nyquist window, so, before conversion to digital form, it is important to employ a low-pass filter in the electronic circuitry to remove all frequency components outside the Nyquist window, thus filtering out noise that would otherwise be aliased. If not, sensitivity is seriously compromised.

3.6 Dynamic range

A second aspect of signal sampling concerns the conversion of the amplitude at each point into digital form. Here we might have preferred to have a large number of very fine digital steps, that is to say, a high dynamic range, so that very weak signals are adequately digitized even in the presence of very strong signals. However, the analog-to-digital converter operates through a series of successive approximations, so the higher the dynamic range, the slower the conversion, putting an upper limit on the sampling rate. It seems we must be reconciled to a limited dynamic range, typically 16 bits (65, 536 steps). This is a particular problem in high-resolution NMR spectroscopy of low-concentration samples in aqueous

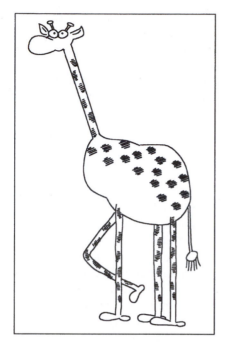
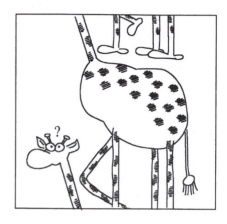

Figure 3.6 The sampling rate in MRI must be sufficiently high that all nuclear precession frequencies fall within the 'Nyquist window'. Any attempt to reduce the width of this window by reducing the sampling rate results in aliasing. In the case shown on the right, aliasing has occurred at the top and bottom of the Nyquist window and parts of the image appear in patently false locations. No actual animals were harmed during these experiments.

solution because water gives a very intense proton signal, that, like all signals, must fall within the range of the converter in order to be properly digitized. This means that the very weak signals are poorly digitized, leading to slight errors on the measured amplitudes. After Fourier transformation (§ 3.7) these errors appears as 'digitization noise'. This problem has still not been resolved satisfactorily, but an entire armoury of different 'water suppression' techniques has been built up to mitigate the dynamic range problem in high-resolution NMR spectroscopy.

Digitization noise is much less of a problem in MRI. Water is most often the material under investigation rather than very weak components in solution, so very fine gradations in the intensity scale are not particularly useful for clinical diagnosis.

3.7 Fourier transformation

Modern high-fidelity music systems often contain a device called a 'graphic equalizer' designed to ensure that the full frequency range of the music is amplified in an appropriate manner. There is usually a digital display showing the signal strength at a series of different audiofrequencies, set out as an array of bright vertical bars (a histogram). The relative heights of these bars change with time in step with the changes in incoming audio signal, and the gain in each 'channel' can be adjusted by the user. For example, one might like to boost the bass at the expense of the treble response. Each vertical bar monitors the component of the audio signal in a particular narrow frequency band, for example, around 256 Hz. One way to derive this information is to build a tuned circuit (a band-pass filter) that accepts signals oscillating at or near 256 Hz but rejects all the rest. With only a small number of different channels, an array of filters can be assembled, each tuned to cover a different narrow frequency range from bass to treble.

Note that the incoming audio waveform (in the 'time-domain') takes the form of wildly varying oscillations, the superposition of many different frequencies all jumbled together. This signal is quite different from the histogram display on the graphic equalizer (the 'frequency-domain'). Yet the two pictures contain the same basic information. One may be converted into the other by the process called Fourier transformation (some of the more sophisticated graphic equalizers use this method instead of band-pass filters). The Fourier transform device is simply asking 'How much of this music signal is actually carried in a band centred at frequency f_1? Display it in channel 1.' Then it repeats the process for a second frequency f_2, and then for each subsequent frequency, displaying the results in the form of a histogram, and it does this fast enough to deceive the eye. This type of presentation allows the operator to make the appropriate adjustments to each frequency channel—something that is impossible to do by direct observation of the incoming time-domain audiofrequency signal.

The same transformation is used in magnetic resonance. The free precession signal is made up of a superposition of many different frequencies—in the case of MRI because there are magnetic resonance signals from regions of the patient in different magnetic fields, and in high-resolution NMR because there are several different chemical species present in the sample. This is an inevitable consequence of exciting the impulse response of the nuclear spin system—all the possible frequencies are excited at the same time. This has been likened to dropping a grand piano from a height onto a hard concrete surface—the resulting 'sound' is virtually indescribable except that it probably comprises all the notes on the keyboard. We would much prefer to hear these notes played one at a time. Fourier transformation provides such a conversion by disentangling the many different frequencies present in the free induction decay. The time-domain signal is converted into a convenient frequency-domain spectrum made up of all the various resonance responses from the nuclear spins.

Fourier showed that any complex pattern can be represented by a superposition of sine waves of the appropriate amplitudes and relative phases. (Strictly the pattern should be repetitive in time, but this is easily arranged for a function that has been stored digitally.) Consequently, any general (repetitive) function may be written as a Fourier series expansion:

$$f(t) = A_0 + \Sigma_n[A_n \cos(\omega_n t) + B_n \sin(\omega_n t)]$$ **3.1**

This expression comprises a zero-frequency component (A_0) and a series of harmonics of the basic frequency ω_1 with their appropriate 'Fourier coefficients' A_n and B_n that determine amplitude and phase. It means that any free precession signal $f(t)$ can be decomposed into a sum (Σ) of regularly-spaced Fourier components. The process of Fourier transformation picks out these different components and assembles them in order of increasing frequency. The result is the NMR 'spectrum' or the MRI map, displayed as discrete responses as a function of frequency. Essentially this is a histogram, analogous to the one displayed on the graphic equalizer mentioned above. If the frequency steps are small enough the histogram is a good approximation to a smooth function. For example, in high-resolution NMR we might observe:

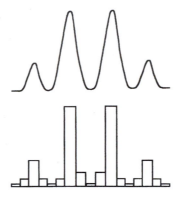

While the *resolution* in the 'ideal' spectrum (top) is determined by relaxation and magnetic field inhomogeneity, the *definition* in the digitized spectrum (bottom) is set by the width of the individual elements of the histogram. Normally the definition should be finer than the resolution.

One might ask why this 'impulse' mode was chosen for magnetic resonance experiments. A quite different 'pedestrian' mode of operation is used in simple optical spectrometers where a prism is slowly rotated so that the different colours are examined one at a time. It was also employed in very early magnetic resonance spectrometers—instead of exciting the impulse response, they swept a weak radiofrequency slowly across the spectrum, detecting each individual response as an absorption of energy from the irradiation field. Unfortunately, the time required to produce a typical spectrum by this sweep method was many minutes. Clearly this is a tediously slow process for the detailed information present in a high-resolution NMR spectrum. Worse still, there are long intervals where no high-resolution signals are observed at all.

This 'slow passage' method of excitation was superseded when it was realized that it offered only poor sensitivity, and when the computer technology for Fourier transformation became available at reasonable cost. The naked eye can take in all the many features of a wide landscape at once, whereas a telescope has only a narrow field-of-view and has to be panned slowly across the scene to gather the same information. This is why Fourier transform spectrometers gather information more efficiently.

For high-resolution NMR spectroscopy we can make an approximate calculation of the sensitivity advantage of the Fourier transform method compared with the old-fashioned frequency-sweep procedure. The rule for obtaining high resolution in the frequency-sweep mode is that the sweep rate must be slow enough to spend a time of the order of the decay time constant (T_2^*) to sweep through a single resonance line. A slow sweep through the entire spectrum would therefore require a time of approximately NT_2^* seconds, where N is the total frequency range of the spectrum divided by the width of a typical resonance line.

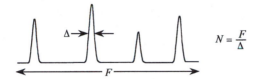

The acquisition of a single free induction decay would require approximately T_2^* seconds. So, neglecting processing time, the Fourier transform method is N times faster than the slow passage scheme for the same signal-to-noise ratio. In the Fourier transform mode we could therefore collect and add together N consecutive acquisitions of the free induction decay in the time employed for a *single* slow-passage sweep. Because multiscan averaging improves the signal-to-noise by the square root of the number of scans, this translates into a signal-to-noise improvement of the square root of N. For a 900 MHz proton NMR spectrometer, N could be as high as 10,000, giving a sensitivity improvement of the order of 100 for Fourier spectroscopy. Even higher enhancements can be achieved for nuclei with wider chemical shift ranges, such as carbon-13. Magnetic resonance imaging almost always employs the Fourier transform technique. In the rare cases where the 'sensitive point method' is used, the parameter N would be set by the number of pixels in one spatial dimension, determined by the width of the image and the required spatial definition.

Fourier transformation is invariably implemented on a digital computer, usually with a program called the Cooley–Tukey fast Fourier transform algorithm,[7] but for our purposes we may regard this simply as a 'black box' that transforms the transient magnetic resonance impulse response into a form that is much more convenient for the user. It converts a time-domain signal into frequency-domain information. In the case of MRI, 'frequency-domain' is equivalent to one of the spatial coordinates, because, in an applied magnetic field gradient, frequency is directly proportional to position. In high-resolution NMR, the frequency domain is simply 'the spectrum'. Processing times for fast Fourier transformation depend on the number of sampling points used to define the time-domain magnetic resonance signal, and are typically measured in milliseconds.

One special requirement of the fast Fourier transform algorithm is that the number of time-domain sample points N must be a power of two; if it is not, the data table is extended to the next higher power of two by appending zeros. Although in principle this slightly falsifies the result, in practice the free precession signal has normally decayed to a very low value at the point where zeros are added, so the difference is minimal. There are alternative methods for converting a time-domain free induction signal into a frequency-domain spectrum or image, but Fourier transformation is the method of choice and is usually taken for granted when describing magnetic resonance experiments.

It is important to be aware of how deficiencies in the free precession signal translate, through Fourier transformation, into possible distortions of the frequency-domain display. The fact that the free precession signal decays with time translates into a line width in the high-resolution NMR spectrum, or into an inherent limit on the sharpness of the MRI image.

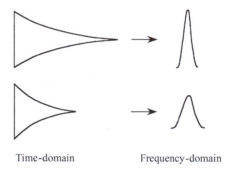

Time-domain   Frequency-domain

A time-domain signal that decays slowly transforms into a narrow frequency-domain signal. This is the 'resolution' of the spectrum or the image. We can think of this as a manifestation of the Heisenberg uncertainty principle—only a signal whose frequency can be monitored for an infinite time transforms into an infinitely narrow resonance response. It is important to make a clear distinction between this limitation on *resolution* and the limit on *definition* imposed by the use of discrete frequency steps in the display.

If signal acquisition is stopped before the free induction signal has completely decayed, this introduces a step function at the end of the time-domain signal, and in the frequency domain the lineshapes are distorted through the introduction of 'wiggles' in the skirts of the resonances. Mathematically this is a convolution of the true lineshape with a sinc function ($\sin x/x$).

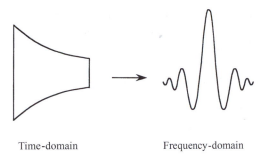

Time-domain   Frequency-domain

Time limitations, particularly in two-dimensional spectroscopy or high-speed imaging, often force us to truncate the signal in this manner. Then it may become necessary to round off ('apodize') the step in the tail of the signal in order to minimize the effect. After Fourier transformation, this eliminates the undesirable sinc-function oscillations at the expense of a slight broadening of the response.

The amplitudes of the first few data points of the free induction signal may be falsified because the receiver has not had time to recover from the effects of the very intense transmitter pulse (also a familiar problem in radar equipment). The result is a displacement and a cyclic distortion of the baseline of the high-resolution NMR spectrum (often called the 'rolling baseline') or wavelike artefacts across the MRI image. If we delay the start of the acquisition operation, thus disregarding these unreliable data points, the phases of signals from different components of the spectrum (or MRI response) have time to diverge, creating an increasing phase error as a function of frequency. This has to be corrected by a software routine before the display stage. Otherwise the loss of a few initial data points is not a serious problem, except for rapidly decaying signals from nuclei with inherently fast spin–spin relaxation (for example, nitrogen-14) where these early data points may represent a large fraction of the total available signal. One remedy is to employ a program (called 'linear prediction') that estimates the amplitudes of the missing early points based on an analysis of the remainder of the free induction decay.

3.8 Display

The most common form of display for MRI is a map recording proton spin density as a function of two spatial dimensions. This could be in the form of intensity contours, or a grey scale, or a colour-coded intensity scale. The use of colour presents a vivid picture, so that a tumour (which may have a higher-than-normal proton density) might then show up as a bright orange or yellow patch on the image. When a grey scale is used, the MRI map may superficially resemble an X-ray picture, although we must remember that MRI examines the proton

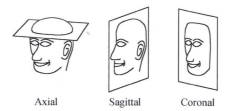

Axial   Sagittal   Coronal

Figure 3.7 The principal directions for MRI slices are axial, sagittal, or coronal, although images in oblique planes can also be computed.

density from a finite slice whereas the X-ray device is looking at the total absorption through the sample, projected onto a plane, so that one feature may appear directly superimposed on another. Furthermore, the factors that determine contrast are quite different in X-ray radiography and MRI.

In general the MRI information is acquired in three spatial dimensions, and a '3D' image may be depicted on a computer monitor, depth perception being enhanced by rotating the image or by some other device. However, it is more practical to view the three-dimensional information as a consecutive series of parallel slices. For example, head scans are commonly displayed as a sequence of axial, sagittal, or coronal slices (Figure 3.7), or even a slice calculated for a skew plane.

In high-resolution NMR spectroscopy the results are displayed in the form of a graph of intensity as a function of frequency—the 'spectrum'. There are in fact two possible forms of response, absorption and dispersion. High-resolution spectroscopy invariably displays the absorption mode, a peak which is symmetrical with respect to the frequency axis. Adjustments have to be made to the phase of the detector in order to obtain pure absorption-mode signals with no admixture of dispersion. The dispersion mode is antisymmetric with respect to frequency and is only used for special purposes, such as magnetic field stabilization (§ 2.2).

For two-dimensional NMR spectroscopy (Chapter 11) one form of display stacks several one-dimensional spectra one-behind-the-other to create the impression of a surface in three dimensions. More commonly, the experimental data are converted into a graph showing intensity contours as a function of two frequency parameters, F_1 and F_2, analogous to geographical contour maps. Three-dimensional NMR information is difficult to display directly; it is normally reduced to two-dimensional slices for ease of examination and for accurate frequency measurements.

Further reading

D. Shaw, *Fourier Transform NMR Spectroscopy*, 2nd ed., Elsevier, Amsterdam (1984).

R. N. Bracewell, *The Fourier Transform and its Applications*, McGraw-Hill, New York (1986).

D. C. Champeney, *A Handbook of Fourier Theorems*, Cambridge University Press, Cambridge (1987).

E. Oran Brigham, *The Fast Fourier Transform and its Applications*, Prentice-Hall, Englewood Cliffs, New Jersey (1988).

A. G. Marshall and F. R. Verdun, *Fourier Transforms in NMR, Optical and Mass Spectrometry*, Elsevier, Amsterdam (1990).

P. J. Hore, *Nuclear Magnetic Resonance*, Oxford University Press, Oxford (1995).

J. C. Hoch and A. S. Stern, *NMR Data Processing*, Wiley-Liss, New York (1996).

4

Relaxation

4.1 Spin–lattice relaxation

In Chapter 2 we considered what would happen if the external magnetic field were to be *suddenly* applied to a sample previously in zero field, and we concluded that the spin system would initially be saturated; both energy levels would be equally populated and no NMR signal would be observed. In a very loose sense the nuclear spins in zero field are 'hot' and need to cool down to the temperature of their environment, the 'lattice'. (The term 'lattice' is now a misnomer, dating back to the early studies of relaxation processes in crystals, where the environment did indeed form a regular lattice.) The process by which some spins drop down from the upper to the lower energy level so as to attain the requisite population distribution is called spin–lattice relaxation. When the spins reach thermal equilibrium with their environment the populations on the upper and lower energy levels are given by the Boltzmann distribution equation which, to a very good approximation, can be written

$$(N_{\text{lower}} - N_{\text{upper}})/N_{\text{lower}} = \Delta E/kT \qquad \textbf{4.1}$$

where ΔE is the energy level separation and k is the Boltzmann constant. Because ΔE is very small in comparison with kT, the excess population in the lower level is very small; most of the spins are equally distributed between the upper and lower levels.

To understand the mechanism of spin–lattice relaxation we have to look for some external interaction that favours downward transitions at the expense of upward transitions. It turns out that the only available interactions that permit this 'thermal contact' between the nuclei and the outside world are extremely weak, so the relaxation process is surprisingly slow. The reason is that the nucleus of the atom is very effectively isolated from its environment, and the violent buffeting that each molecule undergoes through thermal agitation has no direct effect on the orientation of the nuclear spins. If we think of the spinning nucleus as a gyroscope, it would have perfectly frictionless bearings, with no mechanical coupling to the tumbling motion of the molecule; the nuclear spin retains its perfect alignment with the magnetic field as the molecule changes its orientation.

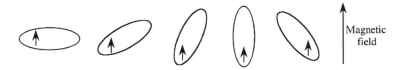

Only very weak magnetic interactions can flip the nuclear spins from one energy level to the other, and then only if these magnetic fields happen to fluctuate at just the right frequency—the Larmor precession frequency. Normally these magnetic interactions arise from the weak magnetic fields generated by other nuclear spins in the same molecule or in very close neighbours. These local magnetic fields are modulated by the chaotic movements of molecules in a liquid. In a certain sense we can think of this in terms of a 'cold' radiation field that favours the downward NMR transitions required for relaxation. It is quite unlike the 'hot' coherent radiation generated by the radiofrequency transmitter which causes upward and downward transitions with equal probability.

Consider the magnetic field at a given site S created by a neighbouring nuclear dipole I. Its intensity depends on two variables—the distance between I and S, and the orientation of the internuclear vector joining I and S. If spin I is part of another molecule, the relative translational motion changes both these parameters, but the internuclear distances are quite large and the consequent magnetic field changes are too weak to affect spin–lattice relaxation appreciably. If I and S are in the same molecule, rapid vibrational motion constantly changes the internuclear distance and hence modulates the local field at S, but this modulation is too fast compared with the Larmor precession frequency to be effective for spin–lattice relaxation. This leaves only the random reorientation of the molecule. The nuclear spins I and S in a given molecule remain always aligned along the main magnetic field but the internuclear vector joining I and S changes its orientation in a haphazard fashion.

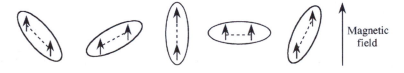

The consequent fluctuations in the local magnetic field at site S cover a range of frequencies near the Larmor precession frequency and constitute the dominant source of spin–lattice relaxation. The frequency match is best for medium-sized molecules in liquids of moderate viscosity. Very small mobile molecules rotate rather too fast for efficient relaxation. Large biomolecules rotate too sluggishly and consequently have long spin–lattice relaxation times.

4.2 Relaxation curves

Newton showed empirically that the rate of loss of heat from a hot body is proportional to the temperature difference between that body and its surroundings. When the temperature difference is large the cooling is fast, but as the hot body approaches the temperature of its surroundings, heat is lost more and more slowly. This can be expressed as a simple differential equation which implies that the cooling curve is a decreasing exponential. In an analogous manner, the rate at which nuclear spins drop back from the excited state to the ground state depends on the deviation of the spin populations from their Boltzmann equilibrium numbers. This recovery curve is also an exponential, and the time constant is called the spin–lattice relaxation time T_1. One definition of T_1 is the time taken for an initially saturated signal to recover 63 % of its full equilibrium intensity. The parameter T_1 is normally measured in milliseconds or seconds, and varies significantly from one substance to another. Addition of a relaxation agent (for example, a gadolinium compound) accelerates spin–lattice relaxation. These paramagnetic materials create local magnetic fields hundreds or even thousands of times stronger than the local fields from nuclear spins, and are therefore far more effective in spin–lattice relaxation. They are widely used as contrast agents in MRI (§ 12.9). Even a low concentration dissolved oxygen from the air (oxygen is weakly paramagnetic) speeds up spin–lattice relaxation to some extent.

Many magnetic resonance experiments involve repeated excitation of the nuclear spins, and this can lead to partial saturation and some loss of NMR response (§ 2.4). Each 90° excitation pulse temporarily equalizes the spin populations on the upper and lower energy levels and care must be taken to allow a sufficient delay between successive excitations for appreciable recovery towards thermal equilibrium through spin–lattice relaxation. When there are chemical sites with quite different relaxation rates, a partially saturated regime may falsify the relative intensities (as seen in the carbon-13 spectrum of panamine in § 11.10). However, in routine operation it is not necessary to wait for *complete* recovery by spin–lattice relaxation. In fact, optimum sensitivity is achieved when the repeated radiofrequency pulses establish a steady-state condition where the spins are slightly saturated. If 90° pulses are used, the best setting for the recycle time (TR) is about 1.3 times the spin–lattice relaxation time T_1. Alternatively, the pulse flip angle may be set to about 70° and the recycle time reduced to the period for which the transient signal is acquired, with no waiting interval. Only 6 % of the maximum possible signal is lost at this flip angle, whereas more than a third of the initial polarization is retained after the pulse. The operating parameters for these partial saturation regimes are not critical, so it is not difficult to set up conditions that ensure near-optimum sensitivity.

On the other hand, saturation can also be put to good use. In MRI, where there are appreciable differences between the T_1 values of different tissues, the contrast of the proton density map can be enhanced according to the different rates of spin–lattice relaxation of different tissues. In a regime where the spins are partially saturated, bright regions indicate fast recovery from saturation and darker parts of the image denote slower recovery. These are known as 'T_1-weighted images'. The effect can be dramatically enhanced by deliberate injection of a paramagnetic 'contrast agent' designed to speed up spin–lattice relaxation and thus highlight some interesting region, as in magnetic resonance angiography.

In high-resolution NMR, 'presaturation' is often used to suppress the strong water signal which would otherwise adversely affect the operation of the spectrometer (§ 3.6). The intense water signal is saturated selectively, leaving the remainder of the spectrum unchanged. There is a wide range of related 'water suppression' techniques; they are particularly important in the study of biomolecules in aqueous solution where the molecules of interest are in low concentration. Often it is not feasible to replace ordinary water with heavy water because of chemical exchange of deuterium.

Saturation is not the only way to disturb the spin populations of the energy levels. If we represent the Boltzmann equilibrium state as a macroscopic vector aligned along the $+Z$ axis of the rotating frame (§ 2.6) then it can be inverted by a 180° radiofrequency pulse. This means that the small excess of spins in the lower energy level are transferred to the upper level; there has been a 'population inversion'. This is an unstable situation and the excess spins in the upper energy level fall back to the ground state at a rate determined by the spin–lattice relaxation time.

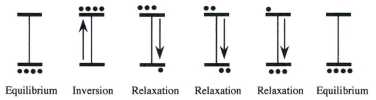

Equilibrium   Inversion   Relaxation   Relaxation   Relaxation   Equilibrium

In fact this is the preferred technique for measuring T_1, called the 'inversion-recovery' method.[1] The NMR signal is monitored by means of a 90° pulse at various intervals TI after the inversion pulse.

$$180° — TI — 90° \text{ acquire}$$

At short values of *TI* the NMR response is inverted. At a longer setting of *TI* it passes through a null condition (equal spin populations on both energy levels), and at still longer values the response becomes positive again, reaching its equilibrium intensity asymptotically at times *TI* much longer than T_1. A graph of the signal recovery is an exponential curve with a time constant T_1. In high-resolution NMR spectroscopy each chemically-shifted response recovers from spin inversion at its own characteristic rate[2] and the resulting spin–lattice relaxation times provide useful structural information, particularly in carbon-13 spectroscopy.

A sketch of spin–lattice recovery curves for different values of T_1 (fast, intermediate and slow) illustrates how MRI can exploit relaxation effects to create T_1-weighted images:

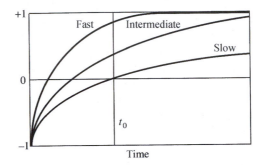

A vertical section through this graph at a chosen time t_0 clearly indicates that quite different NMR intensities will be recorded for tissues with different relaxation times. Indeed it is quite possible for the signal from one species to disappear if it is acquired close to the null condition (as shown for the 'slow' curve above).

In the foregoing we have tacitly assumed that the positive charge carried by the nucleus under investigation has a spherical distribution. This is the case for the proton, but some other nuclear species carry a charge that is flattened (oblate) or elongated (prolate) with respect to the spinning axis.

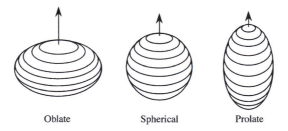

These nuclei are said to possess a *quadrupole moment*. This renders them susceptible to local electric field gradients and this interaction can act as a very effective spin–lattice relaxation mechanism. Not only does this shorten the spin–lattice relaxation time, but it also broadens the magnetic resonance response, rendering such nuclei generally unsuitable for high-resolution studies. Most of the magnetic resonance experiments described below pertain to nuclei with a spherical charge distribution (no quadrupole moment). The hydrogen nucleus with a mass of 2 units (the deuteron) is an exception to this rule because its nuclear charge is only weakly distorted from the 'ideal' spherical shape.

4.3 Cross-relaxation

Newton's law of cooling treats only the simplest possible case—a hot body inter-acting with a thermal reservoir by only a single mechanism. In the same way, our picture of a nuclear spin system relaxing exclusively through a single inter-action with its 'environment' is sometimes an oversimplification. There may, for example, be two separate spin systems A and B, where the spin–lattice relax-ation of B is governed predominantly by its interactions with A, and less by its interaction with a more generalized environment. (This is a quite common occur-rence when B is a carbon-13 spin and A is an attached proton.) This phenomenon is known as 'cross-relaxation' and it gives rise to a remarkable effect, the Overhauser enhancement.[3] When it was first proposed by Overhauser, this effect was greeted with widespread scepticism because it predicted that irradiation of the electron resonance in a system made up of interacting electron and nuclear spins would enhance the NMR signal from the nuclei in a spectacular fashion (many hundred-fold). This runs quite counter to the intuitive view, based on thermodynamic principles, that 'heating' a spin system by radiation should never lead to enhan-ced polarization; normally we expect strong radiofrequency irradiation to destroy the magnetic resonance signal rather than enhance it. Experiments vindicated Overhauser's prediction.[4] It was soon realized that the effect is very general and that there is an analogous (but much weaker) Overhauser effect between two different *nuclear* spins which can provide very useful molecular informa-tion.

Unfortunately there is no simple 'hand-waving' description that explains the nuclear Overhauser effect. The mathematical treatment of the Overhauser en-hancement is analogous to that used to calculate the various electrical currents in a network of resistors driven by a potential difference (Kirchhoff's law). The deviation of nuclear spin populations from equilibrium corresponds to electrical potential, the flux of spins corresponds to electrical current, and the relaxation transition probabilities correspond to electrical conductance.

For the moment we focus on cross-relaxation between protons in relatively small molecules, returning later to the application to macromolecules. For simpli-city we consider a two-spin system which has four transitions between four energy levels.

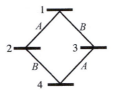

The system is 'driven' by radiofrequency radiation that saturates the two A transitions, equalizing the spin populations on levels 1 and 2, and also the populations on levels 3 and 4. We would therefore detect no signal from the A spins. Cross-relaxation causes a redistribution of these spin populations in such manner as to increase the signal intensity of the B spins. The influence of A on B is known as the 'dipole–dipole interaction' since the two nuclei are behaving like two tiny bar magnets ('dipoles'). The effectiveness of this interaction for cross-relaxation falls off as the sixth power of the internuclear distance. For this mechanism the dominant relaxation process is a simultaneous flip of both A and B protons, causing spins to drop from level 1 to level 4. This 'double-quantum' mechanism is the key to understanding why the B responses are enhanced. In the electrical network analogy the path 1–4 would have a high electrical conductance compared with paths 1–3 and 2–4.

To see how the observed enhancement comes about we assign suitable numbers to the spin populations on the four energy levels; for illustration purposes we can use arbitrary numbers as long as the equilibrium population differences are the same across all four proton transitions, and provided the total population numbers are conserved throughout the manipulations. For convenience we choose an equilibrium population difference of four units.

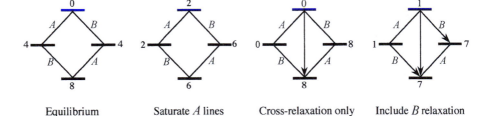

Equilibrium   Saturate A lines   Cross-relaxation only   Include B relaxation

First we apply continuous irradiation to saturate the two A lines. Neglecting relaxation effects for the moment, this maintains equal spin populations across each A line, but has no effect on the population differences across the two B lines (which remain at 4 units). Then we introduce cross-relaxation involving simultaneous flips of both A and B spins. If this were the only relaxation mechanism it would take spins from top level to the bottom level and bring this population difference towards the value (8) characteristic of Boltzmann equilibrium. (The continuous irradiation of the *A* transitions still maintains equal populations on levels 1 and 2, and on levels 3 and 4.) In this (hypothetical) situation the *B* lines would have population differences of 8, corresponding to twice their normal intensities. But the dipole–dipole interaction also affects *B*-spin relaxation directly, and there is also a weak 'zero-quantum' mechanism that allows relaxation between levels 2 and 3. The flux of nuclear spins from level 1 to level 4 is still dominant but the flux from level 1 to 3, from level 2 to 3, and from level 2 to 4 must also be taken into account. These fluxes compete with the 'double-quantum' relaxation and try to pull the *B*-spin population differences closer to the value (4) appropriate to Boltzmann equilibrium. The resulting *B*-spin population differences are reduced to a compromise value of 6, representing a 50 % enhancement of the *B* responses.

This figure of 50 % turns out to be the maximum possible nuclear Overhauser enhancement for proton–proton systems; in reality there are always other 'external' relaxation mechanisms acting on the *B* spins, reducing the enhancement below 50 %. This reduction of the Overhauser effect is sometimes known as 'leakage'; it arises because the dipole–dipole interaction that gives rise to cross-relaxation is short-range and not entirely dominant; other mechanisms eat away at the Overhauser enhancement.

In a practical case, nuclear Overhauser enhancements would be measured for several chemically-shifted responses in the same spectrum, the relative values indicating *relative* internuclear distances. The inverse sixth power dependence on distance ensures that an experimental error of 6 % in the measurement of intensity enhancement translates into only a 1 % error in the derived distance.

In a certain sense the nuclear Overhauser effect bestows the spin population advantage of one nuclear species *A* on a less well-endowed nuclear species *B*. If *A* represents a proton system and *B* represents carbon-13, the protons enjoy a four-fold advantage in spin populations, and the nuclear Overhauser enhancement factor can be as high as threefold in the most favorable situation where the relaxation of carbon-13 relies entirely on the interaction with the protons. This provides a most welcome improvement in the signal-to-noise ratio of carbon-13 spectroscopy and is used almost universally in high-resolution NMR studies of this low-abundance species. Figure 4.1 shows the improvement of the signal intensities in the carbon-13 spectrum of endo-(−)-borneol compared with the same spectrum without irradiation of the protons. The enhancement factors of the proton-bearing carbon sites fall in the range 2.6–2.9, indicating that cross-relaxation is predominantly (but not quite exclusively) determined by the dipolar interaction with the attached protons. The carbon sites carbon-1 and carbon-7, which have no directly-bound protons, show smaller nuclear Overhauser enhancements since they rely to some extent on other relaxation processes.

Signal-to-noise enhancement through the nuclear Overhauser effect has a rival in the alternative technique of polarization transfer (§ 11.8) where the population advantage of spin system *A* is transferred to another spin system *B* in a differential manner. This is one of the principal themes in two-dimensional NMR spectroscopy (Chapter 11).

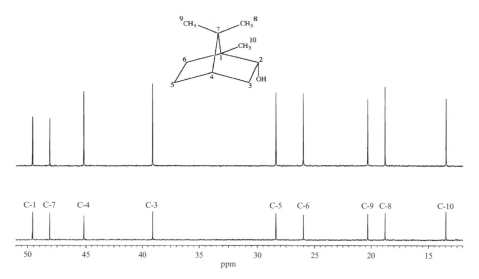

Figure 4.1 The enhancement of intensities in part of the carbon-13 spectrum of endo-(–)-borneol (inset) through the nuclear Overhauser effect. Lower trace: the conventional decoupled spectrum. Upper trace: the spectrum obtained with presaturation of the proton resonances. The experimental enhancement factors are C-1, 1.7; C-7, 1.8; C-4, 3.0; C-3, 2.9; C-5, 2.8; C-6, 2.9; C-9, 2.6; C-8, 2.9, C-10, 2.5. The theoretical maximum enhancement is 2.98. (Spectra courtesy of Toshiaki Nishida).

The treatment outlined above assumes that the molecules under investigation are relatively small so that they tumble rapidly in the liquid phase in comparison with the Larmor frequency. Large biomolecules often fail to meet this requirement as their reorientation can be quite sluggish. In these situations cross-relaxation is dominated by an alternative mechanism in which protons *A* and *B* flip in *opposite directions* (a zero-quantum rather than a double-quantum jump). Then the enhanced signal appears inverted in the spectrum and the maximum enhancement is minus 100 % rather than plus 50 %. For molecules of intermediate size the enhancement may fall between the positive and negative cases and thus be reduced or even disappear, but there are special techniques (for example the 'rotating frame Overhauser effect') which can ensure that the 'true' enhancement is observed.

In applications to large biomolecules such as proteins, many different proton–proton Overhauser enhancements can usually be measured in the same molecule, usually using two-dimensional spectroscopy (§ 11.4). There is little need for accurate determination of interproton distances because the geometry is overdetermined; the cross-relaxation results are simply used as 'distance constraints' on the proposed molecular structure. The key is the rapid fall-off of the Overhauser enhancement according to the sixth power of the interproton distance. For example, if protons on two well-separated units of an extended chain of amino-acids exhibit an appreciable enhancement through cross-relaxation, they must have come within a few Ångstrom units (a few tenths of a nanometre) of each other, indicating that the aminoacid chain has looped back upon itself. This would be a key observation in deciding the tertiary structure of a protein. The nuclear Overhauser effect is one of the most important tools in the armoury of two-dimensional NMR spectroscopy (§ 11.4) particularly for the study of biomolecules.

4.4 Spin temperature

In solid samples an interesting new situation arises. The interaction between nuclear spins is very strong, since each spin experiences strong local magnetic fields from the neighbouring nuclei and there is no motional averaging of these fields. We can now think of the spin system as a separate entity, in a state of internal equilibrium, but still largely isolated from the 'lattice' (all the rest of the sample). This suggests an intriguing new concept—'spin temperature'. It is now permissible to apply the (simplified) Boltzmann expression for the energy level populations

$$(N_{\text{lower}} - N_{\text{upper}})/N_{\text{lower}} = \Delta E/kT^* \qquad \textbf{4.2}$$

to the spin system alone, where T^* now stands for *spin temperature*. In the normal situation where everything is at equilibrium and no radiofrequencies have been applied, T^* and the sample temperature T are of course the same, but by suitable manipulation of the spin populations we can change the spin temperature T^*. The spins can exist at a temperature different from that of the sample, at least on a temporary basis. For example, Equation 4.2 implies that saturation of the spin system ($N_{\text{upper}} = N_{\text{lower}}$) makes T^* infinite. Note that this is only possible in quantum systems where the number of energy levels is restricted (in this case there are usually only two).

The laws of thermodynamics state that there is an absolute minimum of temperature (zero degrees on the Kelvin scale) and that we can never actually reach this point where all motion is completely frozen. As a result, conventional wisdom would rule out negative temperatures on the Kelvin scale. Now suppose we apply a 180° pulse to spins at thermal equilibrium in a solid sample. This interchanges the two spin populations (creating a population inversion), and if we apply Equation 4.2 to that situation, with N_{upper} greater than N_{lower}, we come to the surprising but inescapable conclusion that the spin temperature T^* must be *negative*. To the dismay of those brought up on classical thermodynamics, a negative temperature can indeed exist for this rather special case of strongly interacting nuclear spins isolated from the rest of the world. Naturally the sample temperature remains positive, so some degree of sanity is preserved.

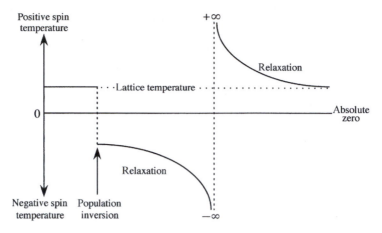

Figure 4.2 Schematic diagram showing the evolution of the spin temperature of nuclei in the solid state after a population inversion. The subsequent spin–lattice relaxation takes the spin temperature to minus infinity, where there are equal spin populations on the upper and lower energy levels. This is equivalent to plus infinity, and relaxation then returns the spin temperature to the that of the lattice, the temperature we would measure with a normal thermometer.

The story becomes even more paradoxical when we examine how these inverted nuclear spins return to thermal equilibrium through the process of spin–lattice relaxation (Figure 4.2). Spins drop down from the upper energy level, thus reducing $(N_{upper} - N_{lower})$, so the spin temperature T^* becomes progressively *more negative*, eventually reaching a temperature of minus infinity as $N_{upper} = N_{lower}$. This 'saturation' condition can just as easily be represented as a spin temperature of plus infinity, and as spin–lattice relaxation continues, T^* starts large and positive and falls exponentially until it reaches the sample temperature again. In a certain sense a negative temperature is very hot! The return to equilibrium never involves passage through the absolute zero of temperature, to the immense relief of conventional thermodynamicists.

It would be a mistake to carry over the concept of spin temperature into NMR experiments in *liquids* because there the spins interact only very weakly and no longer constitute an isolated thermal reservoir in a state of internal equilibrium; consequently the Boltzmann equation (Equation 4.1) cannot be applied to the spin system. Nevertheless some spectroscopists still find it useful to equate saturation with the idea of 'hot' spins, and spin–lattice relaxation with a cooling effect.

4.5 Spin–spin relaxation

Pulse excitation of nuclear spins may be likened to the ringing of a tuning fork, and in both examples the oscillations gradually die away with time. The precessing nuclear spins lose their coherence by a process called spin–spin relaxation and the resultant signal decays with time. So what is the origin of this second relaxation mechanism? Each nuclear spin experiences not only the main applied magnetic field (shielded slightly by the electron cloud), but also tiny local magnetic fields generated by other magnetic nuclei in the immediate environment. These local fields are time-varying due to the relative motion in the liquid phase. (For these purposes it is legitimate to consider even a clinical patient as essentially 'liquid' since the water molecules under investigation are very mobile.)

Think of each nuclear spin as a tiny clock running at the Larmor frequency. In the ideal world all these clocks would run at *exactly* the same frequency—the time-keeping would be perfect. In the real world some clocks run a bit faster or slower than the mean, and if we wait long enough it becomes impossible to tell the 'true' time from any single observation.

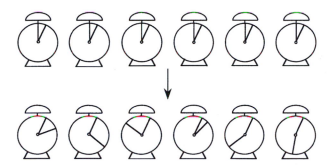

In magnetic resonance, the culprits for this loss of synchronization are the tiny fluctuating local magnetic fields from neighbouring nuclear spins, which slightly perturb the Larmor frequency. Although all the spins are forced to precess in phase at the beginning of an experiment, these time-dependent local fields grad-ually destroy this phase coherence, and the resultant magnetization vector decays with time. The decay follows an exponential curve:

$$M_t = M_0 \exp(-t/T_2) \qquad \textbf{4.3}$$

with a time constant called the spin–spin relaxation time T_2. It is the time taken for the initial signal M_0 to decay to 37 % of its value through spin–spin relax-ation. Once the phase coherence has been lost it cannot be restored, because the time development of each local magnetic field from the neighbouring spins can never be reversed. The relative motion of molecules in a liquid is quite random.

Now, if we try to measure any frequency (say a chemical shift) with the highest possible accuracy, we need to observe it for the longest possible time. If the measurement time is restricted, there is a consequent uncertainty in the observed frequency. In the case of a free precession signal that decays with a time constant

T_2, this translates into a broadening of the NMR response that is inversely proportional to T_2. To take a typical example in high-resolution NMR, if the spin–
spin relaxation time is one second, the full linewidth is 0.3 Hz. For a typical
molecule that moves more sluggishly, T_2 might be one-tenth of a second and the
corresponding linewidth is increased to 3 Hz. Spin–spin relaxation provides a
parameter that allows us to monitor the rate at which a typical molecule rotates
in a liquid. The theoreticians would say that it probes the 'spectral density' of the
reorientational motion.

Spin–spin relaxation determines the *natural* line width, expressed by the for-
mula

$$\Delta\omega = 2/T_2 \qquad\qquad \textbf{4.4}$$

where $\Delta\omega$ is the full linewidth (in radians per second) measured at half-height of
the resonance response. This 'hard core' linewidth can only be observed if all
other line-broadening influences are negligible, for example, in a perfectly uniform and stable magnetic field. It imposes a fundamental limit on the resolving
power of any magnetic resonance technique. In high-resolution NMR, it restricts
the detail with which fine structure can be recorded, while in MRI it can impose
an ultimate limit on the spatial resolution of the images, in situations where all
other blurring influences can be disregarded.

Spin–spin relaxation times can be measured by the spin-echo method (Chapter
9). The most popular scheme involves the generation of a repeated train of spin
echoes in which the echo amplitude decreases exponentially with time constant
T_2. We can sketch typical decay curves for fast, intermediate and slow spin–spin
relaxation:

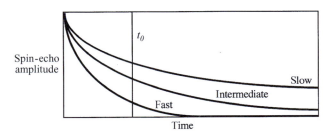

We saw above that differences in the spin–lattice relaxation time T_1 can be
exploited to improve the contrast in MRI images. In a similar manner we can
enhance contrast through the variations in spin–spin relaxation times between
different tissues. In biological tissues T_2 can be much shorter than T_1 and the
range of possible T_2 values for different tissues can be quite large. For example,
cerebrospinal fluid has a typical T_2 value of 300 milliseconds, whereas the liver
has a typical T_2 value of 50 milliseconds. In tumours, the T_2 value of water can be

longer than its value in healthy tissue, and this can serve as an important diagnostic indication.[5] For this reason, 'T_2-weighted' images are very useful in detecting pathology. Signal acquisition is initiated at some appropriate time t_0, giving a different image brightness for each kind of tissue. This is analogous to adjusting the contrast control on a television set.

Experimental measurements of spin–spin relaxation times in high-resolution NMR can provide useful information about molecular structure and motion, and are often used to study the phenomenon of chemical exchange (§ 7.8). When a labile atom moves from one chemical site to another, it carries away a nuclear spin which is then replaced by another spin from another site. This new spin has been precessing for a an arbitrary time at a different frequency. There is therefore a random jump in the observed phase of precession. Each individual nuclear spin experiences a different phase jump, and as a consequence, the ensemble suffers a loss of phase coherence. This shortens the apparent spin–spin relaxation time by an amount that depends on the rate of chemical exchange. We have managed to tag each spin with a completely innocuous label—a change in its precession phase. Unlike other techniques for measuring chemical exchange (for example, deuteration), this method has the virtue it cannot in any way affect the process it is designed to monitor.

Another influence which can shorten the spin–spin relaxation time is the presence of a neighbouring quadrupolar nucleus (such as chlorine-35 or nitrogen-14) that is coupled to the spin being observed—this is known to aficionados as 'scalar relaxation of the second kind'. The spin under investigation undergoes a random jump in the phase of its precession when the quadrupolar nucleus changes its orientation as a result of spin–lattice relaxation. For example, in high-resolution NMR spectroscopy, evidence that a proton is directly bound to nitrogen-14 can be obtained by measuring the spin–spin relaxation time of the proton response.

When we have to deal with the very large molecules characteristic of, say, proteins, the rate of molecular reorientation slows considerably; similar considerations apply to viscous liquids such as glycerine. Local magnetic fields from neighbouring nuclei fluctuate more slowly and have an enhanced effect, significantly shortening the spin–spin relaxation time (T_2). Linewidths are correspondingly increased, and this is one of the reasons why samples of biochemical interest are usually studied at the highest available magnetic fields in order to achieve the greatest separation of the resonance responses from different chemical sites. In the extreme case of a solid substance the local magnetic fields are essentially static, and the spin–spin relaxation time reaches a very short 'rigid lattice' value (§ 10.1).

In high-resolution NMR, and in MRS (Chapter 14) the presence of macromolecules with short spin–spin relaxation times introduces broad features into the spectrum, distorting the baseline and complicating the measurement of the intensities of the responses of interest. This undesirable effect can be minimized by performing a Carr–Purcell spin echo experiment (§ 9.3). By choosing a suitable delay before acquiring the spin echo (typically of the order of 100 milliseconds) we allow the fast-relaxing signal components to decay to low levels without appreciable loss of signal from the slowly-relaxing species (§ 15.2). However, in proton NMR, the echo modulation effect (§ 9.7) may complicate the situation and give rise to spurious intensities.

In MRI, it is the mobile protons, mainly from water, that give rise to the observed signal. Water relaxation can be complicated by the fact that some water molecules are loosely bound to macromolecules. Because there is fast exchange between 'bound' and 'free' water molecules, we observe a weighted average T_2 value. Thus tissues with a relatively low water content tend to have short T_2 values because there is a high proportion of bound water molecules.

4.6 Relationship between T_1 and T_2

It is essential to make a clear distinction between the spin–lattice relaxation time (T_1) and the spin-spin relaxation time (T_2) even though in some substances in the liquid phase they can have approximately the same value. The parameter T_1 governs the behaviour of spin populations and is sometimes called the 'longitudinal' relaxation time because it determines the rate at which the Z-component of magnetization recovers after some disturbance, for example, saturation or population inversion. It also governs how long a spin may occupy the excited state—the 'spin state lifetime'.

The parameter T_2 measures the time constant of the decay of transverse magnetization (the X- and Y-components) and is sometimes known as the 'transverse' relaxation time. It determines how long the precession phases of individual spins remain 'in step' with each other after excitation by a radiofrequency pulse. For this reason T_2 is sometimes called the 'phase memory time'. This term is useful when discussing chemical exchange for it emphasizes how the departure of spins to a chemically distinct site shortens the phase memory time and thus the apparent spin–spin relaxation time. The natural linewidth (the width recorded in a perfectly uniform magnetic field) is inversely proportional to the spin–spin relaxation time.

Now T_1 cannot be shorter than T_2, otherwise we could have a situation where the spin populations had reached Boltzmann equilibrium but there remained some precessing transverse magnetization. Immediately after the initial excitation of the spin system by a radiofrequency pulse the total resultant nuclear magnetization may be represented by a vector of length M. Spin–spin relaxation reduces the transverse components of the vector M, while spin-lattice relaxation increases the component projected onto the Z axis. The magnetization vector never moves outside the surface of a sphere of radius M. In a typical case (with $T_1 = T_2$) the magnetization vector would follow a spiral trajectory from the $+Y$ axis towards the $+Z$ axis as it relaxes towards equilibrium (Figure 4.3).

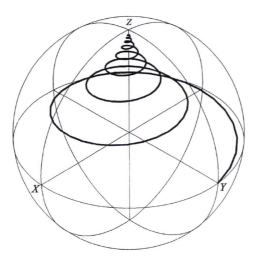

Figure 4.3 Trajectory of the motion of the tip of a nuclear magnetization vector due to free precession in the rotating frame, and spin–spin and spin–lattice relaxation. The relaxation times T_1 and T_2 have been assumed to be equal. A radiofrequency pulse first aligns the vector along the $+Y$ axis. It then changes length and orientation, following a spiral path until it eventually reaches the equilibrium condition along the $+Z$ axis.

If we observe the NMR signal of water containing a relaxation agent such as a gadolinium compound, T_1 is shortened and so is T_2. In this manner we may achieve more rapid polarization (and repolarization) of the sample by enhanced spin–lattice relaxation, but only at the cost of similarly increased spin–spin relaxation and consequent loss of resolving power. For this reason relaxation agents are used rather sparingly in high-resolution NMR, but prove useful in MRI, where image contrast can prove more important than spatial resolution.

The detailed theories of spin–lattice and spin–spin relaxation are quite complex, but need not concern us here. Relaxation merely provides us with two new parameters, T_1 and T_2, that give useful structural information in high-resolution NMR spectroscopy and serve as invaluable tools for enhancing contrast in magnetic resonance images.

Further reading

R. Freeman and H. D. W. Hill, 'Determination of Spin–Spin Relaxation Times in High-Resolution NMR,' in *Dynamic Nuclear Magnetic Resonance*, Academic Press, New York (1975).

E. D. Becker, *High Resolution NMR. Theory and Chemical Applications*, 3rd ed. Academic Press, San Diego, CA (2000).

D. Neuhaus and M. P. Williams, *The Nuclear Overhauser Effect in Structural and Conformational Analysis*, 2nd ed., Wiley-VCH, New York (2000).

5

Sensitivity

5.1 The Boltzmann factor

It is an unfortunate fact that magnetic resonance is not a sensitive technique, that is to say, we need a relatively large amount of material to produce a detectable signal. We have already had a clue to the reason (§ 2.4); most of the nuclear spins in a sample are equally divided between the upper and lower energy levels, with only a tiny excess in the ground state. Because upward and downward transitions are equally probable, one upward jump (absorption of energy) is cancelled by one downward jump (emission), generating no signal in the receiver. Only the small excess population in the lower level (of the order of only 5 nuclei in 100,000) is actually utilized, because this permits net absorption of radiofrequency energy, not matched by equal emission from the upper level. We often loosely refer to this effect as the 'Boltzmann factor' since it is the Boltzmann distribution function that determines the spin populations at equilibrium. Almost all of the tiny nuclear magnets aligned along the magnetic field direction are matched by an equal number that are opposed to the field. This leaves only a very small fraction of spins contributing to the net polarization (§ 2.4). Only under very special circumstances (§ 5.8) can this weak polarization be exceeded.

If magnetic resonance signals are so weak, why not amplify them until they are strong enough to display? The catch is that high amplification also brings to light an undesirable complication—the NMR spectra or MRI displays comprise not only genuine magnetic resonance signals but also some random noise from the electronics used in the detection equipment. If there are too few nuclei contributing to a given resonance line or to a given image pixel, the signal may be completely obscured by this noise. In MRI studies, appreciable amounts of noise are also generated by the sample itself. Hence the pervading obsession in all of magnetic resonance with the need to optimize the 'signal-to-noise ratio'.

This excess population in the lower level, and hence the net polarization, increases in direct proportion to the intensity of the field of the magnet, so high-resolution NMR spectroscopists prefer to work at the highest possible magnetic field (currently 21.14 tesla, giving proton resonance at 900 MHz). On the other hand, to give whole-body access, MRI requires a magnet with a much wider bore, and this limits the achievable magnetic field intensity, normally to 1.5 tesla. There are also regulations governing the maximum magnetic field that may be used with human patients in routine clinical studies, although research with volunteers is not subject to the same restrictions, and experiments can then be performed at fields as high as 7 or even 8 tesla. Increasing the applied magnetic field necessarily implies an increased operating radiofrequency, and since detection is more efficient at higher frequencies, this contributes a further improvement in signal-to-noise. However in MRI this is offset by the fact that image contrast may deteriorate in high polarizing fields, and the radiofrequency attenuation within the human body increases at higher frequencies. As a result of these constraints, it is not yet certain that MRI sensitivity will always improve in step with the strength of the applied magnetic field.

The low Boltzmann factor for magnetic resonance means that we must take all precautions to preserve the polarization we have. Sensitivity requirements often involve repetitive excitation of the nuclear spins and adding together a large number of free induction decays (§ 5.6). Speed is of the essence, so the excitation is repeated without waiting for complete recovery of the polarization through spin–lattice relaxation (§ 4.1). In such cases it can be helpful to enhance the relaxation rate by the addition of a paramagnetic relaxation agent, for example, a gadolinium salt. In MRI, an extension of this idea uses injection of a relaxation agent to enhance the contrast between different parts of the sample; the region that receives this agent recovers its full polarization rapidly and generates a strong signal which appears as a bright feature in the image. In high-resolution NMR spectroscopy, relaxation agents are used only rarely because, unless the dosage is carefully controlled, they can also broaden the resonances and degrade the resolving power. One rather mild relaxation agent for high-resolution NMR is dissolved oxygen gas, which is paramagnetic. Functional MRI of the brain (§ 17.2) exploits the paramagnetism induced in human blood when oxygen is metabolized, leaving paramagnetic deoxyhemoglobin.

5.2 The receiver coil

On a more mundane level, it is important to pay particular attention to those instrumental parameters that improve signal strength. The key importance of the receiver coil has already been emphasized in § 3.2. This coil should have a high quality factor Q, the ratio of the stored radiofrequency energy to the energy dissipated in the coil resistance; a typical value for the Q factor in high-resolution NMR might be 500. The coil quality factor boosts the signal-to-noise ratio in proportion to the square root of Q. A high quality factor is favoured by high conductivity wire. Often strips of copper foil are used, but they are not suitable for aqueous samples containing ions, where dielectric loss is significant, because such coils have a relatively high capacitive coupling to the sample. In MRI, the lossy nature of the patient's tissue normally outweighs the effect of the Q factor of the coil.

The receiver coil should be as close to the sample as possible, that is to say, the 'filling factor' should approach unity; we must not waste any of the space enclosed by the coil. When it is necessary to investigate a very small sample then a smaller coil should be employed. The majority of the inductance should be in the turns of the coil and not in the leads. Tuning capacitors should have low loss. For high-resolution NMR studies where the coil is very close to the sample, the magnetic susceptibility of the wire should be matched to that of air so that there is no distortion of the magnetic field at the sample. This can be achieved by cladding one metal of positive magnetic susceptibility with another of negative susceptibility. For MRI, it is important to tailor the shape and size of the coil to the particular application. Whereas the magnet is normally designed to accept the whole body, the receiver coil needs to fit around the head or a particular limb, or a 'wraparound' surface coil can be employed (§ 3.2).

For high-resolution NMR spectroscopy most applications employ a standard 5 mm diameter glass tube to contain the sample, and a saddle-shaped receiver coil is employed which fits around the sample tube with just enough clearance to allow sample spinning. Some recent developments associated with combinatorial chemistry (§ 16.1) employ a discontinuous flow system where a 'slug' of solution is pumped into the receiver coil, with signal detection while the sample is at rest. This sample is then washed out by a larger volume of pure solvent before inserting a second slug containing a different analyte. This lends itself to computer-controlled automation and permits a more rapid succession of measurements, albeit at the cost of a certain degree of cross-contamination between successive samples. High-performance liquid chromatography is sometimes employed to feed a continuously flowing sample into the NMR receiver coil (§ 15.5).

5.3 The sample

The next major factor determining sensitivity is the sample itself, in particular its volume and the concentration of nuclear spins. In MRI, we might suppose that there is no control over the sample volume; the patient is what he is. But in actual practice there is a direct trade-off between sensitivity and resolution; the size of a voxel (volume element) can be increased, giving higher sensitivity because it contains more nuclear spins, but only at the expense of lower spatial definition.

In high-resolution NMR spectroscopy, sensitivity is roughly proportional to the sample volume and to the concentration of nuclear spins. While these features are beyond our control in MRI, they can be usually be optimized in high-resolution NMR if we have enough material and if its solubility is sufficiently high. In this respect an operating temperature above ambient is often an advantage; it usually increases solubility faster than it decreases the Boltzmann factor. However, many chemical compounds for study are only available in limited quantities; moreover it is more difficult to achieve a uniform magnetic field over a large sample volume. When only limited quantities of material are available it can be advantageous to use a smaller-than-normal sample tube. In one implementation (the 'nano-probe') a small sample is spun very fast about the 'magic angle', an inclination of 54.7° with respect to the main magnetic field direction.[1] With this particular geometry (§ 10.2) spinning suppresses the field distortions caused by discontinuities of magnetic susceptibility, permitting high resolution to be achieved. Another approach employs an extremely small cylindrical sample (typically 77 micrometres internal diameter and 1 mm long) tightly enclosed in a receiver coil surrounded by a liquid of carefully matched magnetic susceptibility.[2] Sensitivity is then determined by the total number of active spins in the sample, and it is eventually limited by solubility rather than by the quantity of material available.

Another important factor that restricts sensitivity is the low natural abundance of certain nuclear species, such as carbon-13 or nitrogen-15. This has greatly limited their application in MRI, even though higher magnetic fields can be used for experimental studies with volunteer patients. However, the concentration of magnetic nuclei can be improved by artificial enrichment of a particular isotope. This can be an advantage in some clinical studies because we can inject an isotopically-enriched substance (for example, glucose artificially labelled with the carbon-13 isotope) which shows up well against the low background signal from natural abundance carbon-13 nuclei. This strategy has been exploited for MRS of brain metabolism using, for example, acetate labelled with carbon-13. Magnetic resonance imaging relies predominantly on proton resonance, but fluorine-19, sodium-23, phoshorus-31 and xenon-129 can be used for specialized applications.

High-resolution NMR is more tolerant of low-abundance isotopes, because the studies are usually carried out at much higher magnetic fields. Often the chemical problem under investigation dictates which nucleus should be employed. Almost every element in the periodic table has at least one isotope with magnetic properties, and has been studied by NMR.

5.4 Thermal noise

As discussed in Chapter 3, the inherent weakness of magnetic resonance signals means that they are usually accompanied by noise—erratic voltage fluctuations that arise principally from the random motion of the electrons in the receiver coil.

For aqueous samples that contain ions, the random thermal agitation of these charged particles also induces a signal in the receiver coil and contributes to the noise. This coupling is capacitive rather than inductive, so it can be minimized by suitable design of the receiver coil. We have to accept a fundamental conflict between the desirable and the undesirable, quantified by the signal-to-noise ratio.

Sensitivity is defined in terms of the minimum quantity of sample that gives a detectable signal. Under normal operating conditions, a high signal-to-noise ratio goes hand-in-hand with good sensitivity, but this is not the case if we introduce a non-linear component or employ a non-linear processing scheme. It is quite possible to devise 'magic' schemes that suppress noise and 'improve' the MRI image or the high-resolution NMR spectrum in a spectacular fashion, but they also suppress weak magnetic resonance responses comparable with the noise. Sensitivity is *not* enhanced by such techniques.[3] As one illustrative example we could consider the method known as 'trigger' detection, where a latent oscillation is set off by a very weak magnetic resonance signal, rather like the initiation of an avalanche. The weak initial signal is thus converted into a very strong final response, and it is easy to fall into the trap of thinking that the sensitivity has been thereby enhanced. But when we focus attention on an initial NMR signal that is so weak that it lies below the level of random noise, we see that now only a noise spike can initiate the avalanche—the weak NMR signal is not enhanced at all. Non-linear data processing schemes fall into the same trap—signals that would have been detected anyway are greatly enhanced in comparison with the noise, but those that were initially weaker than the noise are lost forever. Hence the emphasis on linear systems and linear data processing schemes. The noise level then serves a useful purpose—it indicates the detection limit for that particular experiment.

Let us concentrate, therefore, on *legitimate* methods for improving sensitivity. In high-resolution NMR spectroscopy the problem can be attacked at its source by cooling the receiver coil to a very low temperature (§ 3.2). This has two distinct effects. It quietens down the haphazard motion of the electrons in the wire, an effect inversely proportional to the square root of the absolute temperature, so that a reduction from ambient temperature to the temperature of liquid helium should theoretically offer an eightfold improvement. Cooling also enhances the quality factor (Q) of the coil by decreasing its resistance. Quality factors as high as 20,000 have been achieved at 25 K, to be compared with Q factors of about 500 at room temperature. The signal-to-noise ratio improves in proportion to the square root of Q. These cryogenic techniques for high-resolution NMR studies have been given a new lease of life through the use of high-temperature superconducting materials. However, for radiofrequencies the resistance does not go to zero as it does for direct current. The drawbacks of this method arise from a loss in filling factor of the receiver coil (since it must be thermally shielded from the sample), and a degradation in Q factor when aqueous samples are used, particularly if ions are present. This cryogenic receiver coil technology is still in its infancy and has yet to be widely implemented. To date, sensitivity improvements of approximately fourfold have been achieved, albeit with a rather expensive cryogenic accessory. Note, of course, that these cryogenic probes operate with the sample still at room temperature, so no advantage is gained from the higher polarization that would have been achieved at the low temperature. In any case, cooling is not really an option—in high-resolution NMR the sample is normally a liquid, and in MRI the patient prefers to be kept warm.

5.5 Smoothing

There are actually only two procedures that discriminate between genuine magnetic resonance signals and random noise. The first of these is most simply described as smoothing. The noise response may be fluctuating with time more rapidly than the desired magnetic resonance signal, and may be reduced by a suitable smoothing or filter function, either electronic in nature or through computer software. (In a similar manner, the day-to-day fluctuations in the stock market are smoothed by computing a 30-day moving average, so that the longer-term trends become more evident.) This is a rather crude example of a general mathematical operation called convolution.[4] Let us consider the process of smoothing a noisy magnetic resonance signal by convoluting it with a simple 1:2:1 function. We assume that the magnetic resonance response is represented by a sequence of discrete ordinates plotted as a function of frequency. At some general point along the frequency axis we take 50 % of that ordinate and add to it 25 % of the previous ordinate and 25 % of the following ordinate. A new trace is constructed where this sum replaces the value at that frequency step. The process is repeated for all the frequency increments on the magnetic resonance response (neglecting the first and last). This simple convolution operation reduces the level of high-frequency fluctuations. Processing is very fast and can be cascaded as necessary to increase the degree of smoothing, but eventually it will begin to broaden the responses from genuine magnetic resonance signals.

Noise filtration can also be considered in the time domain. If the free precession signal is acquired for a time much longer than the decay time constant, we accumulate mainly noise in the 'tail' where there is negligible signal. The remedy is to multiply the free precession signal with a decaying exponential curve, the so-called 'sensitivity enhancement' function which de-emphasizes the tail. After Fourier transformation this corresponds to the removal of the high-frequency components of the noise, equivalent to a smoothing operation in the frequency domain. This process cannot be carried too far because it will eventually broaden the high-resolution NMR responses or blur the MRI proton density map. The optimum is a sensitivity enhancement function with a time constant that just matches the decay rate of the free precession signal, the so-called 'matched filter'. This entails only a slight degradation in resolution. This noise reduction technique is used almost universally in NMR and MRI applications. Sensitivity enhancement in the time domain and convolution in the frequency domain are essentially equivalent processes.

5.6 Time averaging

The second property that distinguishes signals from noise is the random, non-reproducible nature of the noise. If two successive free precession signals are acquired, the magnetic resonance signal is faithfully reproduced whereas the noise fluctuates in amplitude and perhaps in sign. If we add N successive free precession signals together (with the correct registration) the true magnetic resonance response increases in direct proportion to N, whereas the noise is sometimes positive and sometimes negative, and to a certain extent is self-cancelling. The noise level only increases as the square root of N, so the signal-to-noise ratio increases as the square root of N. This is known as coherent averaging or time averaging. Note, however, the law of diminishing returns—to double the signal-to-noise ratio we must increase the accumulation time fourfold. In MRI this could place an unacceptable burden on the patient; in high-resolution NMR it could tie up an expensive spectrometer for a long time. In this treatment of sensitivity, it is taken for granted that pulse excitation and Fourier transformation[5,6] are used (§ 3.7). Otherwise, if the old-fashioned frequency-sweep methods are employed, sensitivity suffers because of the very slow rate of data gathering.

The time-averaging technique is degraded if the free precession signals are not combined in exact registration, or if there are inherent instabilities in the system. In MRI this could be exacerbated by involuntary motion of the patient. Time averaging relies on the random nature of noise. It affords little or no benefit if some artefact is masquerading as noise, for then the artefact may well repeat itself in successive scans and will then increase linearly with N, just like a genuine magnetic resonance signal.

5.7 Artefacts

In practical situations, instrumental artefacts may cause more problems for the detection of weak NMR signals than true random noise. Artefacts differ from noise in that, in principle, they are reproducible from one free induction signal to the next. Nevertheless some of these artefacts appear to look like noise and they certainly degrade the sensitivity. Coherent features are the least serious; they comprise the discrete 'spinning sideband' responses caused by spinning the sample in an inhomogeneous magnetic field, and some spurious modulation components from the mains frequency (50 Hz or 60 Hz and their harmonics). Because such sidebands affect all the NMR responses in an identical manner, they can be removed by a data-processing technique known as 'reference deconvolution'.[4]

Decoupling sequences are never perfect (§ 8.5) and the residual imperfections generate weak 'cycling sidebands'. Although there are schemes to reduce the overall amplitude of decoupling sidebands by increasing the complexity of the decoupling scheme (nesting one type of cycle within another), these can cause more harm than good because they 'chop up' the cycling sidebands into many weaker components which then resemble true noise more closely. The devil you know (an identifiable coherent sideband) may be preferable to the devil you don't know.

Mention has already been made of the restrictions imposed by the limited dynamic range of the equipment which converts analog signals into digital form (§ 3.6). Because of the discrete nature of the sampling, this analog-to-digital converter makes slight errors in estimating the intensity of weak signal components. These errors are converted by the Fourier transformation stage into 'digitization noise' which, although deterministic in origin, nevertheless has much the appearance of random noise. This potential problem is avoided by limiting the dynamic range of the incoming magnetic resonance signal, often by suppressing the intense signal from the solvent.

Finally, if the sample is a complex mixture of many chemical components, some of them at very low concentrations, then the NMR spectrum contains a forest of weak unidentifiable signals that have been (rather loosely) called 'chemical noise'. This is a fairly common occurrence in high-resolution NMR of body fluids (Chapter 15).

5.8 Hyperpolarized systems

The foregoing has emphasized the very low intrinsic polarization of magnetic resonance systems, but in recent years increasing use has been made of schemes that generate much higher excess spin populations in the ground state. This is known as *hyperpolarization*. Naturally, when left to themselves, hyperpolarized systems revert to the normal Boltzmann population distribution by spin–lattice relaxation (§ 4.1). Now we normally think of spin–lattice relaxation as a mechanism for causing excited spins to fall back from the upper energy level to the lower level. In complete contrast, relaxation of a hyperpolarized system involves nuclear spins jumping *upwards* from the lower energy level to the upper level until the normal weakly polarized situation is re-established.

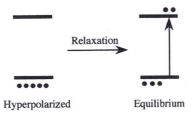

An important practical example is the magnetic isotope xenon-129 which is 26 % abundant in nature. Levels of hyperpolarization as high as 50 % can be achieved, compared with natural polarizations of roughly one part in 100,000, so strong xenon signals are observable despite the low spin density in the gas phase. Because the xenon-129 nucleus has no quadrupole moment, it is suitable for high-resolution NMR, and it has the important advantage that the spin–lattice relaxation time at room temperature is long, typically between 10 and 100 seconds, so a high level of polarization can be retained for an appreciable time.

Preparation of hyperpolarized xenon gas starts with the optical pumping of rubidium atoms by laser light. The energy levels appropriate to optical transitions are so far apart that (in contrast to NMR) the ground state is essentially 100 % populated. An optical pumping experiment can transfer much of this high spin population selectively to another chosen energy level provided that the laser light is circularly polarized. If the rubidium vapor contains xenon gas, 'spin exchange' takes place, transferring part of the polarization to xenon-129.

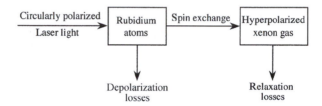

If hyperpolarized xenon is isolated and cooled to the temperature of liquid nitrogen, spin–lattice relaxation is slowed down to times of the order of an hour, allowing the xenon to be transported between different laboratories without appreciable loss of polarization. It is almost an article of faith that magnetic resonance experiments should be carried out at the highest available magnetic field in order to optimize sensitivity. This is *not* the case for a system that has been hyperpolarized; the strength of the signal is then independent of the magnetic field of the spectrometer used for the observation. This permits MRI investigations at low magnetic fields where the complications due to mismatches in magnetic susceptibility are minimized.

High-resolution NMR of hyperpolarized xenon has been used as a probe of porous solids, to measure the rate of diffusion of the gas through a solid material, and to investigate the trapping of molecules within zeolites. For MRI applications, hyperpolarized xenon can be inhaled directly and because the magnetic resonance signal is so strong, it can be used to monitor the process of lung ventilation. In a similar manner, hyperpolarized helium-3 can be used for the same purpose.[7]

Xenon NMR spectra or magnetic resonance images are 'clean' because there is no interference from background signals. The chemical shift of xenon extends over a wide range, and because the 'squishy' outer electron cloud is easily distorted, xenon has the valuable property of being very sensitive to external perturbations. It can, for example, detect the presence of a near neighbour atom although no chemical bond is formed. Hyperpolarized xenon can be used as a 'functionalized biosensor'—if a xenon atom is enclosed within a cage that is attached by a tether to a ligand that binds to a protein, there is an appreciable change in the xenon chemical shift for the bound species. Xenon is lipophilic; it dissolves rapidly in the bloodstream and is transported throughout the body, allowing perfusion imaging of the brain for example, but it has the practical disadvantage for human studies that it acts as an anaesthetic at high concentrations.

5.9 Conclusions

To sum up, there are many factors that influence the sensitivity of a magnetic resonance measurement; some are under our control, while others are intrinsic to the technique itself:

1. The type of magnetic nucleus under investigation
2. The intensity of the main magnetic field
3. The concentration of the material being studied
4. The sample volume (NMR) or the size of a voxel (MRI)
5. The degree of natural isotopic abundance or artificial enrichment
6. The spin–lattice and spin–spin relaxation times (Chapter 4)
7. The duration of multiscan averaging
8. The degree of signal smoothing
9. Design of the equipment, particularly the receiver coil
10. Various instrumental artefacts that have the appearance of noise
11. Special pulse sequences, for example, echo planar imaging (§ 12.7)
12. The Overhauser effect (§ 4.3)
13. Polarization transfer (§ 11.8)
14. Hyperpolarization (§ 5.8)

Further reading

D. I. Hoult and R. E. Richards, *Proc. Roy. Soc. (London)*, A **344**, 311 (1975).
R. Freeman, *A Handbook of Nuclear Magnetic Resonance*, 2nd ed., Addison Wesley Longman, Harlow, Essex, UK (1997).

6

Resolving power

Resolving power is the key factor in both astronomy and microscopy. It is not just a question of making the images big enough to see, but rather of being able to resolve one interesting feature from its near neighbours. A blurred image cannot be improved simply by making it larger. It is the quality of the telescope or microscope lenses that determines the all-important *resolving power* or *resolution*. Magnetic resonance has the same obsession with high resolving power.

In MRI, resolving power implies spatial resolution, the ability to distinguish fine details of the anatomy. In high-resolution NMR spectroscopy it means the ability to separate closely-spaced resonance lines, for example, from two chemically distinct species. But this is only an apparent distinction—both MRI and NMR are principally concerned with the limitations on the uniformity of the applied magnetic field, sometimes called the *homogeneity* of the field. If the magnetic field varies over the volume of interest this blurs the response and hides fine detail in the image or the spectrum.

Resolution should not be confused with *definition*. The picture on a television screen needs to be clear enough (good resolution) that we can distinguish the features of the news presenter, but if you ever happen to sneeze and a droplet hits the screen, it will behave like a primitive microscope and reveal that the screen consists of a raster of discrete coloured dots which limit definition. We normally expect the definition to be much finer than the resolution. The image obtained by MRI or a spectrum recorded by high-resolution NMR is represented in digital form where the digitization steps determine the definition, which in some cases may be coarser than the intrinsic resolution. In MRI we speak of a pixel (picture element) which is derived from a voxel (volume element). We measure only a single intensity for each voxel; any variation of properties across that voxel is lost once and for all. There is now a common technique for hiding some particular detail of a photograph by imposing a cluster of oversized pixels. Similarly, in MRI it may sometimes be necessary to choose a voxel size so large that it obscures the potential resolution, because this gathers signal intensity from a larger number of nuclear spins, thereby improving the sensitivity.

In high-resolution NMR, limits on definition may be imposed by the restricted number of data points available, particularly in multidimensional spectroscopy (Chapter 11). Only when the digital definition is fine enough do we reach the intrinsic resolving power of the instrument. However, in contrast to MRI, employing coarser definition in an NMR spectrum does not improve the sensitivity significantly.

6.1 The natural linewidth

So what are the practical limitations on resolution? First of all there is the fundamental 'hard core' natural linewidth set by spin–spin relaxation as outlined in § 4.5. If the spin–spin relaxation time T_2 is 1 second, then the full-width at half-height of the resonance line can never be less than 0.3 Hz, no matter how hard we work to make the magnetic field more uniform. In practice a natural linewidth of such a small magnitude is unlikely to prove a serious restriction on resolution for most chemical applications of NMR.

In MRI applications, line broadening effects can be more severe than in high-resolution NMR spectroscopy because a fairly large voxel size may be required to ensure adequate signal-to-noise ratio. Furthermore, the spin–spin relaxation times of human tissues can be quite short and may affect the resolving power in some instances.

Natural linewidths begin to assume critical importance for high-resolution NMR samples containing macromolecules, because these sluggish molecules tumble (reorient) quite slowly compared with the intrinsic nuclear precession frequencies, increasing the broadening due to spin–spin relaxation. It is quite common in MRS (§ 14.2) of phosphorus NMR *in vivo* to subtract out broad baseline components so that the intensities of the narrow resonance can be properly evaluated. The proton spectra of certain samples, for example blood, may comprise both broad lines from macromolecules and narrow lines from small molecules. In such cases the responses from the macromolecules can be greatly reduced by performing a spin-echo experiment (§ 9.3) in which signal acquisition is delayed until the fast-relaxing components have died away to a low level. The slowly relaxing components (corresponding to the narrow resonances) still retain most of their intensity.

Magnetic resonance images are also affected by differences in rates of spin–spin relaxation, but this can be put to good use by exploiting the spin-echo technique to introduce a delay before the start of signal acquisition, so that the intensities of various signals depend upon their respective spin–spin relaxation times. This alters the *contrast* of the image—the difference in brightness between signals from adjacent tissues (§ 12.9). These 'T_2-weighted images' are often used in MRI investigations of the human brain. High contrast can be more important than good signal-to-noise ratio for many clinical purposes.

6.2 Instrumental limitations

In general, the natural linewidth is not normally the critical factor; it is more likely that resolution is limited by instrumental shortcomings or some non-ideality of the sample itself. The main factor for high-resolution NMR is the spatial uniformity of the applied magnetic field measured over the effective sample volume. The distribution of magnetic fields translates into a distribution of Larmor frequencies and a broadening of the response. For MRI, lack of uniformity of the main magnetic field begins to degrade the resolving power when adjacent voxels generate responses at the same frequency. This blurs the fine details of the image. There is a second (global) effect if the applied magnetic field varies significantly over the organ of interest. This upsets the desired linear relationship between frequency and position, thus distorting the image that is observed.

Before magnetic resonance was discovered in 1949, hardly anyone was concerned with the design of magnets with a highly uniform field. Early magnetic resonance experiments used any magnet that was available around the laboratory. It was only after the first high resolution proton spectrum was obtained, showing three separate resonances of ethanol,[1] that physicists realized the crucial importance of field uniformity. In a classic paper, Arnold[2] describes the design and construction of a highly homogeneous permanent magnet made of an alloy containing titanium, cobalt and aluminium. The result—resolution approaching one part in 60 million—was a quite remarkable pioneering achievement that made possible the first really high-resolution NMR spectra of protons.

The magnet uniformity problem proves to be more serious for MRI, where the bore of the superconducting solenoid has to be large enough to accept a human patient, and the field must be reasonably uniform over a volume spanning, say, the human head or even the entire torso, if the image is not to be distorted. For high-resolution NMR spectroscopy, the magnet bore can be much narrower (of the order of 5 cm in diameter) while the effective diameter of the sample is only about 5 mm.

The general design principles are essentially the same for present-day magnets built for MRI or NMR. A superconducting solenoid is employed, normally operating at the temperature of liquid helium. A solenoid with uniform windings along its length generates a magnetic field that necessarily falls off at the ends. High field uniformity requires that these end effects be compensated, so an actual solenoid is constructed with several different windings, fed with electric currents calculated to cancel the higher-order variations of field intensity as a function of distance along the axis of the solenoid. In addition, there is a set of superconduct-ing 'correction coils' in which the currents are adjusted during the setting-up procedure to counteract the residual field gradients of the main solenoid. Finally there is a second set of correction coils, operating at room temperature, carrying currents that can be readjusted from one experiment to the next. These correction coils are carefully designed to counteract the existing natural field gradients one at a time, with the minimum interaction between different coils. In MRI, very high currents may be required in the room-temperature correction coils, involving power supplies dissipating many kilowatts. In high-resolution NMR, the correc-tion currents are far weaker and optimisation is often carried out by an automatic program that seeks to maximize the peak height of a standard reference line, usually the deuterium resonance from the solvent. Narrowing the linewidth by improving field uniformity makes the peak height correspondingly taller.

The majority of high-resolution NMR spectra are recorded while the sample is spinning about its long axis,[3] typically at about ten revolutions per second (§ 2.8). A small air turbine is used, often driving a tachometer to monitor and even regulate the spinning speed. This spinning motion forces the nuclei to follow a circular path through the inhomogeneities of the main magnetic field. If the spinning rate is high compared with the instrumental linewidth of the stationary sample, the observed response is considerably narrowed. A typical nuclear spin moves through a range of local magnetic fields and generates a 'spectrum' of precession frequencies. The principal component of this spectrum is at the mean frequency and has a narrow linewidth; the effects of the field gradients transverse to the spinning axis are largely eliminated. The minor components of this spec-trum are frequency modulated at the spinning rate and its harmonics; they give rise to weak 'spinning sidebands' on each side of the main NMR response. The relative intensities of the spinning sidebands can be minimized by increasing the spinning rate and by careful adjustment of the currents in the correction coils, thus reducing the field gradients transverse to the spinning axis.

The chemists who routinely employ high-resolution NMR pay particular atten-tion to optimization of the resolution. This may entail a tedious sequence of manual adjustments to the field correction coils or a protracted automatic com-puter optimization routine. Not only does this make possible the measurement of very small spin–spin coupling constants or very small differences in chemical shift, but it also improves the signal-to-noise ratio by gathering all the available signal components into a narrow response. The integral of each response remains constant, but the peaks become correspondingly taller.

Superconducting solenoids can be designed to give a very high degree of uni-formity for high-resolution NMR. At the highest fields and with sample spinning they can attain a resolving power of the order of one in ten billion (10^{10}). We would hardly expect an astronomical telescope to reach this degree of resolving power. The physically larger solenoids used in MRI must achieve high uniformity over considerably larger effective volumes. In both cases the key is in the geometrical arrangement of the coil windings, and the quality of the superconducting wire itself. It is this high-technology aspect that accounts for a large part of the cost of modern NMR and MRI equipment.

Magnetic resonance imaging inevitably involves the application of magnetic field gradients superimposed on the main (static) magnetic field. Not only must these gradient fields remain stable in time but they should also be extremely linear as a function of distance, otherwise the resulting image will be distorted. As these gradient fields are switched, they can induce eddy currents in surrounding electrical conductors, and these eddy current generate undesirable transient magnetic fields. Schemes are available to minimize eddy currents by shielding the gradient coils, or to correct their effects by suitably shaping the driving current profiles.

Even with 'ordinary' materials (those that are not ferromagnetic) a magnetic field is distorted to some extent as it passes from one material to another because of changes in a property called the *diamagnetic susceptibility*. A perfectly uniform magnetic field has all the lines of force parallel and equally spaced. Any object placed in such a magnetic field slightly distorts these lines of force, for example, by making them slightly less densely packed inside the object; that material is said to be *diamagnetic*. The sketch exaggerates the effect for the purpose of illustration:

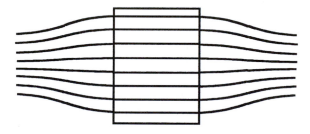

Such a material is said to have a negative magnetic susceptibility and a relative permeability less than unity. Some other materials act to concentrate the lines of force (again exaggerated here):

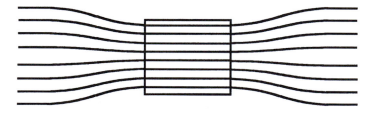

These *paramagnetic* materials have a positive magnetic susceptibility and a relative permeability slightly greater than unity. Most everyday materials are diamagnetic, but they have varying degrees of diamagnetism.

Even if a superconducting solenoid itself generates a perfectly uniform field, the presence of the radiofrequency coil, the field gradient coils, their supports, the shielding, and the sample container, all create some inhomogeneity because of susceptibility differences. The closer to the sample, the more critical are their magnetic susceptibility effects. For high-resolution NMR particular care is taken over the choice of materials that make up the radiofrequency probe, even to the extent of using composite metals for the receiver coil to achieve a magnetic susceptibility close to that of air.

Another limiting factor is the stability of the magnet. It serves little purpose to have a very high spatial uniformity, if the magnetic field fluctuates appreciably in time. Fortunately superconducting solenoids are inherently very stable, since the current is constant and the geometrical stability is high because the coil is immersed in a constant temperature bath of liquid helium at 4.2°K. Mechanical vibrations in the laboratory are damped by carefully designed supports for the solenoid. Residual instabilities and extraneous variable magnetic fields from the environment can be compensated by a servo loop that works to stabilize the ratio of the magnetic field to the Larmor frequency. Nevertheless, it is always important to avoid introducing large iron or steel objects into a magnetic resonance laboratory; not only can they distort the field at the sample site, but if they suddenly collide with the solenoid they present the danger of a catastrophic magnet quench (§ 2.2).

Finally there are effects that act to smear the image or the spectrum. In MRI these may well arise from motion of the patient while the magnetic resonance data are being collected; some of these movements are involuntary, and some are cyclic (for example, the heart beat) and may be circumvented by synchronization of data acquisition with a physiological trigger (§ 12.10). In high-resolution NMR, blurring can result from the loss of registration during time-averaging if there is a slow drift of the magnetic field. This is a fairly common effect in protracted two-dimensional NMR experiments. Some superconducting solenoids are designed to reach higher magnetic fields by pumping on the liquid helium so as to lower the operating temperature below 4.2°K; the field stability may then be less reliable because the pressure can vary with time.

6.3 The patient

In MRI applications the human patient is not an ideal sample; magnetic susceptibility varies throughout the body, and the consequent field distortions are difficult to calculate because they depend on shape in a complex manner. These effects are correspondingly more serious the higher the applied magnetic field, and this may eventually limit the applicability of very high field imaging. Evidence of local field distortion can be demonstrated very vividly by a 'tagging' technique where a regular array of dark lines is superimposed on the image slice in both dimensions, giving a square grid pattern.[4] These lines are generated by a selective saturation sequence employing a regular array of narrow frequency components. In a non-uniform field the grid is distorted in a quantitative manner. The same tagging device can be used to highlight any motion that occurs between the imposition of the tagging sequence and acquisition of the imaging data. This has been exploited to study cardiac motion, for example, by measuring the deformation of the initial square grid observed at mid-systole after tagging at end-systole.

Air passages in the body contain oxygen gas which is mildly paramagnetic, distorting the field in nearby tissues. Blood changes its magnetic susceptibility when it loses oxygen, a fact that is exploited in functional MRI of the brain (§ 17.2). Prosthetic devices, for example, an orthodontic brace, can induce serious distortions of the applied magnetic field through magnetic susceptibility effects. The potential dangers of implanted devices, that may even be ferromagnetic, are addressed in Chapter 13.

6.4 Resolution enhancement

It can often be useful to increase the resolving power beyond that imposed by the instrument itself. In high-resolution NMR it can be brought about artificially by processing the data after acquisition. Resolution in the frequency domain is high if the free precession signal decays slowly in the time-domain; there is a reciprocal relationship between the two domains. If the time-domain NMR signal can be prolonged by multiplication with a rising function of time, then the corresponding linewidths are narrowed and finer detail can be resolved. This 'resolution enhancement' procedure is the converse of the more usual 'sensitivity enhancement' scheme where the time-domain signal is multiplied by a decaying exponential function. An example is shown in § 15.2 where the resolution of a proton NMR spectrum of blood plasma has been artificially enhanced. The penalty for resolution enhancement is a slight decrease in the signal-to-noise ratio, because this kind of data manipulation emphasizes the tail of the free induction decay which carries a disproportionate degree of noise. As always, there is a trade-off between resolution and sensitivity.

Resolution enhancement can also be achieved in the frequency domain. Then the process is called *deconvolution*, a mathematical operation that removes extraneous broadening factors. There is a Fourier transform relationship involved here; multiplication of the time-domain signal by a decaying exponential is equivalent to convolution of the frequency-domain signal with a Lorentzian curve. Deconvolution represents the inverse process. One danger of resolution enhancement or deconvolution is that artefacts in the high-resolution NMR spectrum may be rendered more prominent. For this reason it is advisable to restrict resolution enhancement schemes to magnetic resonance data with adequately high signal-to-noise ratio, thereby lessening the danger that a noise spike might be so enhanced that it is mistaken for a genuine spectral feature. In some experiments, particularly two-dimensional NMR spectroscopy (Chapter 11), time limitations make it impossible to avoid a step function at the end of the time-domain response in the evolution dimension; this introduces sinc-like oscillations on the frequency-domain resonances, and these are aggravated by resolution enhancement.

One of the fundamental concepts of MRI has even been adopted in high-resolution NMR with a view to improving the resolving power. In principle, the blurring effect of field inhomogeneity would be reduced if the sample volume could be made smaller. However, in practice the expected improvement is not achieved because local discontinuities in magnetic susceptibility become increasingly serious for very small samples. On the other hand, it is quite feasible to reduce the *effective* sample volume by selective excitation in an imposed magnetic field gradient followed by signal acquisition in the absence of that gradient. Normally the active volume of the sample is set by the tube diameter (5 mm) and the height of the radiofrequency coil:

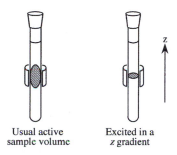

Usual active   Excited in a
sample volume z gradient

Excitation while a magnetic field gradient is imposed along the z axis reduces the effective volume to a thin 'xy' slice, and when that gradient is removed the resolution is improved because the natural gradients in the z direction have much less influence.

Further reading

A. E. Derome, *Modern NMR Techniques for Chemistry Research*, Pergamon Press, Oxford (1987).
E. D. Becker, *High Resolution NMR: Theory and Chemical Applications*, 3rd ed., Academic Press, San Diego, CA (2000).

7

The chemical shift

For those readers mainly interested in clinical applications of magnetic resonance it may be tempting to skip this chapter altogether. This would be a pity, because the chemical shift plays an important part in certain forms of MRI and is crucial to the understanding of MRS, which allows us to follow the metabolism of the human body. However, the main thrust of this chapter is towards chemistry.

The high-resolution NMR spectrum of a chemical compound can be described in terms of two fundamental parameters, the chemical shift (the shielding effect of the extranuclear electrons) and the spin–spin coupling (an interaction between neighbour nuclei). These parameters are intrinsic properties of the molecule under investigation and in no way depend on the type of NMR spectrometer or the way it is operated. The detailed appearance of the spectrum may change according to the strength of the magnetic field, but the chemical shifts and the coupling constants are fixed once and for all. Apart from line broadening effects and perturbations caused by double irradiation, the structure of the high-resolution can be predicted from just these two parameters.

7.1 Chemical shifts

This is the really important parameter for the chemist. An atom consists of a very small central nucleus surrounded by electrons. These electrons are the 'glue' that holds the atoms together, forming a molecule. It is the motion of these electrons in a magnetic field that is responsible for the chemical shift. To understand this mechanism we have to come to terms with the idea that an electron is not simply a very small particle but can be visualized as a kind of diffuse 'cloud' representing the probability that we would find the electron at a particular point in space. We can therefore speak of electron 'density' around the central nucleus. Sometimes we think of an electron as a particle that can be accelerated and made to collide with other particles, sometimes it behaves as a diffuse wave and exhibits interference effects. Physicists call this phenomenon 'wave-particle duality'.

The nucleus is slightly 'shielded' from the applied magnetic field by the electron cloud. A magnetic field causes this cloud to circulate, generating a tiny electrical current which in turn creates an additional magnetic field at the nucleus, opposite in sense to the applied field. Alternatively, we can imagine that the lines of force representing the external magnetic field are slightly deflected by the electron cloud and fail to penetrate it completely, being slightly less closely packed at the nucleus than outside the atom.

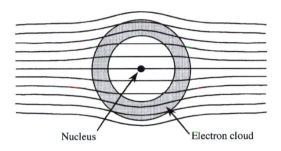

Nucleus   Electron cloud

This reduces the field at the nucleus to a very small extent. The effect is represented by the shielding parameter σ in the expression

$$B = B_0(1 - \sigma) \qquad \qquad \textbf{7.1}$$

where B_0 is the externally applied field and B is the magnetic field at the nucleus. The shielding parameter σ is very small, being expressed in parts per million (ppm). Although the initial measurements of shielding may be made in frequency units (Hz) they are always converted into the dimensionless parts per million units so that they can be readily compared with measurements made by other spectroscopists at a different field strength B_0. If we re-examine a high-resolution NMR spectrum in a second spectrometer at higher magnetic field, it appears 'stretched out' but the chemical shifts remain the same when expressed in parts per million.

Proton chemical shifts span a range of approximately 10 ppm, and carbon-13 shifts about 300 ppm. Because the width of a typical resonance response (expressed in Hz) tends to be roughly the same in all spectrometers, and since chemical shifts (if expressed in Hz) are spread out in proportion to the applied magnetic field, there is always an advantage in operating at the highest possible field B_0. This reduces overlap between responses that have only a very small difference in shielding and makes it easier to interpret the spectrum when fine structure (§ 8.2) is also present.

To describe the position of a given resonance line in a high-resolution NMR spectrum there are two terms in general use that can sometimes seem rather confusing—the so-called 'high-field' and 'low-field' shifts. The problem arises because in Equation 7.1 there are two different magnetic fields—the externally applied field B_0 and the slightly weaker magnetic field B experienced by the nucleus as a result of the shielding effect. The spectrometer transmitter operates at a fixed radiofrequency, so resonance occurs when this frequency and the field at the nucleus B satisfy the Larmor condition. The shielding is acting rather like a handicap in a horse race. To reach the resonance condition we have to increase the external magnetic field B_0 to compensate for the effect of shielding. Thus *low* shielding corresponds to a *low* applied field B_0 to attain the resonance condition, *high* shielding corresponds to a *high* applied field. The accepted convention in the early high-resolution spectrometers was to sweep the applied magnetic field B_0 from a low value on the left of the chart to a high value on the right, so resonances on the left were called 'low-field' resonances; those on the right 'high-field' resonances. Nowadays charts for proton NMR are calibrated in shielding values (σ) running from zero on the left to 10 ppm on the right.

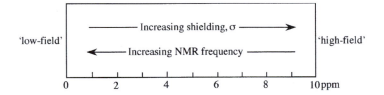

A newcomer to the subject might reasonably expect 'magnetic field' and 'precession frequency' to go hand in hand according to the Larmor condition; we see that there is in fact an *inverse* relationship when we are talking about the externally applied field B_0. This 'high-field/low-field' nomenclature has been retained in modern spectrometers that operate by pulse methods even though they do not sweep the magnetic field at all. Chemists habitually refer to 'high-field' and 'low-field' chemical shifts, visualizing these positions on the standard chart.

There is a slight semantic problem with the term chemical shift. As defined above, it means the magnetic shielding value (σ) of the chemical species in question and this is how the term is commonly used. But chemists are often concerned with *additional* displacements of a resonance line due to some physical or chemical influence, for example temperature, concentration, substituents, molecular association, changes in solvent, or addition of reagents. No explicit distinction is made between the absolute shift (σ) and this 'shift of a shift' $\Delta\sigma$; only the context can serve as a guide to the two possible interpretations. Sometimes $\Delta\sigma$ may be referred to as a 'down-field' or an 'up-field' shift.

7.2 Theory of shielding

If precession of the electron cloud in the applied magnetic field causes the chemical shift, can this effect be calculated? The electrons in an atom or a molecule have a set of energy levels (quantum states) at their disposal, but the gaps between energy levels are so large that only the lowest (the ground state) is appreciably populated at room temperature. The influence of the magnetic field can be quantified in terms of a mixing of the ground state with excited electron states. Unfortunately, the calculation is very difficult in the general case[1] because we do not normally have accurate information about all the excited states (energies and wavefunctions) of the electron when it forms part of a molecule. However, in one particularly favorable situation we can make a rather reliable calculation of the shielding effect. This is the case where there is one excited electron state that is much lower in energy than the rest, so that its influence outweighs that of all the other states. The classic example is the chemical shielding of the cobalt-59 nucleus in symmetrical cobalt III complexes, as these are well-known to have a low-lying electron state which is responsible for the absorption of light in the visible region of the spectrum, giving rise to the colour of these cobalt compounds. The extent of magnetic field-induced mixing of the ground state with this excited state is inversely proportional to the energy of the excited state Δ, so we would expect the chemical shielding to be proportional to $1/\Delta$. Furthermore, because Δ is rather small, the chemical shifts are large, in the case of cobalt-59, more than 1% of the Larmor frequency (three orders of magnitude bigger than proton chemical shifts). The frequency of the first absorption line in the visible spectrum is also directly proportional to the energy Δ, so we anticipate that the chemical shifts observed in a series of different cobalt III compounds should give a straight-line graph when plotted against the wavelengths ($1/\Delta$) observed in the corresponding optical absorption spectra.

Cobalt-59 is 100% abundant in nature, and although it is a quadrupolar nucleus and therefore subject to fairly fast spin–lattice relaxation (§ 4.1), there is no difficulty in recording the NMR response for symmetrically substituted complexes.[2] At a field of 1 tesla, the resonance frequency is near 10.0 MHz. When a series of the cobalt III complexes—potassium hexacyanocobaltate, tris(ethylenediamine)cobalt bromide, sodium hexanitrocobaltate, heamminecobalt chloride, cobalt trisacetylacetonate, potassium trioxalatocobaltate, and tricarbonatocobalt chloride were measured, the expected linear relation to the visible absorption wavelengths was confirmed (Figure 7.1). Corroboration for the theory comes from the temperature dependence of the chemical shifts and the optical absorption peaks. The temperature dependence arises not from any increased population of the excited state (the energy Δ is too large) but from changes in Δ caused by thermal motion of the ligands.

Analogous observations have been made on the relationship of the chemical shielding of nitrogen-15 to the colour of nitrogen compounds.[3] These observations

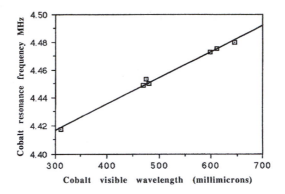

Figure 7.1 Experimental NMR frequency of the cobalt-59 nucleus in a series of symmetrical cobalt III complexes, plotted against the wavelength of the corresponding absorption peak in the visible/ ultraviolet region. When there is a low-lying electronic state, the theory of chemical shielding predicts a linear relationship.

lend considerable credence to the formal theory of chemical shielding[1] but apart from these rather special cases of cobalt and nitrogen shifts, there are still some imponderables that render the computed shielding values rather unreliable. The general solution has so far proved quite intractable.

7.3 The empirical approach

As noted above, chemical shifts can only be calculated in very favourable cases, so the practising chemist is forced into a more qualitative assessments of shielding effects. Ever since the discovery of the periodic table, chemists have focused on *trends* in physical and chemical properties, so it comes quite naturally to treat shielding as an *empirical* parameter. The chemical shift is broken down into four separate influences that are readily visualized and which parallel existing concepts of electronegativity, etc. Once we have abandoned the goal of an absolute calcula- tion of the shielding effect, we need only consider *changes* in the shielding be- tween different chemical compounds. This is a great simplification, for it means that we can neglect the influence of all the electrons in the inner shells of the atom (which are not affected by bond formation), leaving us free to concentrate on the valence electrons and the way they are modified by structural influences. The chemical shift is intimately connected with bond formation and hence with chemistry.

For this reason the hydrogen atom serves as a convenient starting point be- cause it has no inner electron shells at all and has only a single valence electron. In the isolated hydrogen atom this electron forms a spherical cloud; it is called an 's-electron'. This cloud is forced to circulate by the strong applied magnetic field, generating a tiny current, and this creates a weak magnetic field at the nucleus which opposes the intense applied field B_0—this is called a *diamagnetic* effect. In this case of an isolated atom with a spherical electron distribution the calculation of the shielding is straightforward, but not very useful, since we are only really interested in the modification of the shielding when a chemical bond is formed.

Consider now the case that the atom of interest forms part of a molecule that contains another (distant) group which withdraws electrons through an electrostatic effect. To a first approximation we make the assumption that the modified electron cloud retains its spherical symmetry but the electron density is slightly reduced. Thinning the cloud reduces the shielding parameter σ, thus shifting the NMR response towards the 'low-field' end of the spectrum. For example, a carbon-13 nucleus in a molecule containing a nitro group (which withdraws electrons) has a reduced shielding; its resonance is shifted toward low field. On the other hand, a chlorine atom in the molecule is less electronegative than the nitro group, thus preserving more electron density around the carbon-13 nucleus, increasing its shielding and shifting its resonance toward the 'high-field' end of the spectrum. Although this is clearly an oversimplification of the phenomenon, if we measure proton chemical shifts in a series of related compounds containing different electron-withdrawing substituents we find an essentially linear relationship with the electronegativity (electron-withdrawing power) of that substituent. Such simple considerations of local electron density, based on extensive experimental observations on many chemical compounds, often suffice to assign the resonances in a high resolution spectrum.

So far we have sidestepped the question of how chemical bond formation affects the shielding of the two atoms directly involved. Then it is no longer permissible to retain the model of a spherical cloud of electrons. Bonding electrons are largely localized between the two atoms concerned, distorting the spherical symmetry and making the electron cloud less free to circulate in the applied magnetic field. This *paramagnetic* effect is in conflict with the *diamagnetic* effect outlined above. In fact, in anything other than a completely isolated atom, these two opposing influences are *always* involved. It is the interplay between these local diamagnetic and paramagnetic terms that determines the actual chemical shift.

The paramagnetic contribution is most marked for some of the nuclei beyond hydrogen in the periodic table, where bond formation involves electron distributions that have grossly non-spherical shapes ('*p*-orbitals' or '*d*-orbitals'). Because the hydrogen atom has only *s*-orbitals (which are spherical in shape) the range of proton chemical shifts is quite small (not much more than 10 ppm for most compounds) whereas the shift ranges are much larger for carbon-13 (300 ppm), nitrogen-15 (900 ppm), fluorine-19 (300 ppm), or phosphorus-31 (500 ppm). In these last cases the paramagnetic term is dominant.

When the paramagnetic contribution is taken into account, the shielding has different values depending on the orientation of the chemical bond with respect to the magnetic field direction; it is said to be *anisotropic*. The anisotropy of the chemical shielding can be measured directly in a solid sample by making measurements at different orientations in the magnetic field (§ 10.1). It can also be detected in a liquid medium if the molecules can be partially aligned in the direction of the magnetic field (§ 10.6). However, in most liquids the rapid tumbling of the molecules renders their orientations essentially random and masks the anisotropy. We observe only a mean value of the chemical shielding, averaged over all possible orientations, but it is nevertheless non-zero.

The diamagnetic and paramagnetic contributions described above refer to *local* electrons—those involved in the formation of a chemical bond at the site under investigation. There are two further effects that arise from more distant inter-actions. The first is called the 'neighbour anisotropy effect'. Suppose we have a CO group some distance from the site of interest. When this group is aligned along the direction of the magnetic field there is a strong circulation of electrons around the bond (a tiny electric current) and a local magnetic field is induced.

$$
e\!\overset{O}{\underset{C}{\parallel}}\!\nearrow \qquad C\!\!=\!\!O \qquad \uparrow \text{Field}
$$

This makes a small contribution to the field at the nucleus under investigation. On the other hand, when the CO bond lies at right angles to the field, circulation is inhibited and there is a negligible induced field. To a fairly good approximation we can represent this effect in terms of a small magnetic dipole located on the CO group, where the strength of the dipole depends on the orientation of the molecule with respect to the field direction. This induced magnetic dipole creates an add-itional field at the site under investigation and changes its chemical shift. As the molecule tumbles in the liquid all possible orientations are sampled and the strength of the induced dipole varies accordingly, but the magnitude of the shift does not aver-age to zero at the site of interest. Note that the effect only occurs if the distant group has an *anisotropic* electron cloud. Groups with double or triple bonds are the usual culprits. For a spherical electron distribution the strength of the induced dipole is independent of molecular orientation, and its contribution to the shielding disap-pears through averaging due to the rapid tumbling of the molecule in the liquid.

The second type of 'distant' contribution to the chemical shielding occurs in aromatic compounds. We know that certain electrons congregate just above and just below the plane of the benzene ring, forming two clouds having an approxi-mate doughnut-like shape.

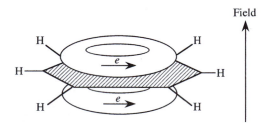

These are called the π electrons. They are relatively free to circulate in the applied magnetic field when it is normal to the plane of the benzene ring, and in this orientation the circulating current induces an appreciable magnetic field acting to oppose the applied field B_0. On the other hand, when the main magnetic field is in the plane of the ring this electron circulation is inhibited. To a good approximation the effect can be represented in terms of a small magnetic dipole at the centre of the benzene ring, aligned normal to the ring. Any protons on the periphery of the benzene ring see an additional magnetic field from this magnetic dipole, augmenting the applied magnetic field B_0 and thereby reducing the shielding. This 'ring current' dictates that all aromatic protons resonate at low field, and the shift can be calculated quite accurately. On the other hand, a proton that approaches the upper or lower sides of the benzene ring experiences an increased shielding. This latter effect is often seen in the folded form of proteins containing the aromatic histidine, tryptophan, or phenylalanine residues.

We see that observed chemical shifts are interpreted in terms of four main influences:

1. The local diamagnetic effect (electron density)
2. The local paramagnetic effect (bond formation)
3. The neighbour anisotropy effect
4. Aromatic ring currents.

The separation into local diamagnetic and paramagnetic effects is to some extent artificial; both are involved when the nucleus forms part of a molecule. It can also be argued that ring currents are only another manifestation of the neighbour anisotropy effect, but the idea of a separate effect called the ring current in aromatic compounds seems justifiable on chemical grounds.

7.4 Referencing

If chemical shifts are to be used for analytical or structural chemistry the numerical values must be readily transferable between one spectrometer and the next, and between different NMR laboratories across the world. This means that some common reference point must be established so that all chemical shifts are related to the NMR frequency of an agreed standard compound. The accepted 'reference' material is tetramethylsilane (TMS), chosen because its proton resonance is a single narrow line that falls at high field, beyond most other resonances, and because it is volatile and hence easily removed from a sample if necessary. For proton spectroscopy tetramethylsilane is assigned the value $\sigma = 10.0$ ppm, defining the high-field end of the spectrum. Thus in a 900 MHz spectrometer a proton with a shielding value $\sigma = 0.0$ lies on the left-hand edge of the chart, at 9000 Hz 'down-field' from TMS. Tetramethylsilane also serves as a reference for carbon-13 spectroscopy. When the chemical considerations preclude the use of TMS, a secondary standard can be used, having a known shift with respect to TMS. For aqueous solutions (where TMS is almost insoluble) the accepted standard is 2,2-dimethylsilapentane-5-sulfonic acid (DSS) where the protons have only a very small chemical shift (17 parts per billion) with respect to TMS.

So far we have considered reference compounds that form part of the sample itself, the so-called 'internal' standards. Special considerations apply to referencing in MRS (Chapter 14) where the focus may be on phosphorus-31 spectra. Chemists have traditionally used phosphoric acid (85 % in water) as a standard reference, but this presents a problem for the study of human or animal spectra *in vivo*. It can only be used as an 'external' reference, sealed into a separate sample tube. An external reference does not experience exactly the same applied magnetic field as the sample or tissue under investigation. The applied field penetrates different materials to different degrees; we say that they possess different magnetic susceptibilities (§ 6.2). These susceptibility effects cause an additional displacement of the response under investigation when measured with respect to an *external* reference; there is no such susceptibility shift when an *internal* reference is employed. To avoid this problem, MRS studies of phosphorus compounds sometimes adopt the narrow resonance response of phosphocreatine as an internal reference standard.

Most high-resolution NMR spectrometers are stabilized by locking the magnetic field to the Larmor frequency of deuterium in the deuterated solvent, often deutero-chloroform $CDCl_3$. This ensures that although the magnetic field of the solenoid may drift with time, the drift is corrected by passing a suitable weak current through a small correction coil. This current is controlled by an error signal derived from the dispersion-mode component of the deuterium resonance, which 'pulls' the field back to exact resonance. One might have been tempted to use this as a chemical shift reference, but it would be unreliable for several reasons—corrections have to be made if the deuterated solvent is changed (say from chloroform to benzene) and there are temperature-induced chemical shifts, particularly when heavy water is employed as the reference. That is why it is important to use the 'internal' tetramethylsilane reference.

With high-resolution NMR spectra all referenced to the same standard, extensive catalogues of chemical shifts have been created with a view to aiding the assignment of spectra of new compounds. This large database can be processed to assess the individual contributions from each substituent; to a good approximation these substituent effects are additive, so we can estimate the chemical shift from tables of substituent shifts. However, corrections may need to be applied for steric repulsions or ring strain. The organic chemists and the biochemists use this empirical information to build up an intuitive 'feel' for the relationship between chemical shift and molecular structure. Occasionally a chemical shift is observed that appears anomalous in terms of the generally accepted rationale; it then receives particular attention. Alternatively there are computer programs that use

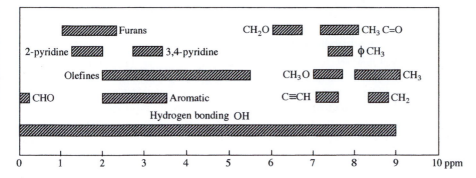

Figure 7.2 Proton chemical shift ranges for some representative organic groups. Note the very wide range covered by the hydroxyl group, attributable to differing degrees of hydrogen bonding.

libraries of substituent shifts to estimate the high-resolution NMR spectrum of an 'unknown' compound.

A typical compound with N chemically distinct sites yields N chemical shifts, often more than enough to resolve a particular structural question. Indeed it quite often happens that the molecular structure is already well understood except for a single ambiguity, for example, an axial or equatorial configuration on a six-membered ring. In such simple cases a single chemical shift measurement may well solve the problem straightaway.

Charts and tabulations of chemical shifts for important nuclear species can be found in several standard texts[4]. Figure 7.2 gives a general idea of the distribution of proton chemical shifts for some commonly-found groups. We can appreciate from the overlap of the bands on this chart that the measurement of a given chemical shift gives only an *indication* of the chemical group involved but does not identify it unambiguously. But remember that in almost all situations there is other information available. Note the very wide range of possible shifts for the hydroxyl group (see § 7.9).

7.5 Nuclei other than hydrogen

Apart from the rare and highly radioactive isotope tritium, the proton has the highest intrinsic NMR sensitivity of all nuclei, and because of its presence in so many chemical compounds and its primary importance in MRI, it is normally the first choice for any investigation. Yet we would be wrong to neglect the other nuclear species. For our purposes these nuclei must possess magnetism, which rules out the abundant isotopes carbon-12 and oxygen-16 which have no magnetic properties. There are four characteristics governing the usefulness of a given nuclear species for high-resolution NMR:

1. Intrinsic sensitivity
2. Natural abundance
3. Lack of a quadrupole moment
4. Chemical interest

The intrinsic sensitivity is mainly determined by the Larmor frequency in a given magnetic field. This frequency is set by the gyromagnetic ratio (γ) and determines the degree of polarization (§ 2.4), and, in addition, the efficiency with which the radiofrequency signal can be detected.

In § 4.1 we noted that in some nuclear species the positive charge on the nucleus is distorted from the 'ideal' spherical shape—these nuclei are said to possess a quadrupole moment and they are very sensitive to local electric field gradients. This additional coupling of the nucleus to its environment greatly enhances spin–lattice relaxation with the result that quadrupolar species have very broad lines, making them generally unsuitable for high-resolution NMR spectroscopy (but see deuterium below). We therefore concentrate on those nuclear species that have a spherical charge distribution and are impervious to local electrostatic field gradients. They are known as spin-$\frac{1}{2}$ nuclei.

There are two very interesting nuclear species that have reasonable intrinsic sensitivities but suffer from low abundance in nature, carbon-13 (1.1 %) and nitrogen-15 (0.37 %). In a 1 tesla magnet, carbon-13 has a resonance frequency of 10.7 MHz and nitrogen-15 has a resonance frequency of 4.3 MHz. This puts them at a significant disadvantage with respect to proton NMR, but the signal-to-noise ratio of their spectra can be greatly improved by artificial isotopic enrichment, either specific or general. Many modern studies of proteins often employ two-dimensional spectroscopy (Chapter 11) where the samples have been labelled with carbon-13 or nitrogen-15 (or both) to simplify the corresponding proton spectra. This highlights another very common method for circumventing the problem of low sensitivity—indirect detection of one nuclear species (X) by polarization transfer from protons to X and then back to protons (§ 11.7). Low natural abundance is not necessarily a universal drawback. It has been claimed that Providence got the natural abundance of carbon-13 just about right—if it had been much higher, carbon-13 spectra would have been hopelessly complicated by carbon–carbon coupling.

Both carbon-13 and nitrogen-15 benefit from having wide chemical shift ranges (300 and 900 ppm respectively) due to the large paramagnetic contributions to shielding from the p-electrons involved in chemical bonding (§ 7.2). This makes assignment and interpretation of the spectra much simpler than for proton NMR. The Fourier transform technique ensures good sensitivity for carbon-13 spectroscopy, aided by appreciable signal enhancement through the nuclear Overhauser effect (§ 4.3) and considerable simplification by broadband decoupling of protons (§ 8.5). It is even feasible to pick out those molecules that have two adjacent carbon-13 spins and detect their spectra in a selective manner even though they represent only one molecule in every 8000. A third low-abundant nuclear species is silicon-29, which is 4.7 % abundant in nature and has a resonance frequency of 8.46 MHz in a magnetic field of 1 tesla. This is a key nucleus for several types of solid-state NMR, particularly the study of zeolite structures.

Two other nuclear species, fluorine-19 and phosphorus-31, enjoy 100 % abundance in nature, have high intrinsic sensitivities, wide ranges of chemical shifts, and no quadrupole moments. We may compare their properties at a magnetic field of 21.14 tesla where the proton has a Larmor frequency of 900 MHz. Fluorine has a resonance frequency of 846.7 MHz, but has a rather restricted chemical interest, while phosphorus (at 364.3 MHz) is similarly restricted for chemical investigations but finds an important niche in MRS (Chapter 14). For this application much lower magnetic fields are employed, for example 1.5 tesla, where the phosphorus frequency is 25.9 MHz. It is used to monitor compounds such as adenosine triphosphate, phosphocreatine and inorganic phosphate, which are so important for the study of metabolism in humans and animals (§ 14.2).

Finally the deuterium nucleus, which would appear to fail one of the four requirements listed above owing to its quadrupole moment, in fact gives quite well-resolved high-resolution spectra because the quadrupole moment is exceptionally weak. It has a resonance frequency of 138.3 MHz at 21.14 tesla, and a natural abundance of 1.5 %. However, the deuterium chemical shift range expressed in practical units (Hz) is 6.5 times narrower than that of the proton. Isotopic enrichment is easily accomplished and there are interesting applications that employ specific deuteration as a means of simplification of the spectra of hydrogen compounds. High-resolution proton NMR typically employs fully deuterated solvents (chloroform, acetone, benzene or dimethylsulfoxide, for example) to avoid contamination of the spectrum of interest with an intense response from the solvent. This custom has been exploited in field regulation systems where the main magnetic field is 'locked' to the frequency of the deuterium resonance of the solvent.

While the species mentioned above are some of the 'popular' nuclei, it is important to remember that essentially every element in the periodic table has at least one magnetic isotope and can be investigated by NMR spectroscopy. To give just two illustrative examples, the quadrupolar nucleus sodium-23 has been used for MRI purposes, and xenon-129 (natural abundance 26.4 %) can be artificially 'hyperpolarized' by a laser technique to give strong signals even though, as a gas, the density of spins is quite low (§ 5.8). The xenon atom has a diffuse outer electron cloud that is extremely sensitive to its immediate environment.

7.6 Solvent effects

The empirical treatment of the chemical shift mentioned above refers to shielding influences within the molecule under investigation (*intra*molecular effects). There are some weaker *inter*molecular shifts caused by the solvent that are difficult to quantify and are now generally regarded as just a nuisance. We can regard the

solvent effect as a distortion of the electronic structure due to collision or transient association with the surrounding solvent molecules.[5] Fortunately most solvent
shifts are relatively small, of the order of 0.2 ppm or less for proton NMR. Note
that a solvent effect can be detected simply by changing the concentration of the
solute. If the solvent has a high dielectric constant (for example, acetonitrile) and
the molecule under investigation possesses an electric dipole, there is an electrostatic contribution called the 'reaction field' which can contribute to the solvent
shift to the extent of several parts per million.

The exploitation of solvent shifts has been largely limited to their use in separating chemical shifts that are accidentally coincident. Replacing the usual chloroform solvent with benzene often introduces specific solvent shifts that serve to
resolve such ambiguities. For example, the methyl group protons of steroids normally have almost coincident chemical shifts but the individual resonances can be
separated in benzene solution. Otherwise NMR spectroscopists try to work with
the same solvent (often deuterochloroform) and disregard the solvent shift. When
it is important to make careful comparisons of chemical shifts between different
compounds, dilute solutions in the same solvent are used, thus largely eliminating
the effect the solvent shift unless there is some specific molecular association.

The widespread use of an internal reference standard (tetramethylsilane) has
the effect of minimizing solvent shifts because they affect the reference material in
a similar manner to the substance under investigation. Only the site-specific
solvent effects remain, and these are normally quite weak.

7.7 Lanthanide shift reagents

Much larger 'external' effects can be caused by addition of certain paramagnetic
substances since they create an intense local magnetic field. When this is done
deliberately, the paramagnetic substance is called a 'shift reagent'[6] and considerable research has gone into finding compounds that induce very large shifts
without significantly broadening the observed resonances.[7] These reagents are
designed to form transient complexes with the molecule under investigation and
the influence on chemical shifts can be regarded as another manifestation of the
neighbour anisotropy effect discussed in § 7.3, the paramagnetic centre acting as
an intense magnetic dipole that changes its strength according to the orientation
of the molecule in the magnetic field. Physicists would say that the paramagnetism arises from an unpaired electron spin that has an 'anisotropic g-tensor'. The
induced shifts are largest for nuclei closest to the site of the paramagnetic ligand,
decreasing rapidly with distance. They have the effect of 'stretching out' the observed spectrum over a wide range of frequencies, simplifying the assignment in
crowded proton spectra and providing information about the conformation of the
molecule. The magnitude of the chemical shift dispersion can be controlled by
changing the concentration of the added shift reagent. The most commonly-used

shift reagents are the lanthanides, often chelated ions of europium, praeseodymium or ytterbium.

One interesting application of shift reagents is the study of optical isomers, the left- and right-handed forms that occur with certain molecules. Written on paper, the two structures look the same, and they have identical chemical shifts. Viewed in three dimensions, the two structure are different, being related as mirror images; they are said to be *chiral* molecules. A paramagnetic ligand that is itself chiral[8] interacts more strongly with one form than with its mirror image, thus lifting the degeneracy of the chemical shifts.

7.8 Fast and slow chemical exchange

A chemical molecule need not have a rigid structure—it may have two or more different conformations in space and in general each conformation possesses its own characteristic chemical shifts. The classic example is the pair of protons of a methylene group that is attached to an asymmetric site. Even if there is completely free rotation about the intervening C–C bond, these two protons have different chemical environments and therefore different shifts; they are said to be 'non-equivalent' methylene protons. Usually steric repulsions dictate that there are three possible conformers in a 'staggered' arrangement, related by 120° rotations about the C–C bond; let us call these forms *A*, *B* and *C*.

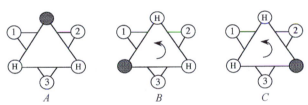

A   *B*   *C*

The asymmetric environment is represented in the background as three different substituents labelled 1, 2 and 3. Usually the rate of interchange between these three conformers is fast in comparison with the chemical shift differences. In this limit, if we fix our attention on one particular methylene proton, it precesses for a short while at a frequency characteristic of conformer *A*, then jumps to a frequency appropriate to conformer *B* or *C*, only remaining at each site long enough to precess through a very small angle. Its precessional motion is rather jerky, but it can be described as precession at a 'pure' frequency that is the average of the chemical shifts of sites *A*, *B* and *C*, with superimposed small random phase excursions that give the observed resonance line a slight broadening. In the general case where the populations of the three conformers are different, the observed frequency is the *weighted mean* of the three chemical shifts.

This is a general result, fast chemical exchange gives rise to a single response at the weighted mean frequency of the individual chemical shifts. Analogous behaviour is observed in the case of an unstable molecule, where an atom or group of atoms detaches itself and moves to a chemically distinct site in another molecule, to be replaced by identical atom or group. A proton that jumps rapidly between two sites spends too little time at either site to establish the intrinsic frequencies of the two different environments—instead it is 'fooled' into precessing at the weighted mean frequency. We shall see below (§ 7.9) that if the relative populations of the sites change, then the observed resonance is displaced towards the NMR frequency of the site with the increased population.

The opposite case, where the rate of exchange is slow in comparison with the chemical shift difference, is treated in more detail under two-dimensional spectroscopy in § 11.3. In this limit, the proton has plenty of time to precess through several revolutions before it jumps to another site. Well-defined responses are observed at the characteristic frequencies of each site, although there is a slight line broadening attributable to the finite lifetimes in each site. There are, of course, some intermediate situations where the rate of exchange is comparable to the differences in chemical shift. Under these circumstances the response is broad and may or may not show two peaks.

Slow chemical exchange can be studied by 'saturation transfer'.[9] If a nuclear spin moves from one chemically distinct site 'I' to another site 'S', then saturation of the NMR response of site I leads to partial saturation of the response from site S. In effect we have 'tagged' the nuclear spins by disturbing the Boltzmann distribution—in the case of complete saturation by equalizing the populations in the upper and lower energy levels. Although only one nuclear spin in roughly 100,000 is affected, this is enough to cause a loss of NMR signal intensity at the saturated site, and this loss can be transferred to the second chemical site by exchange. Saturation of the chosen NMR response is usually implemented by a frequency-selective 90° radiofrequency pulse (§ 2.9) and the results are often recorded by difference spectroscopy in order to highlight the intensity changes.

In general, *any* disturbance of the spin populations from their equilibrium values can be used as a 'marker' to monitor chemical exchange. This includes population inversion by a selective 180° radiofrequency pulse, enhancement by the nuclear Overhauser effect (§ 4.3) or by polarization transfer (§ 11.8) or even hyperpolarization (§ 5.8). Although these techniques permit the rate of chemical exchange to be evaluated, the most common application is to *identify* two NMR responses that are involved in slow chemical exchange. For example, if a ligand binds strongly to a protein, saturation of the NMR response of the free ligand (often in excess concentration) can be used to identify the corresponding response in the complex (§ 16.2).

7.9 Hydrogen bonds

However difficult it might be to *estimate* the chemical shift for a given chemical situation, the *observed* shift is pretty well constant, being perturbed only slightly by the physical conditions or by weak intermolecular interactions. There are some important exceptions to this rule, the most notorious being the OH proton, for example, the hydroxyl resonance of ethanol. Depending on the solvent, the ethanol concentration, or the sample temperature, the OH response can appear somewhere within a spectral range spanning several parts per million (Figure 7.2). This phenomenon involves hydrogen bonding. An OH proton that forms part of a hydrogen bond has an intrinsic chemical shift at low-field (low shielding value σ) while the 'free' OH proton has an intrinsic shift at high-field. There is fast chemical exchange (§ 7.8) between these two sites, and what we observe is a mean resonance frequency, weighted according to the relative amounts of hydrogen-bonded and free molecules. Whenever an NMR frequency shows such extreme sensitivity to the physical conditions (solvent, concentration, or temperature) there is a strong presumption that hydrogen-bonding is implicated.

7.10 Isotope shifts

When we examine the periodic table we see that each chemical element exists in several isotopic forms, for example, the hydrogen nucleus is normally a proton, but there is a small natural abundance of deuterium where the nucleus contains one proton and one neutron. The chemical properties are virtually the same, this is why they are called *isotopes* because both occupy the same slot in the periodic table. However, the mass of the deuterium nucleus is twice that of the proton, and its intrinsic magnetism is quite different. Each isotope has its characteristic nuclear precession frequency in a given magnetic field; the deuterium frequency is roughly 6.5 times lower than that of the proton. Now both the hydrogen and the deuterium atoms have the same electronic structure, and we might have expected that chemical shifts observed for protons and deuterium nuclei to be the same, once allowance has been made for the different operating frequencies (by expressing the shifts in parts per million) but if hydrogen bonding is involved there are small discrepancies of the order of 1 ppm. This is known as the *primary* isotope effect.

When hydrogen is attached to another magnetic nucleus, for example carbon-13, substitution of the heavier isotope deuterium slightly reduces the frequency at which the C–H bond vibrates, and because the vibration does not follow a pure sinewave (it is said to be *anharmonic*) the average length of a C–H bond is slightly greater than that of a C–D bond. This gives rise to a slight change in the chemical shift of the carbon-13 resonance—the *secondary* isotope effect. Thus the carbon-13 shielding (σ) in deuterochloroform is about 0.3 ppm higher than that in ordinary chloroform. Secondary isotope shifts can sometimes be used to solve an assignment problem; for example, deuterating a given carbon site slightly shifts the carbon-13 resonance to high-field. Isotope shifts are most evident when a proton is replaced by a deuteron, because of the large proportional change in nuclear mass; the effect of substituting nitrogen-15 for nitrogen-14 would be correspondingly smaller. Because hydrogen exhibits a much smaller range of chemical shifts than the heavier nuclei, the secondary isotope shifts are correspondingly smaller for proton NMR but they are nevertheless measurable—of the order of a few parts per billion.

7.11 Implications for MRI

Although the majority of magnetic resonance images are from water, we cannot always escape the effects of chemical shifts. In § 1.4 we likened the nucleus to a spy, reporting on the NMR frequency at the particular value of the magnetic field at his location in space. If an MRI scan detects responses from both water and fat in human tissue, then there are two types of spies, and they operate different transmitters, broadcasting on slightly different frequencies. One spy can be said to be using the 'wrong' frequency and reporting a 'false' position. The spy nucleus only senses a single parameter, the local magnetic field, and cannot distinguish the contributions from the applied gradient and the chemical shift. The MRI proton density map (§ 12.1) consists of two superimposed images (water and fat) slightly displaced from one another, which is undesirable for routine clinical investigations. If a three-dimensional image is acquired by applying successive gradients in all three directions, then this displacement occurs in all three spatial dimensions. One remedy is to employ such intense applied field gradients that they overwhelm the chemical shift difference, to the extent that they hide the chemical shift displacement within a single pixel.

Certain more sophisticated imaging techniques actually exploit chemical shift differences, deriving an image from some chosen chemical substance while rejecting the rest. This 'chemical shift imaging' or 'spectroscopic imaging' (§ 14.9) supplements the information obtained from MRS and proves very useful for monitoring the distribution of various metabolites or drugs within the human body.

Further reading

L. F. Johnson and W. C. Jankowski, *Carbon-13 NMR Spectra*, Wiley, New York (1972).

G. C. Levy and G. L. Nelson, *Carbon-13 Nuclear Magnetic Resonance for Organic Chemists*, Wiley, New York (1972).

F. W. Wehrli and T. Wirthlin, *Interpretation of Carbon-13 NMR Spectra*, Heyden, London (1976).

R. K. Harris and B. E. Mann, *NMR and the Periodic Table*, Academic Press, London (1978).

H. Günther, *NMR Spectroscopy: Basic Principles, Concepts, and Applications in Chemistry*, Wiley, Chichester, UK (1995).

E. D. Becker, *High Resolution NMR. Theory and Chemical Applications*, 3rd ed., Academic Press, San Diego, CA (2000).

8

Spin–spin coupling

8.1 Interactions between spins

We now come to a second important aspect of high-resolution NMR spectra—
the fine structure. While the chemical shift is the main factor determining the
frequency of the response from a particular chemical site, each response may
also exhibit some fine structure representing interactions with neighbouring
magnetic nuclei. If we imagine we are 'sitting' on a particular nuclear spin, we
would know whether a nearby spin is 'up' or 'down', because this creates a weak
additional magnetic field at our location, either positive or negative. When we
consider the ensemble of similar nuclear spins in the sample there are essentially
equal numbers of 'up' and 'down' neighbours. Instead of a single response at
the chemical shift frequency there are two responses, one slightly above and
the other slightly below the chemical shift frequency. The electrons that make
up the chemical bonds between two sites serve as a conduit for this magnetic
interaction.

This 'spin–spin coupling' gives rise to a characteristic pattern for each chemically distinct resonance response. Often this pattern is a symmetrical 1:1 doublet,
1:2:1 triplet or 1:3:3:1 quartet, where the relative intensities are governed by the
binomial coefficients. Spin–spin coupling is transmitted through the valence electrons and is therefore a *molecular* property and cannot be altered by changing the
external conditions. The magnitude of the spin–spin interaction is defined by the
coupling constant (J) measured in Hz. In contrast to the chemical shift, the spin–
spin coupling is *independent* of the strength of the applied magnetic field B_0.
Consequently, small spin–spin splittings can only be resolved in a very uniform
magnetic field; increasing the strength of the field does not help. The magnitudes
of proton–proton coupling constants usually lie in a range up to about 20 Hz, but

couplings involving heavier nuclei can be much larger. The vast majority of coupling constants are positive but a few carry a negative sign; for most purposes the sign is irrelevant.

Coupling constants can be calculated theoretically in some favorable cases. For coupling between nuclei separated by three chemical bonds (the so-called 'vicinal couplings'), the Karplus relationship[1] has gained widespread acceptance.

$$^3J = A + B\cos\phi + C\cos2\phi \qquad \textbf{8.1}$$

where ϕ is the dihedral angle between the terminal bonds.

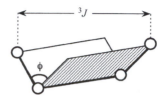

In practice it turns out that the form of the angular dependence is well represented by the general shape of the Karplus curve but the theoretical predictions for the coefficients A, B and C give a rather poor fit to experimental measurements. For this reason NMR spectroscopists tend to treat A, B and C as empirical parameters, obtained by fitting a trial version of the Karplus expression to a series of measurements of coupling constants in substances where the dihedral angles are known from other evidence. This resulting parameters A, B and C are then used to derive dihedral angles in new cases. Vicinal couplings provide a valuable indication of molecular conformation, widely used for probing the detailed arrangement of adjacent aminoacid residues in biological macromolecules.

8.2 Spin multiplets

So how are these characteristic patterns generated, and why are the relative intensities related to the binomial coefficients? Spin–spin coupling between protons splits each chemically-distinct response into a doublet, a triplet, or a quartet. These 'spin multiplets' serve as a very useful signature that tells us about the number of adjacent spins. Suppose we observe the resonance of a proton (A) with just one adjacent proton (X) having two possible spin states ↑ and ↓. Proton X generates a tiny magnetic field at site A, either positive or negative, depending on whether X is aligned along the field (↑) or opposed to it (↓). This splits the A resonance into a doublet with a splitting equal to J_{AX} (Hz) the spin–spin coupling constant.

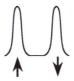

For these purposes the populations of states ↑ and ↓ are essentially equal (they would differ only by about 1 part in 10,000 for protons) so we observe a symmetrical doublet. Spin coupling is a reciprocal effect; if we record the X resonance, it is also a doublet of splitting J_{AX} reflecting the two possible spin states (↑ and ↓) of the A proton.

Now suppose that the proton A under investigation has two different neighbours, X and Y. Then the A response is a doublet of doublets because two coupling constants J_{AX} and J_{AY} are involved, giving four lines of equal intensity for the A resonance.

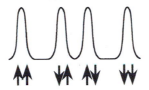

Such a pattern often occurs in chemical compounds where the neighbour is a methylene group (CH_2) with a local environment that is not symmetrical, so that X and Y have different chemical shifts and different coupling constants to the observed proton A. The CH_2 protons are said to be 'chemically and magnetically non-equivalent'. In many other cases the methylene group has a symmetrical environment and X and Y have the same chemical shift and equal couplings to A. They are chemically and magnetically equivalent. We would then write the system as AX_2 and note that although there are still four possible combinations of the spin states of the two methylene protons, the ↑↓ and ↓↑ states have the same effect on A. The A response is a triplet with intensities 1:2:1 and splittings J_{AX}.

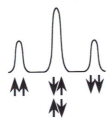

This is the result of letting J_{AX} equal J_{AY}.

Another common case is a neighbour methyl group (CH_3) where the three protons are equivalent. There are eight possible combinations of spin states of these three protons, depending on how they are aligned with respect to the magnetic field direction, but the ↑↑↓, ↑↓↑ and ↓↑↑ states have the same effect on the observed A proton, and the same is true of the ↑↓↓, ↓↑↓ and ↓↓↑ states. This is how the binomial coefficients become involved; there is only one way to select the case of all spins up, but there are three ways to select two spins up and one spin down.

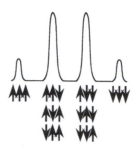

Consequently the observed response in the presence of a neighbouring methyl group is a 1:3:3:1 quartet of splitting J_{CH}.

In practice the simplest illustrative spectra for the basic spin multiplet patterns occur in carbon-13 spectroscopy. Figure 8.1 shows part of the carbon-13 spectrum of endo-(–)-borneol with splittings due to C–H couplings. There are two singlets

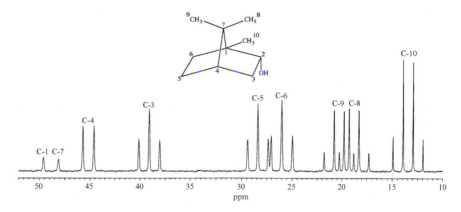

Figure 8.1 Part of the 125 MHz carbon-13 spectrum of endo-(–)-borneol showing the CH splittings. There are two singlet responses from the quaternary carbon sites carbon-1 and carbon-7; they are weak owing to partial saturation. Site carbon-4 shows a 1:1 doublet. The CH_2 sites carbon-3, carbon-5 and carbon-6 generate 1:2:1 triplets. The methyl groups carbon-8, carbon-9 and carbon-10 form 1:3:3:1 quartets, two of which are interpenetrating. For simplicity all the long-range CH couplings have been hidden within the linewidth. These different multiplet patterns serve as an aid to assignment. (Spectrum courtesy of Toshiaki Nishida.)

at low field from carbon atoms carbon-1 and carbon-7. These sites have no directly attached protons so spin–lattice relaxation is slow, there is partial saturation and the intensities are lower than those in the rest of the spectrum. Carbon atom carbon-4 carries a single proton and gives a 1:1 doublet. The sites carbon-3, carbon-5 and carbon-6 each carry two equivalent protons and show the expected 1:2:1 triplets. The remaining sites (carbon-8, carbon-9 and carbon-10) are methyl groups and show 1:3:3:1 quartets; those from carbon-8 and carbon-9 interpenetrate. In fact, this spectrum is oversimplified because there are also some long-range C–H couplings, but these are quite small and are hidden within the line-width. Carbon-13 multiplet patterns such as these are helpful for assignment purposes, supplementing the chemical shift evidence, but for more routine applications, carbon-13 spectra are recorded in the decoupled mode (§ 8.5) where this fine structure is absent; each chemically distinct site is a singlet. An example of proton-decoupled endo-(–)-borneol is shown in § 4.3.

We can extrapolate from these examples to predict that a spin multiplet arising from coupling to N equivalent protons is made up of $N + 1$ equally-spaced lines with relative intensities given by the binomial coefficients. Alternatively, Pascal's triangle (where each new row is derived from the previous row) can be used to predict the more complicated cases:

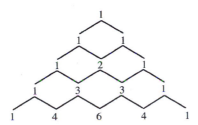

For example, the carbon-13 resonance of methane (CH_4) is a quintet with relative intensities 1:4:6:4:1. These rules are only valid for nuclei with spin-$\frac{1}{2}$; more complex relationships apply to coupling to nuclei that have a quadrupole moment, such as deuterium, but in many cases such splittings are 'washed out' as we shall see below.

Couplings are multiplicative; we can deduce the overall spin multiplet pattern at site A by introducing the various couplings to A one-at-a-time, in any order. For example, if the neighbours of A are a single proton and a methyl group, the A pattern is a doublet of quartets (or a quartet of doublets). Remember that it is the number of spins in the *environment* of a particular site that matters, not the number of equivalent nuclei at the site under observation. A methyl group can quite easily have a doublet structure, but an *adjacent* proton will be a quartet.

In proton systems, a given nuclear spin may be coupled to several other sites, rendering the multiplet patterns quite complicated. The 800 MHz proton

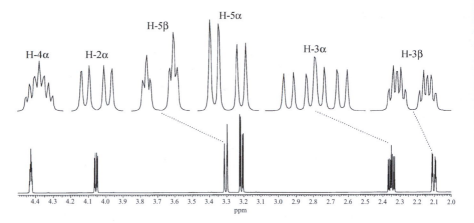

Figure 8.2 Part of the 800 MHz proton NMR spectrum of *cis*-4-hydroxy-L-proline showing the different patterns of proton–proton splittings (expanded tenfold in frequency in the upper trace). The solvent is heavy water, so the exchangeable protons have been deuterated. See Figure 8.3 for the coupling constants and their assignments. (Spectrum courtesy of Toshiaki Nishida.)

spectrum of *cis*-4-hydroxy-L-proline (Figure 8.2) is an example of a rich network of proton–proton couplings in a small molecule. The spin multiplets are shown on an expanded frequency scale and their values are set out schematically in Figure 8.3. It is interesting to note that not all the proton–proton pairs in this molecule exhibit spin–spin splitting; however we must be careful not to conclude that these couplings are zero; they are merely too small to be resolved. The two geminal couplings (between protons on the same carbon atom) are indicated as negative. Most proton–proton couplings are positive, but in fact the sign of a coupling constant is not evident in the conventional spectrum and must be determined by double-resonance experiments.

The response from hydrogen-4 in proline reflects coupling to four different sites, but only seven lines are apparent. This comes about because two small couplings are equal and two larger couplings are almost equal and twice as large. We can construct a 'tree' that shows the cascade of four splittings.

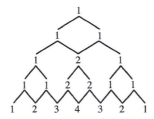

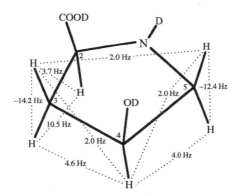

Figure 8.3 A schematic diagram indicating the various proton–proton couplings found in *cis*-4-hydroxy-L-proline. Note that certain proton sites, for example hydrogen-4, show as many as four different couplings. The two geminal couplings (between pairs of protons at sites 3 and 5) are known from other evidence to carry negative signs, but this has no influence on the form of the high-resolution spectrum.

This particular case results in a seven-line pattern but in fact, because of degeneracies in frequencies, it is actually made up of sixteen different lines. The response from H3β (above the ring) also shows couplings to four different proton sites. A multiplet of this kind is commonly written as 'dddd' meaning 'a doublet of doublets of doublets of doublets'.

The magnitudes of spin–spin couplings cover a wide range of values. The coupling in molecular hydrogen H_2 is the largest proton–proton coupling; this splitting is not observable in hydrogen itself but can be inferred by measuring the splitting in the monodeuterated molecule HD. Couplings can be classified according to the number of intervening bonds—^1J (direct coupling), ^2J (geminal coupling), ^3J (vicinal coupling), ^nJ (long-range coupling where $n > 3$). As a general rule, the magnitude of coupling constants falls off as the number of intervening bonds, but there are several exceptions. For routine spectral assignment purposes an accuracy of ± 0.1 Hz in the measurement of a coupling constant is quite sufficient. There are special techniques available to measure coupling constants to much higher accuracy if necessary.

8.3 'Splitting' and 'coupling'

The terms 'splitting' and 'coupling' need to be carefully distinguished. Both are given the symbol J and are measured in Hz. Although in many situations the experimentally observed spin–spin splitting is equal to the coupling constant, there are some special cases where this splitting may be modified or even vanish. Spin–spin coupling is a property of the molecule and cannot be manipulated if the molecule has a fixed structure. We examine below how spin–spin splittings may increase, decrease or disappear altogether.

Spin coupling generates spin multiplet patterns only if the neighbouring spins have sufficiently long lifetimes in each state ('up' or 'down'). If a given neighbour nucleus is in a chemical group undergoing chemical exchange at a rate fast compared with the coupling constant, it does not cause any splitting. We can picture this in rather simple terms. The spin A experiences additional magnetic fields due to coupling to a neighbour X—a small positive field when X is in state ↑ and a small negative field when X is in state ↓. If the lifetime of X in these states is long (in comparison with the reciprocal of the coupling constant) then spin A precesses for quite a long time at one frequency before X is replaced by another nuclear spin in a different state. As a result, there are two distinct A frequencies— the response is a doublet. On the other hand, if X is subject to fast chemical exchange (§ 7.8), the ↑ state makes rapid random jumps to the ↓ state, thereby reversing the sign of the induced magnetic field at site A and causing this nucleus to execute a rather jerky precessional motion, switching between fast and slow precession many times in one revolution. As a result we observe only the arithmetic mean frequency—the chemical shift of A without spin–spin splitting. The jerkiness of the motion translates into a slight line broadening of the A response. For sufficiently fast jumps between spin states even this slight broadening becomes unobservable. We could say that the splitting has been 'washed out'. Later we will examine how a similar result can be achieved artificially by radiofrequency irradiation (§ 8.5).

The methyl group of methanol is good example of loss of multiplet structure through fast chemical exchange. Although the methyl group is coupled to the hydroxy proton it normally shows no splitting because of fast exchange of the OH proton. Because each 'new' hydroxy group may be carrying a proton in either a ↑ or a ↓ state, the local field at the methyl group reverses sign in half the exchange events and the splitting is washed out. In contrast, carefully purified methanol at low temperature *does* show a splitting (a doublet on the CH_3 response and a quartet on the OH resonance) because the rate of exchange is now slow in comparison with the coupling constant.

Several organic molecules contain nuclei with a quadrupole moment, that is to say, the charge carried by the nucleus is not spherical but elongated or flattened along one axis (§ 4.2). Such nuclei are strongly coupled to local fluctuating electrostatic fields, and they usually have very short spin–lattice relaxation times (§ 4.1). (A notable exception is the deuteron [heavy hydrogen] which has only a small quadrupole moment.) Fast spin–lattice relaxation means that the quadrupolar nucleus jumps rapidly between states, so fast that its splitting at the site of a nearby proton or carbon-13 spin disappears, just as with fast chemical exchange. For this reason we can safely ignore the presence of these quadrupolar species—chlorine-35, chlorine-37, bromine-79, bromine-81 or nitrogen-14—even though they are abundant isotopes and spin–spin coupling to such nuclei undoubtedly exists. We can also ignore abundant nuclei with no magnetism—carbon-12 and oxygen-16 being the prime examples. This leaves a magnetically 'quiet' background for the observation of proton and carbon-13 responses in many organic compounds.

There is another type of interaction between nearby magnetic nuclei called the dipole–dipole interaction. This is an important effect in NMR investigations of solid samples (§ 10.1) but the dipole–dipole splitting vanishes in normal liquids because of the rapid reorientation of the molecules. However, in partially aligned molecules in the liquid state a scaled-down version of the dipole–dipole splitting is observable. Since this dipole–dipole interaction has the same physical character as the spin–spin coupling, the experimentally observed splitting is determined by the (algebraic) sum of the two interactions. In this manner spin–spin splittings observed when there is no alignment appear to be increased or decreased if the molecules become partially aligned. This has become an important tool in the study of macromolecules partially aligned in a solvent containing bicelles (§ 10.6) because the additional contribution to the splitting is dependent on the spatial relationship between the two interacting protons.

One might well inquire why the three protons within the methyl group do not split each other's resonances; after all, each has two close magnetic neighbours and it can be inferred from deuterium substitution experiments that there is indeed a spin–spin coupling between these protons. Once again we draw a distinction between *coupling*, which is a molecular property, and *splitting*, which is something we observe in the NMR spectrum. There is an important general rule that we do not observe splittings due to coupling between equivalent nuclei. In the next section (§ 8.4) there is another illustration of this rule for the case of two coupled protons with the same chemical shift.

8.4 Strong coupling

It may come as a real disappointment to learn that the simple rules for the structure of spin–spin multiplets outlined above are in fact only approximations. They apply in cases where the chemical shift difference is large in comparison with the relevant coupling constant,

$$|\delta_A - \delta_X| \gg |J_{AX}| \qquad \textbf{8.2}$$

Fortunately, at the high magnetic fields employed for high-resolution NMR spectroscopy, this inequality is usually satisfied, and the spectra are made up of the simple multiplet patterns described above, often called 'first-order' multiplets. When this is not the case, the nuclei are said to be strongly-coupled and the spectra become more difficult to analyse. Relative intensities are no longer given by the appropriate binomial coefficients, splittings are no longer necessarily equal to coupling constants, and new responses may appear in the spectrum.

The simplest case of strong coupling is a system of two coupled protons, where the chemical shift difference is comparable with the coupling constant. The accepted notation labels this an *AB* spectrum to distinguish it from the weak-coupling limit, where it would be called an *AX* spectrum. It is a straightforward matter to calculate the changes in the form of the spectrum as the chemical shift is reduced from a high value to zero (Figure 8.4). The spectrum is made up of two doublets of splitting J_{AB}, but as the chemical shift is reduced, the intensity pattern changes. The outer lines lose intensity at the expense of the inner lines until, when the chemical shift approaches zero, the outer lines become vanishingly small. When the chemical shift is exactly zero (an A_2 spectrum) the outer lines

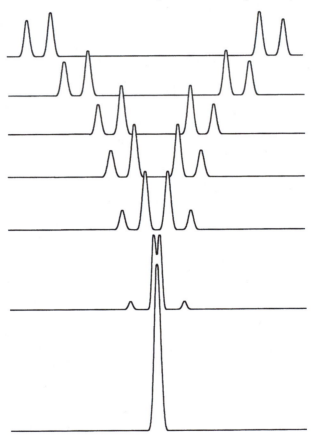

Figure 8.4 Simulation of '*AB* spectra' of two coupled protons as a function of the chemical shift difference. In the top trace the shift is ten times the coupling constant and the intensities are only slightly perturbed from the weakly-coupled limit. As the chemical shift is reduced, the outer lines get weaker; the spectroscopist would say they take on the character of 'forbidden transitions'. In the lowest trace, where the chemical shift is identically zero, the outer lines disappear completely and the inner lines coalesce. This is called an 'A_2 spectrum'.

disappear completely, leaving a singlet at the chemical shift frequency. Note that this is a good example of the rule mentioned above—when the two protons are equivalent no spin–spin splitting is observed, even though we know that the coupling exists. More complex groupings of strongly-coupled spins generate correspondingly more complicated high-resolution spectra. Analysis is best left to a numerical computer program that fits the observed spectrum and finds the appropriate chemical shifts and coupling constants.

8.5 Decoupling

Sometimes spin multiplet structure can prove an embarrassment. This is particularly true in high-resolution NMR spectroscopy of carbon-13 because the coupling to directly-attached protons is so large (normally in the range 125–175 Hz) that it causes extensive overlap with adjacent chemically-shifted responses. The result is often impossible to disentangle. The remedy is 'decoupling'—the application of a sequence of intense radiofrequency pulses at the proton frequency, designed to flip the protons between ↑ and ↓ states so rapidly that the carbon-13 spins 'think' they are no longer coupled to the protons. Then each chemically distinct carbon-13 site gives just a single resonance line and the spectrum is very simple to interpret. This is called *broadband* decoupling because it must remove all the CH splittings from the carbon-13 spectrum and do so for the entire range of proton chemical shifts (about 10 parts per million).

The broadband decoupling sequence has to be carefully designed so that the motion of the proton magnetization is cyclic, for all possible proton chemical shifts. This might be described as 'stirring' the proton states, and for efficient decoupling the rate of stirring must be fast compared with the coupling constant. Consider the simplest case of a single proton coupled to a single carbon-13 spin. The normal carbon-13 spectrum consists of a doublet of splitting J_{CH}, representing two possible proton spin states ↑ and ↓. If the decoupling sequence causes the proton to follow a cyclic trajectory from ↑ to ↓ and back to ↑ repeatedly, the two carbon-13 lines are forced to undergo a similar cyclic interchange between their extreme frequencies (Figure 8.5). If this 'stirring' of the protons is fast enough it leaves only a singlet response at the carbon-13 chemical shift and the spin–spin splitting disappears. An analogous 'averaging' of magnetic interactions occurs in many aspects of magnetic resonance, for example the line narrowing that occurs with a spinning sample (§ 6.2). However, this decoupling technique necessarily involves the introduction of weak 'cycling sidebands' on each side of the decoupled resonances.

A small deviation from exact cyclicity of the motion leaves a weak 'residual splitting' on the carbon-13 resonance, which may or may not be small enough to be hidden within the linewidth. This deviation from ideality is usually greatest at the extremes of the proton chemical shift range where the decoupler frequency is furthest from resonance, or when the decoupling power is too low. But a

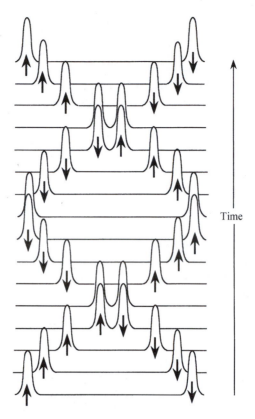

Time

Figure 8.5 Schematic diagram showing how two carbon-13 lines from a CH group move when a cyclic decoupling sequence is applied to the proton. The small arrows represent the two possible spin states of the proton. If the cycling is fast enough, we observe only a singlet carbon-13 response at the mean frequency (the carbon chemical shift).

high-power decoupler heats the sample and could affect it chemically, for example, by denaturing a protein. This problem is particularly critical at high applied magnetic fields or where it is necessary to decouple nuclei with large chemical shifts ranges (carbon-13 or nitrogen-15, for example) while observing protons. It also causes concern in MRI or MRS, where the organs in question must be protected from excess heating (§ 13.4).

For these reasons there has been an extensive search for effective decoupling techniques that work at low radiofrequency power. Many different radiofrequency pulse sequences have been tried; only the most commonly used ones are described here. The analysis is based on decoupling protons while observing carbon-13, but the conclusions apply quite generally. The key is to find a scheme that continuously inverts the proton spins over a wide range of proton NMR frequencies. A simple 180° pulse is very inefficient for this purpose, the decoupler frequency has to be very close to the proton precession frequency to achieve good inversion. It was soon discovered that a composite $180°$ pulse[2] was far more effective. A composite radiofrequency pulse is a 'sandwich' of several pulses, so designed as to compensate the inherent imperfections of each individual pulse. (The idea is related to the use of the compensated pendulum in early chronometers.) A good example is a three-pulse sandwich made up of a positive $90°$ pulse followed immediately by a reversed $180°$ pulse and then a positive $270°$ pulse. This composite pulse can be used as a broadband inversion element[3] that is particularly insensitive to instrumental shortcomings, which is important because broadband decoupling involves the repeated application of a very long train of inversion pulses where even a small imperfection can cause a large cumulative effect.

Let us write the symbol R for a composite $180°$ pulse. Two such pulses in the same sense ($R\ R$) force the protons to execute a cycle, but the resonance offset causes a slight overshoot beyond the ideal $360°$ rotation. This error is largely compensated by applying the next pair of composite pulses inverted in phase, creating the 'magic cycle' known as MLEV-4:[4]

$$R R \bar{R} \bar{R}$$

where $\bar{R}$ denotes rotation in the opposite sense. It can be shown theoretically that the efficiency of such a magic cycle is unaffected by cyclic permutation of one of the elements, that is to say,

$$R R \bar{R} \bar{R} \quad \text{and} \quad \bar{R} R R \bar{R}$$

are equally effective. The same is true for a magic cycle where all the rotations are reversed, that is to say,

$$R R \bar{R} \bar{R} \quad \text{and} \quad \bar{R} \bar{R} R R$$

also have the same efficiency. However, these four different forms of the magic cycle leave different residual imperfections, often equal in magnitude but opposite in sign. Further improvements in broadband decoupling can therefore be achieved by constructing a 'supercycle' (MLEV-16) made up of a sequence of permuted or phase-inverted magic cycles:[4]

$$R R \bar{R} \bar{R} \quad \bar{R} R R \bar{R} \quad \bar{R} \bar{R} R R \quad R \bar{R} \bar{R} R$$

If we adopt the shorthand notation where $90°(+X)\ 180°(-X)\ 270°(+X)$ is written as $1\ \bar{2}\ 3$, this explains why this sequence has come to be known as WALTZ-16. Supercycles greatly improve the performance of decoupling schemes, and have been widely used in high-resolution NMR spectroscopy.

When it is necessary to cover an extremely broad band of frequencies, the composite pulse elements are replaced by what is known as an 'adiabatic sweep'. This entails ramping the frequency of B_1 from far below resonance to far above resonance at a relatively slow rate (the adiabatic condition). The effective field (the resultant of B_1 and the resonance offset ΔB) swings in an arc from the $+Z$ axis of the rotating frame through the $+X$ axis to the $-Z$ axis, and the nuclear spins remain 'locked' along this effective field throughout. Whatever their resonance frequency, the proton spins are carried from the ↑ state to the ↓ state very efficiently. Above a certain threshold decoupler level the performance is quite insensitive to the radiofrequency intensity or its spatial inhomogeneity. Decoupling over a frequency range spanning hundreds of kHz can be readily implemented by these adiabatic decoupling sequences.[5] They find good use in experiments to decouple carbon-13 or nitrogen-15 while observing proton spectra, particularly in very high-field magnets.

At the opposite extreme, decoupling can be rendered extremely frequency-selective so that a multiplet splitting is removed from a chosen chemical site while all the rest of the spectrum remains unaffected. This 'selective decoupling' mode often employs an unmodulated radiofrequency source at a relatively low power level. It is used to identify which pairs of nuclei are coupled together, although the same information can also be obtained by two-dimensional spectroscopy (Chapter 11).

9

Spin echoes

9.1 Time reversal?

Imagine a slow-motion movie of a wineglass falling onto a hard concrete floor
and smashing into hundreds of small slivers. Now imagine the same film run in
reverse so that the wineglass appears to reconstitute itself from its parts. Even
small children recognize that this cannot represent the real world. All our experience confirms that large numbers of glass fragments *never* spontaneously converge
with just the right timing and in the correct geometry to form a wineglass (Figure
9.1). Disorder does not lead to order, unless there is some deliberate outside
intervention. We cannot reverse the direction of time.

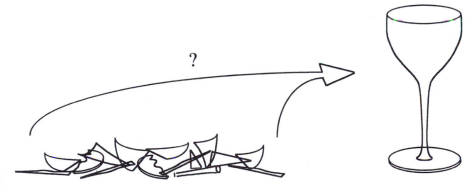

Figure 9.1 Experience confirms that the shards from a shattered wineglass never spontaneously
come together to form the intact wineglass again. Although we can make a movie film of the glass
breaking, and run the film backwards, we all know that this is not realistic. It is not possible to
reverse the direction of time.

One of the most intriguing phenomena in magnetic resonance is the spin echo, because, superficially, it appears to break this rule. We can contrive a situation where, for several seconds, a magnetic resonance sample in a strong magnetic field generates no response at all but then, suddenly, without any external stimulus, a signal begins to grow, reaches a peak, and then decays away to nothing. Have the individual nuclear spins suddenly decided to precess in phase? All our experience would suggest that they normally do just the opposite. Whenever an ordered state is created it degenerates into a disordered state—free precession signals decay with time and eventually disappear. Not only does the spin echo seems to present a challenging paradox, but it turns out to have many important applications in high-resolution NMR and in MRI.

In § 2.8 and § 6.2 we examined the problems arising from the fact that the applied magnetic field is never entirely uniform in space, even when measured across a relatively small 'volume of interest'. This is one of two factors contributing to the decay of the free precession signal, which in turn determines the observed width of a typical resonance response. The other factor, spin–spin relaxation (§ 4.5), is a fundamental physical phenomenon arising from the random fluctuations of the local magnetic fields from nearby nuclear spins. The decay of the observed signal due to spin–spin relaxation can never be reversed by any manipulations we may devise because we have no control over the randomly fluctuating local magnetic fields from neighbouring nuclear spins. On the other hand, the effects of magnetic field non-uniformity *can* be reversed, as was first realized by Hahn.[1]

Imagine breaking the sample down into a mosaic of small volume elements. Although the variation of the magnetic field across the sample is in fact continuous, it is a reasonably good approximation to 'digitize' the problem in this way. Each volume element is small enough that we may assume that the magnetic field within it is uniform, but slightly different from the fields in neighbouring elements. On the other hand, each volume element is large enough that it contains a very large number of nuclear spins, so our pictorial description in terms of a classical magnetization remains valid (§ 2.6). We initially assume that there is no large-scale motion or diffusion, so the field within each volume element remains constant in time. Abragam[2] has coined the term *isochromat* to denote the magnetization from one such volume element. We can represent these individual isochromats as vectors and sum them to obtain the overall magnetization of the sample. Note that this is a vector summation, so if the isochromats point in all possible directions, the resultant macroscopic magnetization is zero. This is the situation when the sample has been left for a long time with no radiofrequency excitation. An isochromat is manipulated by allowing it to precess in the *XY* plane through the influence of a field gradient (imposed or natural) and by radiofrequency pulses which rotate it about the *X* axis.

When the magnetic resonance signal is excited, all the isochromatic vectors have the same phase, but as free precession occurs, different isochromats gradually get out of phase with one another and the overall resultant magnetization decays with time. Eventually the dispersal of individual phases is so complete that the macroscopic signal goes to zero. Nevertheless, if we were able to examine any one small volume element alone, there would still be an appreciable magnetic resonance signal. The loss of phase coherence due to non-uniformity of the applied magnetic field is on a macroscopic scale (millimetres), not on the scale of individual molecules (nanometres). Locally the nuclei still continue to precess in phase until dispersed by spin–spin relaxation.

Hahn[1] realized that phase dispersal on this macroscopic scale could be reversed in an experiment involving a sequence of two radiofrequency pulses separated by a short interval, which we shall call τ. The initial decay of the signal during τ is reversed after the second pulse, giving a maximum response at time 2τ called a 'spin echo'. Hahn's original experiment is a little complicated to demonstrate pictorially, but a simpler illustration of the spin echo phenomenon emerges if we consider the effect of applied field gradients rather than a natural distribution of fields due to spatial inhomogeneity of the magnet.

9.2 Gradient-recalled echoes

This is a technique widely employed in MRI (§ 12.1), where magnetic field gradients are required to define the location of the nuclear spins within the sample, but we cannot afford to let isochromats get out of phase and mutually interfere. Suppose we apply an intense field gradient along the z direction, so strong that we can readily neglect the non-uniformity of the magnet by comparison. (We shall use lower-case x, y and z for the direction of applied field gradients, and capital X, Y and Z for the axes of the rotating reference frame.) Think of the sample as being divided into a series of slices parallel to the xy plane. Initially the magnetization vectors from all these slices are aligned in the same direction of the rotating reference frame ($+Y$). The field gradient induces a progressive increase in precession frequency as a function of distance along the z axis, and after a fixed time the vectors form a helix. Let us call this time τ.

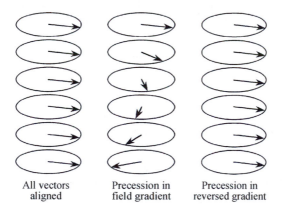

| All vectors aligned | Precession in field gradient | Precession in reversed gradient |

If we then reverse the direction of the applied field gradient, isochromats in the planes that originally precessed clockwise now precess anticlockwise, *each at the same rate as before*. After an equal period of free precession in the reversed gradient, all isochromats come back into alignment to form a strong resultant, the *gradient-recalled echo*. If the magnitude of the gradient remains constant, the echo occurs at time 2τ. Isochromats that wound into a helix during the first interval τ, unwind again during the second interval τ.

Gradient-recalled echoes are widely used in MRI because the application of a field gradient is an essential ingredient of the method. In the general case it is the product of the gradient strength and its duration that matters, so a helix of vectors formed in a weak gradient over a long period can be 'unwound' with a strong gradient in a correspondingly shorter time. The amplitude profile of the gradient pulse need not of course be rectangular; indeed a trapezoidal shape is the norm, often with 'pre-emphasis' to counter the effects of eddy currents (§ 12.2).

Gradient reversal appears to behave rather like time reversal as far as the spins are concerned. The initial 'disorder' is only apparent; since it was created by a known perturbation it can be undone by exactly reversing that perturbation. Disorder is sometimes represented by the concept of 'entropy', but it would be quite wrong to use this term to describe the dispersal of spin isochromats; entropy should be reserved for the loss of coherence due to spin–spin relaxation, which creates disorder on an atomic scale, and this can never be reversed.

9.3 The Carr–Purcell echo

This example of a single dominant field gradient represents a special case; spin echoes can also be generated in the more general case where there is some haphazard distribution of local magnetic fields (several different gradients) due to the lack of exact spatial uniformity of the applied field. Such naturally-occurring gradients cannot be reversed, but an equivalent effect can be achieved with what is known as a refocusing pulse. Each volume element of the sample is represented by an isochromat initially aligned along the $+Y$ axis of the rotating reference frame. Owing to their different precession frequencies these individual vectors fan out in the XY plane of the rotating frame so that eventually their resultant dwindles to zero. For the purposes of illustration we may consider just two representative vectors precessing clockwise—one fast (f) which accumulates a large precession angle, and the other slow (s) which accumulates a smaller angle.

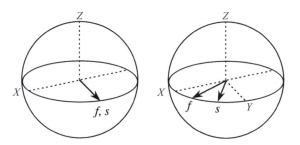

After a suitable interval τ an intense radiofrequency pulse induces a 180° rotation of all isochromats about the $+Y$ axis. This rotates the fast and slow vectors into mirror image positions with respect to the YZ plane. They then continue to precess at the same rate in and the same sense as before (clockwise). If we wait an equal time τ after the 180° pulse, the fast vector catches up with the slow vector as it reaches the $+Y$ axis, and both are in exact alignment once again.

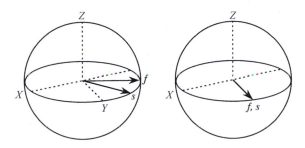

Similar arguments apply to *all* the isochromats; they are all refocused along $+Y$ at time 2τ and we observe a strong resultant signal. The motion is analogous to the opening and closing of a fan. An alternative description maps the phase evolution of a typical set of isochromats, emphasizing the analogy with the re-focusing of divergent rays of light by a suitable lens.

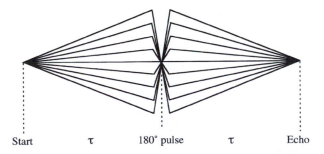

This is the spin echo experiment of Carr and Purcell.[3] Beyond the focus point at 2τ the isochromats fan out again and the resultant signal decays once more, but a further 180° pulse, for example at time 3τ, will bring them to a new focus at time 4τ. If the process is repeated at regular intervals we observe a regular sequence of spin echoes, called a Carr–Purcell echo train.

Several analogies have been proposed to help visualize the echo phenomenon. We might picture the evolution of isochromats in terms of a horse race where, at the halfway point, each horse is suddenly required to make a 180° turn and gallop back to the starting line; the fastest horses then have the farthest to go, and they all bunch together at the end of this unconventional race. An alternative analogy imagines a colony of ants, all starting from the same point on the rim of a pancake and marching purposefully, say, anticlockwise around the edge. If we flip the pancake through 180°, and if the single-minded ants continue to march anticlockwise and at the same speeds, they will eventually come together again at the starting point (Figure 9.2).

At the beginning of this chapter an apparent paradox was proposed in which an ensemble of nuclear spins seemed to organize itself spontaneously so as to generate an observable NMR response. It was of course a trick. The system had been prepared by a 90° excitation pulse followed τ seconds later by a 180° refocusing pulse. An unwitting observer of the spectrometer output display would see only noise until, suddenly, at time 2τ a spin echo is formed.

If we monitor the amplitudes of the peaks of successive echoes in a Carr–Purcell train, they decrease exponentially with a time constant equal to the spin–spin relaxation time T_2. Although a free induction signal decays quite quickly owing to the non-uniformity of the magnetic field, the echoes persist for a much longer time (Figure 9.3). This allows us to measure the natural decay of the NMR signal in a situation where it would normally be completely masked by the more rapid decay due to field inhomogeneity. Where a long train of echoes can be

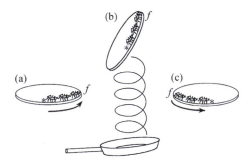

Figure 9.2 Hahn's analogy for the formation of a spin echo. (a) Several ants start at a fixed point (*) on the rim of a pancake and march purposefully anticlockwise, the fastest being labelled f. (b) The pancake then undergoes a 180° flip, and we assume that all the ants cling to their positions. (c) If the ants again march anticlockwise at the same rates, the fastest is now behind the slower ones and, after an equal interval, they all reach a focus at the original starting point.

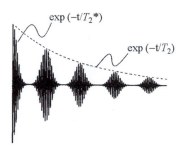

Figure 9.3 A 'train' of four successive spin echoes. The echo envelope is defined by the decay constant T_2^* representing losses due to non-uniformity of the applied magnetic field. The decay of the peaks of the echoes gives a measure of the spin–spin relaxation time T_2 which is appreciably longer than T_2^*.

generated in this manner, it offers a significant gain in sensitivity compared with the acquisition of a single free induction decay. Alternatively, it provides an array of different kinds of magnetic resonance information in a short time. Multiple echoes are used in MRI to make a two-dimensional proton density map in a single 'shot' instead of having to examine each trace one at a time. This important technique, known as 'echo planar imaging', is described in § 12.7.

9.4 Diffusion

The above description of spin echo formation implicitly assumed that the nuclear spins were stationary—they did not change precession frequency by moving from one voxel to another during the experiment. If there is motion in the sample, such as macroscopic flow or diffusion, this upsets the timekeeping of the nuclear spin isochromats; refocusing is inhibited, and the spin echo is attenuated. We concentrate here on random molecular diffusion; the question of concerted motion in a flowing sample is examined later (§ 9.8).

The rate of molecular diffusion can be measured by applying equal magnetic field gradients before and after the 180° refocusing pulse of a spin echo experiment, with the two gradient pulses separated by a fixed interval Δ.[4] These applied gradients are made sufficiently intense that they completely dominate the effect of natural inhomogeneity of the applied field, so that essentially all dephasing of isochromats occurs during the first narrow gradient pulse. Normally the combined effects of the 180° pulse and the second matched gradient would bring these isochromats back to a focus (Figure 9.4), but if molecular diffusion occurs during the intervening interval Δ, isochromats move into slightly different locations find themselves in the 'wrong' local field at the time of the second gradient pulse. As a consequence, the echo amplitude is attenuated by an amount that depends on the rate of diffusion.

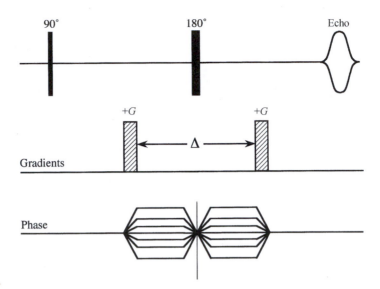

Figure 9.4 Measurement of molecular diffusion by a spin-echo experiment. The gradient pulses ($+G$) are so strong that all natural field gradients can be neglected. Phase dispersion caused by the first gradient pulse would be exactly refocused by the second equal gradient pulse except for diffusion that occurs during the Δ interval. The consequent attenuation of the echo allows the rate of diffusion to be measured.

Molecular diffusion can be treated as a 'random walk' problem, where the molecules make small jumps in haphazard directions. If a given molecule diffuses over a sufficient distance through a non-uniform field its precession frequency will change enough to inhibit refocusing by a 180° pulse. Hahn[1] showed that the consequent loss of echo intensity is proportional to the cube of the interval τ. In the simple sequence

$$90° - \tau - 180° - \tau - \text{echo}$$

the interval τ can be of the order of one second, giving rise to a significant loss of echo amplitude through diffusion. However, echo loss through diffusion occurs independently in each τ interval, as if the nuclear clock were reset by the refocusing pulse; the dephasing it is not cumulative. Consequently, if we set up a multiple-echo Carr–Purcell train with short τ intervals, it is largely immune to the effects of molecular diffusion, allowing the spin–spin relaxation time to be measured.

Chemical exchange (§ 7.8) also affects the refocusing process, by moving a typical nuclear spin to an alternative site where the precession frequency is different, replacing it with another spin with a random precession phase. Spin echo experiments can thus be used to measure the rate of chemical exchange, even for cases where exchange has no detectable effect on the width of the observed resonance response. This may be thought of as a shortening of the apparent spin–spin relaxation time, sometimes called the 'phase memory time'.

9.5 The Hahn echo

Hahn discovered the echo phenomenon by accident when his pulse transmitter malfunctioned and applied two (equal) pulses instead of one. It is greatly to his credit that he was able to analyse what had happened, because a 90° refocusing pulse generates a spin echo of a quite complicated form, where the individual isochromats converge onto a strange figure-of-eight pattern rather than onto a point focus. Hahn called this the '8-ball' echo. The phenomenon can be understood by following the motion of a typical set of isochromats (excited by a 90° pulse about the $+X$ axis) as they diverge in the non-uniform magnetic field (Figure 9.5). For simplicity of illustration we suppose that these isochromats attain a uniform distribution around a circle, and without prejudice to the argument we may truncate the distribution so that no isochromats precess further than $\pm 180°$. It is convenient to divide these isochromats into two groups, the 'slow' group of vectors that have precessed through angles in the range $-90°$ to $+90°$, and the 'fast' group that have precessed through angles between $\pm 90°$ and $\pm 180°$. (This distinction will also turn out to be important below when we discuss the stimulated echo.)

The clearest picture emerges if we represent this distribution by the locus of the tips of the magnetization vectors, rather than following all the vectors individually. Thus at time τ this locus is a great circle in the XY plane (Figure 9.5(a)). The second 90° pulse rotates this circle about the $+X$ axis, producing a circle in the XZ plane (Figure 9.5(b)). It is instructive to calculate the motion of this locus at times $\tau/4$, $\tau/2$, $3\tau/4$ and τ after the second 90° pulse. The faster-moving sections of the locus cause the loop to fold over on itself, eventually reaching the figure-of-eight pattern on the surface of the unit sphere (Figure 9.5(f)). Only those vectors that precessed through exactly $\pm 90°$ in the first τ interval actually reach the $-Y$ axis at the time of the Hahn echo. The remaining isochromats contribute only part of their magnetization to the echo because it is the component along the $-Y$ axis which matters. Vectors at the poles make no contribution at all. It turns out that the total spin echo intensity represents just half the available magnetization (assuming no losses due to relaxation). We may speculate now on what happens to that 'lost' magnetization.

9.6 The stimulated echo

One's natural reaction is to prefer the 'cleaner' picture of spin echo formation afforded by the Carr–Purcell scheme, and consequently neglect the Hahn

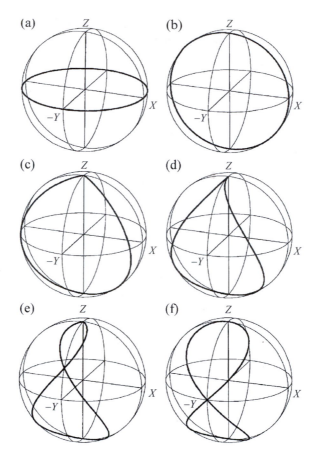

Figure 9.5 Formation of the Hahn spin echo. (a) The bold circle in the equatorial (XY) plane represents the locus of the tips of magnetisation vectors dispersed in a non-uniform magnetic field. (b) At time τ, a 90° radiofrequency pulse rotates this locus into the XZ plane, leaving the fastest vectors near the $+Z$ axis and the slowest vectors near $-Z$. During the subsequent time evolution represented by (c) through (f) the spread in rates of free precession causes the two halves of this locus to fold over onto each other, eventually forming a figure-of-eight (f) with a resultant aligned along the $-Y$ axis. This is the '8-ball' echo.

sequence. But there is an interesting twist to the Hahn scheme—if a third 90° pulse is applied to the spins at a later time (not *too* late of course, because of relaxation effects) a new kind of echo appears. Hahn called this the *stimulated echo*, and it turns out to be a very useful phenomenon. The pulse sequence may be written

$$90°—\tau—90°—T—90°—\tau—\text{(stimulated echo)}$$

where T must be longer than τ. Then we observe the '8-ball' spin echo at time 2τ and a stimulated echo at $2\tau + T$.

So how does this unexpected second echo come about? Immediately after the initial $90°$ pulse, all isochromats are aligned along the $+Y$ axis of the rotating frame and after free precession for an interval τ they become dispersed around the XY plane, reflecting the distribution of values of the local magnetic field. The second $90°$ pulse rotates this distribution into the XZ plane (Figure 9.6(a)). We are now concerned only with the Z-components of these vectors, which have different magnitudes (Figure 9.6(b)). Their X-components eventually give rise the '8-ball' echo as described above, and as time goes on, these transverse components fan out and relax, leaving a zero resultant along the $\pm Z$ axes. If we resolve all the remaining isochromats along the $\pm Z$ axes, this leaves just two resultant vectors, one along $+Z$ and the other along $-Z$ (Figure 9.6(c)). The former originates from the group of fast-moving isochromats whereas the latter originates from slow-moving vectors. Individual isochromats near the poles make strong contributions to these resultants while isochromats near the X axis have little effect. If we neglect relaxation effects, the resultant along $+Z$ has the same magnitude as the resultant along $-Z$.

At this point all the information is stored as Z-magnetization, represented by nuclear spins either at equilibrium (aligned along $+Z$) or with a population

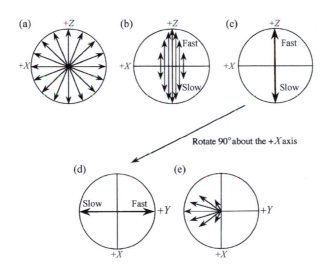

Figure 9.6 Formation of a stimulated echo. (a) Dispersed magnetization vectors in the XZ plane at time τ, just after the second $90°$ pulse, equivalent to the locus shown in Figure 9.5(b). (b) After the magnetic field non-uniformity has dispersed all transverse components of magnetization, only the Z-components are retained, representing spin populations at equilibrium ($+Z$) and after a population inversion ($-Z$). (c) These individual vectors are combined into just two resultants, representing 'fast' and 'slow' groups. (d) The third $90°$ radiofrequency pulse at time $\tau + T$ rotates these vectors into the XY plane. (e) Each individual vector 'remembers' its original characteristic precession frequency and amplitude and comes to a partial focus at time $2\tau + T$, forming the stimulated echo.

inversion (aligned along $-Z$). One might be forgiven for thinking that this lack of *phase information* would preclude the formation of a spin echo. But as demonstrated below, this is not the case. Each isochromat retains a memory of its original characteristic precession frequency throughout the experiment. Although temporarily aligned along the $\pm Z$ axes, these isochromats will soon be allowed to precess freely once again. A population disturbance of the right form can indeed generate a stimulated echo.

At time $T + \tau$ the third $90°$ pulse rotates the $+Z$ resultant to the $+Y$ axis and the $-Z$ resultant to the $-Y$ axis (Figure 9.6(d)). Since the magnitudes of these two vectors are the same, there is zero induced NMR signal at this time. The individual isochromats are now once again free to precess in the XY plane at their characteristic frequencies, identical to those they possessed during the first τ interval. But remember that these vectors now have different magnitudes, reflecting the losses suffered when the Z-components were selected (Figure 9.6(b)). Let us follow the motion of the two strongest vectors first. The vector along $-Y$ does not move at all (it was stationary during the first τ interval) whereas the vector along $+Y$ precesses through $180°$ in the second τ interval. Consequently, these two vectors come into alignment along the $-Y$ axis at time $T + 2\tau$, making a large contribution to the stimulated echo. The rest of the slow group fan out as illustrated in Figure 9.6(e), making smaller contributions to the stimulated echo; and vectors that precess through $\pm 90°$ have no effect at all. On the other hand, vectors in the fast group precess through angles between $\pm 90°$ and $\pm 180°$, and at time $T + 2\tau$ superimpose themselves exactly on the corresponding slow vectors (Figure 9.6(e)). Together they constitute the stimulated echo.

The stimulated echo remained something of a scientific curiosity for a long time, then it found an important application in MRS (§ 14.8) in a technique called STEAM (stimulated echo acquisition mode), where the fact that the spin isochromats are stored during the interval T in the form of a population disturbance is turned to advantage because these components are only attenuated by relatively slow spin–lattice relaxation, not by spin–spin relaxation.

9.7 Echo modulation

A $180°$ pulse refocuses the effects of different precession frequencies. One contribution to the intrinsic frequency of the nuclei is the chemical shift (Chapter 7), which arises from the shielding of the applied field by the extranuclear electrons. Consequently, chemical shift effects are refocused in a spin echo experiment in the same way as applied field gradients or magnetic field inhomogeneity. But there is another interaction—the spin–spin coupling that gives rise to the multiplet structure of high-resolution NMR spectra (§ 8.1). Here the behaviour is more complicated, causing a new phenomenon called echo modulation.[5]

Consider the simplest case of two coupled protons I and S. The NMR response from proton I is centred at a frequency given by the chemical shift of I but is split into a doublet by the coupling constant J. We can represent these two responses by two vectors precessing at the appropriate frequencies. These vectors may be labelled α and β because they correspond to the two possible states of the S spin. Let us call the faster vector α and the slower one β, so that α accumulates the larger precession angle.

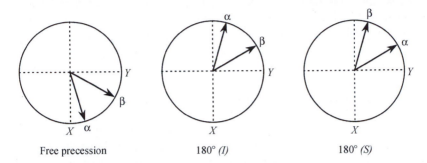

| Free precession | 180° (I) | 180° (S) |

In the Carr–Purcell scheme a 180° pulse is then applied. We may think of it as a cascade of two 180° pulses, one applied only to the I spins and one to the S spins, essentially simultaneously. The first rotates the two I-spin vectors into mirror image positions with respect to the Y axis. The second flips the S spins, interchanging their spin state labels α and β. In the next τ interval both vectors precess clockwise towards the $+Y$ axis, but the slower vector β is now handicapped because it subtends a large angle with respect to $+Y$, whereas the faster vector α has a head start since it is closer to $+Y$. The result is that at time 2τ the vector α overshoots the $+Y$ axis while β lags behind. The effect of chemical shift has been cancelled, but the α and β vectors have continued their initial divergence, and since their frequencies differ by J Hz, at the time of the spin echo they have reached angles of $+2\pi J\tau$ and $-2\pi J\tau$ radians with respect to the $+Y$ axis.

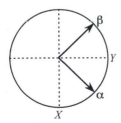

Modulated echo

The echo amplitude is the resultant of these two vectors, $2\cos(2\pi J\tau)$. If a series of spin-echo measurements is set up so that we can monitor the echo amplitude as a function of time $t = 2\tau$, we observe an amplitude modulation of the echo described by $2\cos(\pi J t)$.

Note that the key feature is the 180° pulse applied to the S spins. If this is absent, for example, in a system where S is a different nuclear species (the *heteronuclear* case), then the vectors α and β refocus exactly along the $+Y$ axis and there is no echo modulation. On the other hand, if we wish to modulate the echoes in the heteronuclear case we can deliberately apply a $180°$ pulse to the S nuclei at just the right moment.

Echo modulation is important in many high-resolution NMR experiments because it allows the two I-spin vectors to be prepared in a diametrically opposed configuration by allowing them to diverge by $\pm 90°$ if the time τ is set equal to $1/(4J)$. We shall see later that this is the first step in many polarization transfer (§ 11.8) and multiple-quantum experiments (§ 11.9).

9.8 Compensation effects

In the description of the Carr–Purcell spin echo, we chose to apply the $90°$ excitation pulse about the X axis, but the $180°$ refocusing pulse about the Y axis. This has an important practical advantage when we use a repeated sequence of refocusing pulses to generate multiple echoes. In the alternative experiment where both pulses are applied about the same axis any errors in the length of the $180°$ pulse (due to miscalibration or non-uniformity of the radiofrequency field) are cumulative and the echo amplitudes are falsified. Meiboom and Gill[6] demonstrated the importance of symmetry in the evolution of spin echo sequences, and showed that an error in the length of a $180°$ pulse can be compensated on even-numbered echoes if there is a $90°$ phase shift between the excitation and refocusing pulses. Any error on the first echo arising from an incorrect $180°$ pulse is then compensated on the second echo, and this compensation is repeated for all subsequent even-numbered echoes. This Carr–Purcell–Meiboom–Gill (CPMG) scheme is widely used for measuring the natural decay of the magnetic resonance signal (§ 4.5) by monitoring the exponential decrease in the echo peaks.

It turns out that this type of compensation is an important general property of even-numbered echoes.[7] Another type of instrumental shortcoming can be a *cumulative* phase error on successive echoes. With the Meiboom–Gill modification, the symmetry of the phase evolution diagram is such that these phase errors are compensated on all even-numbered echoes. An equivalent compensation can be achieved with gradient-recalled echoes in MRI. The problem arises when the signal from blood is being monitored, with some of the blood flowing through the applied field gradient and thus changing its precession frequency continuously. The problem is analysed in detail in § 12.11, where it is shown that the NMR signals from both stationary and flowing nuclear spins can be refocused on even-numbered gradient-recalled echoes.

Further reading

R. Freeman, *Pulsed Magnetic Resonance: NMR, ESR and Optics*, Chapter 10, ed. D. M. S. Bagguley, Oxford University Press, Oxford (1992).

10

NMR in solids

Ice and water are the same chemical substance, yet one is a solid and the other a liquid. We all recognize the difference from their bulk properties, but it is the nature of the molecular motion that really distinguishes these two states of matter. The molecules of liquid water are in continuous rapid motion in all possible directions. Although water molecules are too small to be seen under an ordinary microscope, their chaotic translational motion can be made evident by sprinkling a fine powder on the water surface. These small solid particles are large enough to been seen under the microscope yet small enough to be buffeted in a random manner by the water molecules (Brownian motion). More important to the NMR spectroscopist is the 'tumbling' motion—a chaotic, stepwise reorientation of the molecules which has a very profound effect on the NMR spectra.

In the solid state the translational and rotational motions are largely 'frozen' and we have a regular, rigid-lattice structure. The physical properties may then be different in different directions. For example, a crystal will shear more easily along certain planes than along others, and the magnetic resonance properties are similarly 'anisotropic'. In some cases, motion may persist in the solid state (for example, the rotation of methyl groups) but these examples become rarer as the temperature falls, and all movement would disappear completely if the absolute zero of temperature could be reached.

There are certain other states of matter that have properties intermediate between those of a liquid and those of a solid. For example, when water forms part of a tendon, where the collagen fibres are aligned along the tendon axis, the motion of the water molecules becomes anisotropic. Although the rapid tumbling motion persists unabated, there is a slight preponderance of molecules aligned in the direction of the collagen fibres. Another important example is that of liquid crystals—where the molecules are aligned in some particular direction but are otherwise free to move in a similar way to those in a normal liquid. All these motional effects can be studied by NMR methods.

10.1 The dipole–dipole interaction

The apparent obsession with liquid samples for high-resolution NMR spectroscopy persisted for many years because solids generate very broad NMR responses, obscuring almost all the interesting chemical shift effects. The problem arises from new types of interaction that make their appearance in the solid state. First of all, each nuclear spin experiences intense local magnetic fields from its neighbours—the 'dipole–dipole' interaction. The nucleus acts as a magnetic dipole, and at a distance equivalent to a typical chemical bond (one Ångstrom unit, equal to one-tenth of a nanometre) generates quite an intense local magnetic field—of the order of 1 gauss (0.0001 tesla). The variation of magnetic field intensity around a dipole can be represented by the spatial distribution of the lines of force.

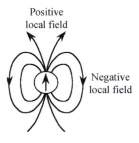

Positive local field

Negative local field

In a solid each nuclear spin is surrounded by a fixed matrix of neighbour spins, and it experiences local magnetic fields determined by the number, positions, and distances of all these dipoles. Furthermore, the neighbour spins are in a random arrangement of 'up' or 'down' states, so each contribution to the local field may be positive or negative. The result is a broad, mostly featureless NMR response. The local magnetic fields that arise from the dipole–dipole interactions in a solid interfere with the exact timekeeping of a given nuclear spin, that is to say, the spin–spin relaxation time T_2 is much shorter than in a liquid. On the other hand, the lack of motion in a solid means that the local fields from nearby dipoles fluctuate rather slowly and are therefore ineffective for spin–lattice relaxation (long T_1). Saturation is therefore more of a problem in solid samples.

Another phenomenon that makes its appearance in a solid sample is the fact that the magnitude of the chemical shielding depends on the orientation of the molecule with respect to the applied magnetic field. This 'chemical shift anisotropy' is always present but is masked in liquid samples by rapid molecular tumbling. Spin–spin coupling (§ 8.1), so important in liquid samples, also persists in the solid state but is very often masked by the much larger dipole–dipole splittings. This interaction is also anisotropic. Finally, unless we are dealing with a nucleus carrying a charge that has spherical symmetry, there is a phenomenon called the nuclear quadrupole interaction where the nucleus is affected by local electric field gradients. A detailed discussion of chemical shift anisotropy and quadrupole interactions is beyond the scope of this book.

In a liquid all these interaction are 'washed out' because the molecules execute rapid, random, reorientational movements caused by the buffeting they receive from their neighbours. We can think of the nucleus as being supported on completely frictionless bearings, so that when a molecule containing a pair of nuclear dipoles rotates in a magnetic field, the dipoles always stay aligned along the magnetic field direction.

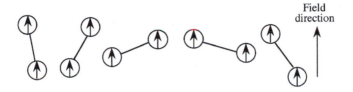

Field direction

As a consequence, the interaction between the two dipoles varies rapidly with time, and the average value is zero. In a similar manner, the interaction between any quadrupole moment and local electric field gradients is 'washed out' in a liquid. Note, however, that the fluctuating components of these interactions act as relaxation mechanisms (§ 4.1). Chemical shielding and spin–spin coupling lose their anisotropy in the liquid state but leave non-zero values.

A solid can be a single crystal, a polycrystalline powder, or have an irregular (amorphous) structure. A single crystal sample generates an NMR spectrum with a discernible structure which changes as a function of the orientation in the applied magnetic field. However, it is a considerable practical disadvantage to have to grow a single crystal for NMR purposes, so the majority of investigations make do with polycrystalline powders where the crystallites take on all possible orientations. We observe only the superposition of the spectra from individual crystallites with all possible alignments with respect to the main magnetic field. Note that in many applications of NMR, particularly those addressing materials science, dissolving the sample in a solvent is not an option, for that would destroy some essential features of the solid-state structure.

Consider, for simplicity, two close protons (A and B) completely isolated from all other interactions. The local magnetic field induced at site A by the dipole at site B depends on the angle θ which the vector A–B makes with respect to the applied field.

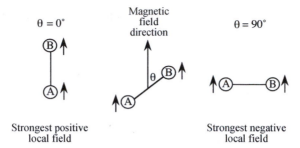

Strongest positive   Strongest negative
local field   local field

The maximum positive local field occurs for $\theta = 0$, when the two dipoles lie one behind the other, while the maximum negative local field (which is only half the intensity of the maximum positive field) occurs for $\theta = 90°$ when the two dipoles lie broadside to one another. Between these extremes there is a continuum of local magnetic fields as a function of the inclination angle θ. Zero dipolar field corresponds to $\theta = 54.7°$. Note that crystallites with completely random orientations are much more likely to be aligned near $\theta = 90°$ than near $\theta = 0°$. (For the same reason, there are many more parcels of land (or sea) one kilometre square near the equator than there are near the north or south poles.) The number of spins in a given local field can be represented by the graph:

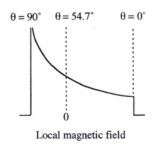

Local magnetic field

This diagram represents the case where both spins are aligned parallel to the main magnetic field. For the equally probable case of opposed spins (one aligned along the main field and one opposed to the field direction) all the local fields change sign and the curve is reversed left to right. When we combine the two cases the distribution of local fields has two peaks.

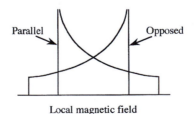

Local magnetic field

In practice we never have a completely isolated pair of spins; they are surrounded by many other magnetic nuclei, but if these neighbours are not too close then their influence can be approximated by a random distribution of local magnetic fields represented by a Gaussian broadening function. This lack of structure may seem surprising at first, but becomes clear if we consider a simple case. Suppose that a very close pair of protons 'HH' is surrounded by six proton neighbours with octahedral symmetry.

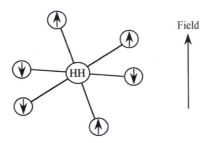

While all six neighbours are at the same distance from HH, the inclinations of the internuclear vectors with respect to the applied magnetic field are all different. Furthermore, the spin states of these neighbours are random; for the case illustrated, there are twenty possible configurations of three 'up' spins and three 'down' spins. When we take into account the other possible combinations of 'up' and 'down' neighbours, there are 64 possible local dipolar fields at site HH, all different. Then we have to take into account local fields from the next-nearest neighbours, and so on. The result is a broadening function that is a very close approximation to a Gaussian curve. We observe a broad 'powder pattern'.

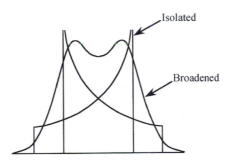

This is known as a 'Pake doublet' after its inventor.[1] Careful fitting of the experimental lineshape allows the internuclear distance to be determined with quite good accuracy. Unfortunately there are not too many solid samples that have a tight group of protons relatively isolated from all neighbours. Consequently, for many years, magnetic resonance work on solids was rather neglected and high-resolution NMR of liquids stole all the limelight.

10.2 Magic angle spinning

It was the introduction of some ingenious new experimental techniques that gave solid-state NMR its new lease of life. The first of these was the discovery that the dipole–dipole interaction averages to zero when the sample is made to spin rapidly about an axis subtending 54.7° with respect to the direction of the applied magnetic field. Perhaps this remarkable phenomenon[2] came as a surprise to some scientists because the critical orientation 54.7° is now universally known as the 'magic angle'. Chemists will recognize this as one-half the tetrahedral angle—the angle between two C–H bonds in aliphatic compounds.

Consider an isolated pair of magnetic dipoles connected by a vector that makes angle θ with respect to the magnetic field. We have already seen that if θ is the magic angle the dipole–dipole interaction is zero; if θ is a smaller angle, the induced local magnetic field is positive and if θ is greater than the magic angle the local field is negative. Now consider an internuclear vector making an *arbitrary* angle β with respect to the field. When this vector is rotated rapidly about an axis inclined at the magic angle, the dipole–dipole interaction varies cyclically between positive and negative extremes.

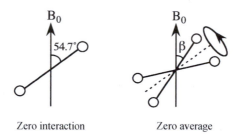

Zero interaction   Zero average

The time-averaged interaction is zero. If we extend this analysis to a solid with many different dipole–dipole interactions, they all average to zero and the original broadening effect disappears, leaving only narrow resonances at the chemical shift frequencies. Magic angle spinning (MAS) also generates modulation components at the spinning rate and its harmonics, and these give rise to spinning sidebands in the spectrum. The faster the spinning, the greater the frequency spread of the sidebands and the lower their intensities. If the spinning sidebands are not to be too obtrusive, the spinning rate has to exceed the linewidth of the stationary sample by an appreciable factor. The technology to accomplish spinning rates of several thousand rotations per second in a stable regime requires considerable practical ingenuity. If air is used to drive the spinner turbine it becomes unreliable when the speed of sound is reached; air has to be replaced by helium to achieve very fast spinner rates. (Note that these speeds are orders of magnitude faster than the spinning rates employed in liquid-phase high-resolution spectroscopy.)

10.3 Multiple-pulse methods

Then came a breakthrough that to some extent sidestepped these rather demanding mechanical problems. Waugh, Huber and Haeberlen[3] had the idea of *manipulating* the magnetic dipoles themselves so that their motion mimicked rotation of the sample about the magic angle. A sequence of four intense radio-frequency pulses is applied in a cycle that is repeated rapidly compared with the rate of spin–spin relaxation. Each pulse is a 90° rotation about the $\pm X$ or $\pm Y$ axes of the rotating reference frame. This pulse sequence has the effect of placing the magnetization vector along the $+X, +Y$ and $+Z$ axes for equal durations 2τ, switching rapidly between these three orientations.

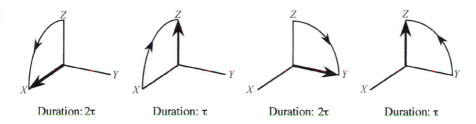

| Duration: 2τ | Duration: τ | Duration: 2τ | Duration: τ |

The motion is a sequence of rapid jumps between the X, Y and Z axes, rather than a continuous rotation. After a trivial reordering, the sequence can be written as a regular cycle where the magnetization vector jumps between the Z, Y and X axes, spending an equal time at each orientation. This is equivalent to a simple rotation about the magic angle 54.7°.

The cycling rate can be made sufficiently fast by employing very short, intense radiofrequency pulses and short residence times along each axis. The rather cumbersome method of magic angle spinning (§ 10.2) has thus been replaced by an essentially equivalent manipulation of the spins that is not governed by the same practical constraints on the rate of rotation. This particular 'magic cycle' is known as 'WAHUHA' after the three authors on the original paper.[3] More sophisticated sequences have now been developed based on the same principle.

10.4 Dipolar decoupling

There are many situations that are intrinsically favorable to high-resolution NMR in the solid state because of the low natural abundance of nuclei such as carbon-13, nitrogen-15 or silicon-29. For such samples, neighbours of the same nuclear species are relatively rare and therefore well separated, allowing the mutual dipolar broadening to be neglected to a first approximation. Nature has conveniently provided a dilute system of nuclear spins well suited to high-resolution studies in the solid state.

However, the dipolar broadening by the abundant protons remains, and its influence needs to be eliminated. This 'heteronuclear' interaction can be decoupled by the application of intense radiofrequency irradiation at the proton frequency. Because the protons are tightly coupled among themselves by strong proton–proton dipolar interactions, the proton flipping benefits from a cooperative effect, making heteronuclear dipolar decoupling quite efficient. Complex sequences of the kind used in high-resolution NMR of liquids (§ 8.5) are not necessary in this situation. There remains the problem of poor sensitivity for these low-abundance species but the natural density of spins in a solid is relatively high compared with experiments in solution.

10.5 Cross-polarization

A critical factor determining the sensitivity of a magnetic resonance experiment is the degree of polarization of the spin system (§ 2.4) that is to say, the excess population of spins in the ground state, for these are the only spins that contribute to the observed NMR signal. If we are interested in naturally-abundant carbon-13 in a solid sample, the inherent sensitivity is poor, not only because of the low natural abundance of carbon-13 but also because of the relatively weak polarization. Yet in the same sample there is almost always an abundant proton system with high polarization. It was Hartmann and Hahn[4] who showed how to exploit this *embarras de richesses* by transferring polarization from the protons to carbon, a process called 'cross-polarization'. The trick is universally known as the Hartmann–Hahn experiment.

This is a rare case where thermodynamic principles govern the mechanism of sensitivity enhancement—we can analyse the problem in terms of energy exchange between 'hot' and 'cold' nuclear spins. In a solid the protons are tightly-coupled among themselves by the strong dipole–dipole interactions; they constitute a thermal reservoir where all the protons are in equilibrium. Consequently, we can invoke the Boltzmann relationship (Equation 2.2) between the temperature T, the energy gap ΔE, and the spin populations in the ground state (N_{lower}) and the excited state (N_{upper}). For magnetic resonance the energy level separation ΔE is always very much smaller than kT (k is the Boltzmann constant). To a very good approximation (§ 2.4) we can write:

$$(N_{\text{lower}} - N_{\text{upper}})/N_{\text{lower}} = \Delta E/kT \qquad \textbf{10.1}$$

This equation demonstrates that the excess population in the ground state is always very, very small. For a tightly-coupled system of protons (fast spin–spin relaxation) well isolated from the outside environment (slow spin–lattice relaxation) we can use this expression to define a 'spin temperature' (§ 4.4) which may well be different from the 'lattice temperature'—the temperature of the sample measured with a conventional thermometer. To take just one illustrative example, when the protons are saturated, the populations in the ground and excited states are equalized. Since ΔE is non-zero, the only way that Equation 10.1 can be satisfied is with an *infinite* spin temperature, but of course the rest of the sample ('the lattice') remains at ambient temperature.

Hartmann and Hahn considered the situation where the proton spins are first excited by a 90° pulse about the $+X$ axis of the rotating reference frame. The proton magnetization can be represented by a single vector aligned along the $+Y$ axis. Then a constant radiofrequency field B_1 is applied along the $+Y$ axis. It is strong in comparison with all local magnetic fields—so strong that it dominates all other possible perturbations that might otherwise have caused a spread of nuclear precession frequencies. Consequently, the proton magnetization is held fixed along the $+Y$ axis; it is said to be 'spin-locked'. It remains locked until the strong radiofrequency field B_1 is extinguished.

Now as far as the protons are concerned they 'see' only the magnetic field B_1, yet their energy level populations still correspond to having been polarized in the usual main magnetic field B_0, which is about five orders of magnitude more intense than B_1. The protons are therefore *hyperpolarized*—the ground state has an excess spin population far greater than would be expected in such a low magnetic field. In terms of the Boltzmann expression Equation 10.1 they have an extremely low spin temperature, the lattice temperature multiplied by the factor B_1/B_0. This is not of course a stable situation; eventually relaxation processes deplete the excess proton spin population to the very low value characteristic of polarization in the weak field B_1, but these processes involve weak interactions with the environment (the lattice) and are very slow in the solid state. There is plenty of time for some interesting manipulations. The very cold proton reservoir can be exploited to cool down the carbon-13 spins, thereby enhancing their polarization.

Cross-polarization involves the establishment of thermal contact between the proton and carbon spin systems. Under normal circumstances proton and carbon spins cannot 'talk' to one another because their nuclear resonance frequencies are quite different. Communication is achieved by applying a second radiofrequency field B_2 at the carbon-13 frequency, with an intensity defined by the Hartmann–Hahn matching condition:

$$\gamma_H B_1 = \gamma_C B_2 \qquad \textbf{10.2}$$

In practice, since the gyromagnetic ratio of the proton (γ_H) is four times that of carbon-13 (γ_C), matching requires that the radiofrequency B_2 be four times stronger than B_1. At this condition, protons and carbon-13 nuclei precess at equal rates in their respective rotating reference frames, providing a common 'communication channel' between the two spin systems. This allows magnetic energy to be exchanged between the two species through a 'flip-flop' mechanism where carbon-13 makes a downward transition for each upward proton transition (and vice versa). The total energy of the system is conserved, but because of the discrepancy between the two spin temperatures, the 'cold' protons cool the 'hot' carbon-13 spins. The polarization of the carbon-13 nuclei is boosted giving a correspondingly increased NMR response. Since there is a very large reservoir of magnetic energy in the proton spin system, this transfer of polarization has only a very minor effect on the protons and it is possible to make multiple transfers to the carbon-13 spins, increasing their polarization step by step by a large factor. The process is only terminated when spin–lattice relaxation erodes the proton polarization. Cross-polarization (CP) by this method has proved very effective for enhancing the NMR signals of low-abundance nuclei in solids. When combined with magic angle spinning, the technique is abbreviated CP-MAS.

10.6 Partially-aligned liquids

Molecules in a true liquid have all possible orientations in space with equal probabilities and all their physical properties are independent of the direction in which the property is measured—they are said to be *isotropic* liquids. Solids present a complete contrast, many physical properties depend on direction—they are intrinsically *anisotropic*. Intermediate between these two extreme cases are materials that exhibit the rapid random thermal motions characteristic of a liquid but the molecules nevertheless have a preferential orientation. Partially-aligned liquids tend to be made up of flat or rod-like molecules. They include 'thermotropic' liquid crystals (used in display devices) which lose this preferential alignment when heated above a certain temperature, reverting to a normal liquid. If a small molecule is dissolved in a liquid crystalline medium, it too can acquire a degree of alignment through collisions with its aligned neighbours.

Strong magnetic fields may sometimes induce a slight preferential alignment in a liquid that would otherwise be isotropic. Of particular interest in biochemistry are cell membranes, which are made up of aligned 'amphiphilic' molecules that are attracted to water at one end and repelled by it at the other. Because an intense magnetic field can affect the degree of alignment, some concern has been expressed that the permeability of a cell membrane to certain chemicals might be altered during an MRI experiment (§ 13.1) although there is no concrete evidence that this actually happens.

In partially-aligned systems the dipole–dipole interactions do not average to zero as they would in a truly isotropic liquid and the high-resolution NMR spectrum reflects these additional splittings which have the same general character as the spin–spin splittings in conventional high-resolution spectra. Random thermal motions are still present, so the degree of alignment (the 'order parameter') is usually quite small and the dipole–dipole interactions are scaled down in proportion. These properties have been successfully exploited for the study of the three-dimensional structure of proteins. Whereas most of the information about internuclear distances comes from measurement of the nuclear Overhauser effect (NOESY) outlined in § 11.4, these results can be supplemented by measuring the dipole–dipole splittings induced by weak alignment of the protein in an environment of disk-shaped molecules called bicelles. The scaled dipole–dipole splitting is of the same order as the spin–spin splitting, and either adds to it or subtracts from it. This is another case where the experimentally observed splitting is not equal to the spin–spin coupling (§ 8.3). This complementary information about the spatial relationship between the two interacting protons often results in a considerable improvement in the quality of the structural determination.[5]

The scaled-down dipole–dipole splitting in a partially aligned system has been put to good use for the determination of the structure of small molecules dissolved in a liquid crystal matrix. Unfortunately, some of these spectra can be incredibly complex and difficult to assign because so many different dipole–dipole splittings may be involved. One remedy would be to investigate the proton NMR spectrum of a molecule that has been almost completely deuterated, so that most of the proton–proton interactions are eliminated, leaving a greatly simplified spectrum. There is an ingenious alternative approach. Suppose we are interested in the spectrum of aligned benzene molecules where there are six interacting protons. There are special techniques that permit the excitation of 'multiple-quantum' transitions that involve two or more protons jumping together, thus violating the normal selection rule $\Delta m = \pm 1$. In the general case, the multiple-quantum spectrum would consist of all possible 'many-quantum jumps' $\Delta m = 0, 2, 3, 4, 5$ and 6. The $\Delta m = 6$ spectrum is quite independent of the dipolar interactions and simply gives a single line at a frequency determined by the sum of the chemical shifts of all six protons. Excitation and detection schemes can be devised[6] that can select the $\Delta m = 5$ spectrum and largely suppress the rest. This yields a doublet representing just one dipole–dipole splitting, almost as if the benzene molecule had been deuterated at four locations, leaving only two interacting proton sites. The interpretation is then straightforward.

Further reading

C. A. Fyfe, *Solid State NMR for Chemists*, C.F.C. Press, Guelph, Ontario, Canada, (1983).

P. T. Callaghan, *Principles of Nuclear Magnetic Resonance Microscopy*, Clarendon Press, Oxford (1991).

E. O. Stejskal and J. D. Memory, *High Resolution NMR in the Solid State*, Oxford University Press, Oxford (1994).

11

Two-dimensional
spectroscopy

11.1 Correlation by double resonance

Experiments that irradiate the sample with two radiofrequency fields are known as double resonance, and by convention the second radiofrequency is labelled B_2. Irradiation with B_2 perturbs the system and the resulting change is monitored by the radiofrequency B_1. The essential property of double resonance investigations is that they *correlate* what happens at one chemical site with what happens at another, thereby establishing that there is an interaction between them. This normally indicates that the two sites are in the same molecule and relatively close to one another.

Let us start with a simple example. When a hydrogen atom detaches itself from a molecule and moves to a different chemical site, it carries with it a proton spin which acquires a different precession frequency at the new site. If the exchange rate is slow in comparison with the chemical shift difference between the two sites, two separate resonance responses are observed. Suppose we invert the spin populations at the first site by means of a selective 180° pulse (§ 2.9). The chemical exchange carries these inverted spins to the second site, thus opposing the signal from the spins already at that site, and reducing the intensity of that response. Each atom involved in the exchange has thus been 'tagged' by a population inversion of its nuclear spin. This double resonance experiment not only identifies which two sites are involved, but also provides a means for measuring the rate of exchange.

Now consider a related case where the spin–lattice relaxation of protons at the first site (I) is largely determined by the magnetic interaction with a protons at a nearby site (S). If we apply a selective 180° pulse that inverts the spin populations of S, cross-relaxation changes the intensity of the NMR response from site I. (For rapidly tumbling molecules it *increases* the intensity, while for slowly moving molecules it *decreases* the intensity.) The mechanism for this nuclear 'Overhauser effect' is examined in detail in § 4.3. Once again the double resonance experiment identifies the two interacting sites and provides information about the rate of cross-relaxation. For the large molecules of interest in biochemistry, this nuclear Overhauser experiment is widely used to establish constraints on the inter-proton distances.

Double resonance experiments can also exploit the spin–spin coupling mechanism. If two protons I and S are coupled, the four observable transitions ($I1$, $I2$, $S1$ and $S2$) necessarily share energy levels:

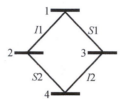

A selective irradiation experiment can be devised where a radiofrequency pulse at the I-spin frequency causes intensity changes on the S-spin response. The intensity of a given NMR response is proportional to the population difference between the lower and upper energy levels. For illustration purposes the proportionality constant is irrelevant, so we can represent the populations very schematically:

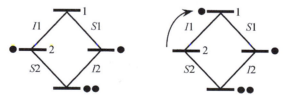

Equilibrium populations   Population inversion

Here we have chosen population numbers so as to make the population difference across each transition one unit for a system at equilibrium. A 180° radiofrequency pulse applied selectively at the frequency of transition $I1$ interchanges the spin populations of energy levels 1 and 2, and because these energy levels are shared with the S spin, this enhances the response $S2$ by withdrawing spins from level 2, and reduces the intensity of the response $S1$ by augmenting the spin population of level 1. By contrast, if the selective radiofrequency pulse had been applied at the frequency of the $I2$ response, the sense of the intensity changes observed at the S site would be reversed—$S1$ would be increased and $S2$ decreased.

We could perform this experiment by systematically stepping the radiofrequency through a frequency range that spans both I responses, plotting the changes in the response at site S at each step. Most of the traces will be blank. Only if the perturbation frequency happens to hit one of the I-spin responses do we see an S-spin spectrum (one positive peak and one inverted peak). If we stack the consecutive traces as a function of the irradiation frequency, the result is a pattern of four resonances forming a square of side J_{IS} , with intensities that alternate positive and negative:

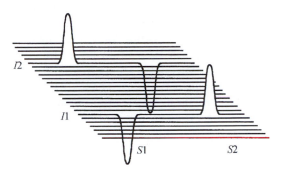

We shall see in § 11.5 that this exactly matches the pattern obtained by one of the important techniques of two-dimensional spectroscopy. Note that these responses disappear through mutual cancellation if the spin–spin coupling constant J_{IS} is smaller that the line width.

These three double resonance techniques all have the property that they *correlate* the NMR responses from two chemical sites that interact in some way, either through chemical exchange, cross-relaxation or spin–spin coupling. Perturbation of one site 'lights up' the response at the other, thereby identifying them both. All three experiments have their equivalents in two-dimensional spectroscopy, as we shall see below.

11.2 NMR in two frequency dimensions

We might describe the double resonance experiments outlined above as operating in a 'pedestrian' mode—a full examination of all the possible irradiation frequencies would require that the measurement be repeated many many times, stepping the frequency of B_2 in rather small increments across the NMR spectrum. This wastes precious spectrometer time, because in many of these scans no NMR signal is observed at all. There is even a stronger criticism—even if we were lucky enough to find just the right irradiation frequency at the first attempt, we would only observe a single correlation, while in general there are many such correlations waiting to be discovered. Two-dimensional spectroscopy allows us to gather all the requisite information continuously, no spectrometer time is wasted viewing empty space, and nothing is missed.

The reader will have noticed that the word 'correlation' has been given a rather special meaning here. Let us take the analogy of a relay race viewed by an observer at some distance. Several runners, distinguishable by their characteristic team colours, start the first leg of the race and become strung out around the race track according to their respective athletic abilities. Then there is a short period of utter confusion during which batons are exchanged, and a new set of runners start the second leg of the race. The observer would notice a strong *correlation* between the colours worn by front runners in the first leg and those of the leaders in the second leg, a pattern repeated throughout the entire range of abilities. This of course presupposes that each athlete successfully passed the baton to a teammate.

Two-dimensional NMR spectroscopy operates in a similar manner.[1] Spins from many different chemical sites precess at their characteristic frequencies during an initial period called the 'evolution' time. Then follows a brief 'mixing' time, during which some type of magnetic resonance information is transferred between particular pairs of spins. During the next period (called the 'acquisition' time) all the new precession frequencies are measured. For spin pairs where no transfer occurred the frequencies during evolution and acquisition are the same and we learn nothing of interest. But for interacting sites we notice a frequency change between evolution and acquisition; this indicates correlation between the two sites. Correlation is not a black-or-white concept—there is a continuous gradation between strong correlation and none at all. We might liken these intermediate cases to those unfortunate relay runners that fumble the baton without actually dropping it.

Everything hinges on this crucial instant of handover; relay races would otherwise offer no particular interest. The same is true of two-dimensional NMR spectroscopy. At the interface between the evolution period and the acquisition period some vital piece of information is passed between certain pairs of spins—it may be an apparently minor shift in the phase of the precessing magnetization—but it is essential to the correlation. There are many such transfers taking place at the same instant, yet each 'connection' is made without error, and the resulting spectrum tells us exactly what they were. This is why the concept of 'correlation' has been given particular emphasis.

Measurement of the frequencies during the acquisition period (t_2) is straightforward—Fourier transformation (§ 3.7) of the free precession signal separates all the signal components and assembles them in the form of a high-resolution NMR spectrum. It would serve no useful purpose to apply the same method to the evolution period because this would not provide the all-important correlation information. The receiver is not active during evolution. The 'baton' that is passed in this 'race' is simply the phase of the nuclear precession at the end of the evolution period. In order to convert this into an evolution *frequency*, the experiment is repeated several times, methodically incrementing the length of the evolution time (t_1) in small steps (so that the phase increments are not too large). The time development of this phase angle is equivalent to a frequency. The various precession frequencies during the evolution period are separated by a second stage of Fourier transformation, this time as a function of t_1.

This information is most conveniently displayed as a two-dimensional chart that shows frequencies from the evolution period (the F_1 axis) plotted against frequencies observed during the acquisition period (the F_2 axis). Pairs of nuclear spins that do not interact at all give rise to responses that lie on the principal diagonal ($F_1 = F_2$), providing no correlation information. Pairs of sites that interact in some way still show some diagonal responses but also some new ones that lie off the principal diagonal, the so-called 'cross-peaks'. If a pair of cross-peaks are observed at frequency coordinates (f_I, f_S) and at (f_S, f_I) it indicates a two-way interaction between sites I and S—a correlation. In general, the intensity of these cross-peaks in relation to the parent diagonal peaks is an indication of the strength of the interaction.

The representation of peak intensities as a function of two frequency variables (F_1 and F_2) presents something of a challenge. One scheme is to stack consecutive one-dimensional traces one behind the other; this gives a pleasing three-dimensional impression but has the disadvantage that some peaks may be obscured behind others that lie nearer the front of the display. The most general display mode is a graph with frequency axes F_1 and F_2, and intensities represented by contours; this makes the extraction of exact intensities more difficult but allows the frequencies to be measured accurately.

It was Jean Jeener who first discovered the principle of two-dimensional spectroscopy and he notes in the abstract of his report[2] that it offers an alternative to existing double-resonance experiments with the advantage that it gathers the information much more efficiently. However, it is not a short-duration experiment, because multiple scans with incrementation of t_1 are unavoidable, but each scan acquires strong NMR signals that contribute to the overall signal-to-noise ratio. The sensitivity is comparable with that of a one-dimensional experiment of the same overall duration. Two-dimensional spectroscopy has now superseded most of the 'pedestrian' double-resonance experiments, except in very simple situations where only one or two correlation need to be established. By providing a clear pictorial representation of the interactions between nuclear spins, it is ideally suited to the way in which an organic chemist visualizes molecular structure.

11.3 Exchange spectroscopy (EXSY)

Chemical exchange describes the phenomenon where an atom (or group of atoms) leaves a molecule and attaches itself to a different site in another molecule, or (alternatively) flips between two chemically distinct conformations of the same molecule. Let us imagine that we are sitting on a particular nuclear spin as it hops between two different chemical sites that have a chemical shift difference Δ Hz. If the rate of exchange is slow in comparison with Δ then the nuclear spin will precess through several revolutions before being forced to switch to the other frequency by a random exchange event. Now a frequency is only perfectly defined if it can be monitored for an infinite time; shortening the lifetime of nuclear precession causes a broadening of the observed resonance response. Consequently in this 'slow exchange' regime we observe separate responses from the two sites, but their resonance responses get broader as the lifetimes are shortened by chemical exchange.

Slow exchange can be conveniently studied by two-dimensional NMR, where it is usually known as exchange spectroscopy (EXSY). The basic pulse sequence[3] may be written:

$$90° - t_1 - 90° - t_{mix} - 90° \text{ acquisition } (t_2)$$

The evolution period t_1 serves to encode the various precession frequencies. As t_1 is incremented, the final phase ϕ of each precessing NMR signal increases, and the rate of increase depends on the relevant precession frequency. It is this phase angle ϕ which determines what happens next because it determines how much magnetization remains along the Y axis. The second 90° pulse creates Z magnetization that has a cosine dependence on ϕ.

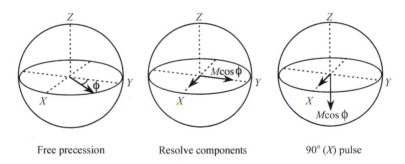

Free precession   Resolve components   90° (X) pulse

Only the component $M\cos\phi$ is affected by the 90° pulse about the X axis. As nuclear spins from site I move to site S during the fixed mixing period (t_{mix}) they carry with them a population disturbance proportional to $M\cos\phi$. The third 90° pulse converts this into a new signal at site S. Consequently, as t_1 is incremented, the sequence of signals detected during the acquisition period is modulated by this changing population disturbance. A spin that started life precessing at the frequency of the I site finishes at the frequency of the S site and contributes to a cross-peak in the two-dimensional spectrum at coordinates (f_I, f_S). Transfer of spins in the opposite direction (from S to I) gives rise to a second symmetrically related cross-peak at coordinates (f_S, f_I).

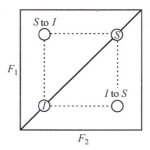

For a molecule with many different chemically-distinct sites, two-dimensional EXSY spectrum may display several such cross-peaks, and their relative intensities reflect the corresponding rates of the various chemical exchange processes.

Only slow exchange generates cross-peaks in a two-dimensional spectrum, but for the sake of completeness we also examine here the 'fast exchange' regime (§ 7.8) where the exchange rate is much faster than the chemical shift difference Δ. Our chosen nuclear spin precesses through a small angle at a rate appropriate to site A then quickly hops to site B and precesses through another small angle at the new rate before hopping back again, and so on. The overall result is a slightly jerky precession at the arithmetic mean frequency of sites A and B, assuming that there are equal numbers of A and B sites. If there are more A sites, they make a proportionately larger contribution to the precession frequency—the observed mean resonance frequency is weighted according to the populations at the two sites. As the exchange rate gets faster, the precession angle between jumps gets smaller and smaller, the motion appears smoother and the observed resonance line gets narrower.

Fast chemical exchange is responsible for the remarkable chemical shift variations that are observed when hydrogen-bonding occurs (§ 7.9). The relative populations of hydrogen-bonded and 'free' sites are very sensitive to temperature or concentration, so the NMR signal from an OH group may appear anywhere within a chemical shift range spanning several parts per million as the relative populations of the two sites are changed. Such extreme variability in a chemical shift is almost always evidence for hydrogen bonding.

The chemical exchange phenomenon has proved very useful in MRS (Chapter 14) where NMR signals from metabolites are monitored *in vivo*. One early example makes use of the observed change in the chemical shift of the phosphorus-31 resonance from inorganic phosphate as a function of the acidity of the solution. A dynamic equilibrium is established where there is fast exchange between $H_2PO_4^-$ and $HPO_4^{2-} + H^+$. The phosphorus resonance response appears at the weighted mean frequency and the equilibrium is disturbed by the addition of hydrogen ions (H^+). Thus the phosphorus-31 chemical shift is a measure of the acidity of the solution. Lactic acid is the most probable source of H^+ in this situation. In one famous early metabolic study[4] of McArdle's syndrome, a glycogen phosphorylase deficiency, the patient's muscles became slightly alkaline during exercise whereas they would normally have accumulated lactic acid. This was taken as an indication of a pathological inability to convert glycogen into lactic acid in this patient whose illness had previously defied diagnosis.

11.4 Cross-relaxation (NOESY)

If the spin–lattice relaxation of a given nuclear site is affected by the dipole–dipole interaction with adjacent nuclear spins, then any disturbance of the populations of the latter gives rise to a change in the NMR intensity at the first site. This 'cross-relaxation' experiment (§ 4.3) is usually known as the 'nuclear Overhauser effect'[5] and its magnitude depends on the proximity of the two sites. For small molecules that change their orientation relatively fast in the liquid phase the effect is an enhancement of the observed intensity; for macromolecules that are too large to tumble sufficiently rapidly, the result is a decrease in intensity. The critical reorientation rate is determined by the nuclear Larmor frequency, so it is a function of the intensity of the field of the magnet.

The two-dimensional version of this cross-relaxation experiment follows the recipe outlined above for slow chemical exchange. The mechanism for this nuclear Overhauser spectroscopy (NOESY) is quite analogous to EXSY, involving the transfer of spin population between interacting sites during the mixing period, followed by detection of the corresponding pair of cross-peaks. Where necessary, the rate of build-up of the Overhauser effect can be measured by performing a sequence of experiments at different settings of the mixing time.

The intensity (or rate of build-up) of a NOESY cross-peak indicates how close the two nuclear spins are in space. The magnetic dipole–dipole interaction decreases as the *cube* of the internuclear distance, while the cross-relaxation effect falls off as the *sixth power* of the distance. This is a very steep fall-off indeed, and makes it possible to take some important shortcuts in the interpretation of cross-peak intensities. Indeed, many investigators rely solely on the presence or (apparent) absence of a cross-peak, arguing that an observed cross-peak establishes that the two protons in question must lie within a distance of not much more than half a nanometer (five Ångstrom units). This simple proximity test is usually referred to as a 'distance constraint' and used to supplement molecular dynamics calculations. This rather cavalier use of the experimental data is justified by the fact that there are normally so many cross-peaks in the NOESY spectrum from a protein system that the geometrical problem is considerably overdetermined.

The two-dimensional NOESY experiment has proved to be a powerful tool for determining the way in which a protein chain folds back upon itself; when a cross-peak *is* observed, the two protons *must* be in reasonably close proximity. Care must be exercised with molecules whose rate of tumbling in the liquid phase is neither 'fast' nor 'slow' but in fact close to the nuclear Larmor frequency, for then the Overhauser effect may be near zero. Fortunately, there is an elaboration of the experiment ('ROESY') which ensures that the Overhauser effect is not masked in this manner, whatever the rate of molecular tumbling. The remarkable success of high-resolution NMR applied to biochemistry owes a great deal to the widespread application of two-dimensional nuclear Overhauser spectroscopy of protons.

11.5 Correlation spectroscopy (COSY)

In the sections above we have adopted a rather broad definition of the term 'correlation'. The experiment we now examine was initially known as chemical shift correlation but is now universally known simply as correlation spectroscopy (COSY). The COSY acronym is normally restricted to homonuclear systems, usually protons, while the equivalent heteronuclear correlation experiment is now generally known as 'heteronuclear single-quantum correlation (HSQC)' as we shall see later in § 11.7. Those of us who generally discourage the use of acronyms are nevertheless forced to admit that the terms EXSY, NOESY, COSY and HSQC serve as a convenient shorthand to distinguish these widely-used two-dimensional experiments. In this context correlation may be taken to mean 'identify responses from two different nuclear sites that are connected by spin–spin coupling'. Since spin–spin couplings are relatively short-range, this is a powerful method of testing for proximity of nuclei, particularly in large molecules. We shall see later that small coupling constants generate only weak cross-peaks in correlation spectra.

A two-dimensional COSY spectrum represents NMR intensities as a function of the two frequency axes F_1 and F_2, both spanning the entire range of chemical shifts (in the case of proton systems about 10 parts per million). The diagonal peaks are all centered on the principal diagonal $F_1 = F_2$ at frequencies determined by the appropriate chemical shifts. They merely provide the same information as the conventional (one-dimensional) proton spectrum. Spin–spin coupling gives rise to the cross-peaks, and these are the important diagnostic feature. Cross-peaks occur in symmetrical pairs—one above and to the left of the principal diagonal, the other at the mirror-image position, below right. Spin coupling between a site I and a site S generates cross-peaks centered at coordinates (δ_I, δ_S) and at (δ_S, δ_I) where δ_I and δ_S are the chemical shifts.[6]

Our task is to explain the mechanism behind the formation of cross-peaks in a two-dimensional COSY spectrum. If we simply describe it as 'coherence transfer' we are merely stating the result, without any real appreciation of the mechanism. Formal mathematical treatments in terms of the density matrix or product operators give little insight into the physical behaviour of the nuclear spins. The simplest visualization invokes the concept of a transient population disturbance on the energy levels shared by the coupled spins. We consider the simplest possible case of a spectrum from two weakly-coupled spins I and S, with chemical shifts δ_I and δ_S and a coupling constant J_{HH}. The conventional spectrum consists of four lines with frequencies (in Hz):

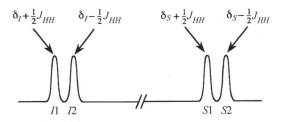

These lines can be labelled $I1$, $I2$, etc., according to the topology of the energy-level diagram shown above (§ 11.1). The pulse sequence for COSY experiments is deceptively simple,

$$90° — t_1 — 90° \text{ acquisition } (t_2)$$

Consider the mechanism that gives rise to transfer from I to S, arguing that the reverse process can be deduced by symmetry considerations. The first 90° pulse excites nuclear magnetization from both $I1$ and $I2$, represented by two separate vectors of length M. They precess at their respective frequencies and accumulate phase angles ϕ and ψ at the end of the evolution period t_1. These angles depend on the length of the evolution period, being defined by

$$\phi = 2\pi(\delta_I + \frac{1}{2} J_{HH})t_1 \quad \psi = 2\pi(\delta_I - \frac{1}{2} J_{HH})t_1$$

Initially we follow the fate of the $I1$ and $I2$ vectors separately. After free precession for a time t_1 they can be resolved into components along the $+X$ and $+Y$ axes:

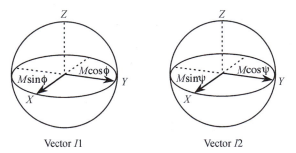

The second 90° pulse can be considered to be a cascade of two selective 90° pulses, one applied at the I site and the other at the S site, essentially simultaneously. The former pulse rotates the $M\cos\phi$ component into the $-Z$ axis. Now a vector M aligned along the $+Z$ axis represents spin populations at equilibrium, while a vector M directed along $-Z$ corresponds to a population inversion. Consequently, the vector $M\cos\phi$ along $-Z$ represents a *partial* population inversion. (We shall return later to the other component $M\sin\phi$ which was not affected by the second radiofrequency pulse.) These population disturbances affect energy levels 1 and 2.

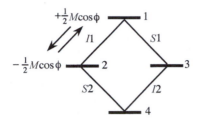

Energy level 1 gains some nuclear spins at the expense of energy level 2. Because the two S transitions share these levels, after excitation by the second selective 90° pulse we observe a *loss* of intensity $+\frac{1}{2} M(\cos\phi)$ for line $S1$ and an equal *gain* in intensity for line $S2$. As the evolution time t_1 is incremented, these intensity changes are modulated at a frequency $(\delta_I + \frac{1}{2} J_{HH})$ Hz. Fourier transformation as a function of t_1 locates this response in the F_1 dimension. Consequently, we observe a 'down-up' pattern of two lines at frequencies $S1$ and $S2$ in the F_2 dimension, on a trace at the frequency of $I1$ in the F_1 dimension.

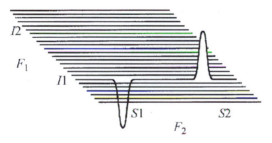

Now consider the fate of the other vector that precessed at the frequency of line $I2$ during the evolution period, accumulating a phase angle ψ different from ϕ. The selective 90° pulse converts the component $M\cos\psi$ into a partial population inversion between energy levels 3 and 4 which are also shared by the two S-spin lines.

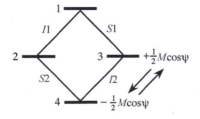

Consequently there is an increase in intensity of S1, as additional spins are added to level 3, and an equal loss in intensity of S2, as spins are removed from level 4. These intensity changes are modulated at the precession frequency $(\delta_I - \frac{1}{2} J_{HH})$ during the evolution period. We observe an up–down pattern at the frequencies S1 and S2 in the F_2 frequency dimension, on a trace at the frequency of $I2$ in the F_1 dimension.

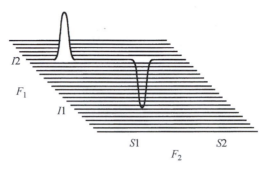

Combination of these two separate results creates a COSY cross-peak in the form of a square of side J_{HH}, consisting of four absorption lines alternating in intensity in both frequency dimensions.

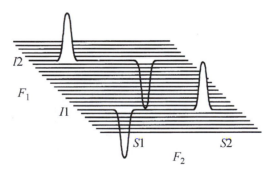

This is the same pattern that was obtained in the double resonance experiment outlined in § 11.1, sometimes called *pseudo*-COSY. An analogous argument accounts for population transfer from S to I, which gives rise to a similar cross-peak on the other side of the principal diagonal. The details are easily worked out by substituting I for S and S for I in the description above.

Because of the 'up–down' pattern of intensities within a cross-peak, if J_{HH} is small compared with the linewidth, adjacent positive and negative lines approach one another and mutually interfere. Consequently, coupling constants significantly smaller than the linewidth give vanishingly weak cross-peaks. This is why the COSY technique is a good indicator of proximity of the nuclear spins involved; only resolvable couplings give strong cross-peaks. Most two-dimensional spectra record the cross-peak in the form of a contour diagram:

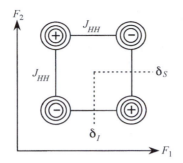

Not all the available magnetization appears as cross-peaks. Recall that at the end of the evolution period, magnetization components $M\sin\phi$ and $M\sin\psi$ remained along the $+X$ axis. These are quite unaffected by the second 90° pulse and continue to precess at the same frequencies during the evolution and acquisition periods, giving rise to a diagonal response centered on the line $F_1 = F_2$. The coupling to S splits each I line into a doublet so the final result is again a square pattern of side J_{HH}, but because the magnetization vectors lie along the X axis rather than the Y axis of the rotating reference frame, all four lines appear in the 'dispersion mode'. A simulation of the complete two-dimensional COSY spectrum for this simple two-spin case is shown in Figure 11.1

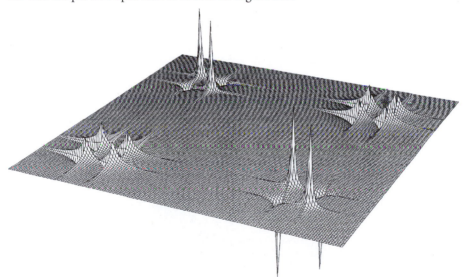

Figure 11.1 Simulation of a two-dimensional correlation (COSY) spectrum for a system of two coupled protons. The spin–spin coupling splits each group into four responses in a square pattern. Two such groups lie along the principal diagonal running from the lower left to upper right; these responses are in the dispersion mode in both frequency dimensions. The remaining two groups, called 'cross-peaks', lie off the principal diagonal and consist of four absorption mode responses with alternating intensities. (Simulation courtesy of Michael Woodley.)

A coupled two-spin system is of course the simplest possible case. In general, the diagonal and cross-peaks of a COSY spectrum have a more complicated multiplet structure because the I and S nuclei are also coupled to other sites. However, we may designate these as 'passive spins' for they are not involved in the transfer between sites I and S but merely introduce additional splittings on the basic square patterns described above. A passive spin P coupled to both I and S, with the magnitudes of the coupling constants in the order J_{IP}, J_{SP}, J_{IS} would generate a cross-peak pattern of the form:

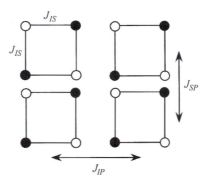

These passive splittings always generate lines of the same phase, so they are easily distinguished from the 'up-down' patterns characteristic of the two active spins. Figure 11.2 illustrates a typical COSY cross-peak from one of the protons in nicotine[7] where there is a large active splitting and three smaller passive splittings.

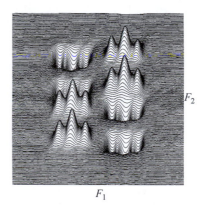

Figure 11.2 A typical experimental COSY cross-peak representing coherence transfer between two protons in nicotine. The 'up-down' features in both frequency dimensions arise from the 'active' coupling of 7.9 Hz which is responsible for the coherence transfer. A 'passive' coupling of 4.8 Hz splits the response again in the F_2 frequency dimension, and passive couplings of 2.2 and 1.7 Hz introduce additional splittings in the F_1 dimension. (Reproduced from F. Del Rio-Portilla and R. Freeman, *J. Magn. Reson.* A **108**, 124 (1994) with the permission of Academic Press.)

A typical COSY spectrum has a string of responses along the principal diagonal, one for each chemically distinct site in the molecule. Figure 11.3 shows part
of the 800 MHz COSY spectrum of the antibiotic erythromycin A. This is a
contour map where the positive peaks are represented by open contours while
negative contours are filled (black). It was recorded using a very popular modification of the conventional COSY sequence, called 'DQ-COSY' where the signals
are filtered through double-quantum coherence (§ 11.9). This has two advantages—it displays the diagonal peaks in absorption rather than dispersion, which
makes it easier to detect cross-peaks close to the diagonal, and it eliminates the

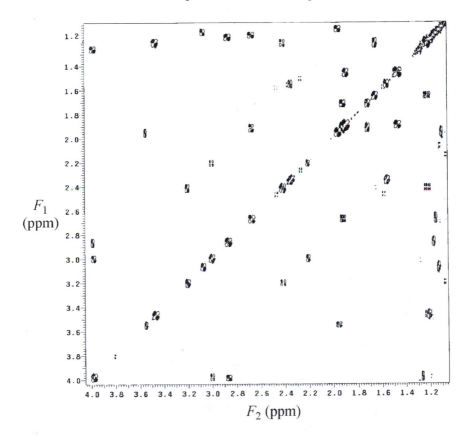

F_1 (ppm)

F_2 (ppm)

Figure 11.3 Part of the 800 MHz COSY spectrum of protons in erythromycin A recorded with
double-quantum filtration so that the peaks lying along the principal diagonal $F_1 = F_2$ appear in
the absorption mode. These diagonal peaks indicate the proton chemical shifts. Cross-peaks
appear in pairs, symmetrically-related with respect to the principal diagonal; each pair indicates a
coupling between the appropriate proton sites. Both diagonal and cross-peaks show the characteristic square pattern with alternating intensities (open and filled contours). Additional splittings due
to passive couplings are discernible on some cross-peaks, for example, at $F_1 = 2.7$ ppm, $F_2 =$
1.9 ppm. (Spectrum courtesy of Toshiaki Nishida.)

undesirable responses from isolated protons, in particular solvent peaks. Note the distinctive 'up–down–down–up' square patterns from both diagonal and cross-peaks in this two-dimensional spectrum. On a few cross-peaks the additional splittings by passive couplings can be clearly resolved. Each pair of symmetrically-related cross-peaks establishes that two protons are correlated—they have a resolvable spin–spin coupling. This is a powerful aid to the assignment of the experimental high-resolution spectrum.

11.6 Hartmann-Hahn experiments

Two-dimensional COSY spectra only involve a single-step transfer, for example from I to S or from S to I, but there is a useful variant of this technique that invokes a different correlation mechanism. In § 1.4 we likened the nuclear spins within a molecule to spies, each transmitting information about the chemical environment in the form of a characteristic frequency. Because they lack a common frequency, spies at different locations within the molecule cannot communicate among themselves unless some new form of contact can be devised. The Hartmann–Hahn experiment[8] achieves this by forcing two coupled spins (I and S) to rotate at identical frequencies in a *radiofrequency* field so intense that the difference in chemical shifts is irrelevant. This provides the common communication channel between the two 'spies'. In a sense, they behave like two coupled pendulums, exchanging energy back and forth in a cyclic manner. In the Hartmann–Hahn scheme, the transverse precessing magnetization components from I and S are prepared in opposition and the difference magnetization oscillates back and forth between the two sites. Figure 11.4 shows the time development of the Hartmann–Hahn interchange between the two proton sites of the molecule of uracil.

By choosing a suitable value for the mixing period we can achieve maximum transfer from one site to its neighbour. In contrast to the COSY technique, this transferred magnetization can move on to further, more distant sites in the same coupling network. For this reason the technique has been called TOCSY (total correlation spectroscopy)[9] or alternatively the HOHAHA (homonuclear Hart-mann–Hahn) experiment. The resulting cross-peaks have all component lines in the same sense, in contrast to the alternating-intensity pattern characteristic of cross-peaks in COSY spectra. Two-dimensional TOCSY spectra correlate all the nuclear spins in the same coupling network, but the available intensity is 'diluted' by being spread over many different sites.

Figure 11.5 shows the TOCSY spectrum of erythromycin A covering the same frequency region as the COSY spectrum shown in Figure 11.3. All cross-peaks have the same sign, reflecting the fact that there is net transfer of magnetization in a TOCSY experiment, in contrast to the differential transfer observed in a COSY spectrum. Although this avoids the mutual cancellation between compon-ents of a COSY cross-peak when the couplings are small, TOCSY cross-peaks only

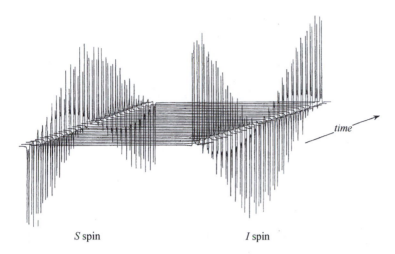

time

S spin   *I* spin

Figure 11.4 Spectra recorded at 10 millisecond intervals showing the cyclic interchange of magnetization between two coupled protons (*I* and *S*) of uracil during a Hartmann–Hahn experiment. The response of proton *S* is initially inverted (front trace). As the contact time is progressively increased, inverted magnetization migrates from site *S* to site *I*, leaving the *I* signal inverted and the *S* signal upright after 140 milliseconds (middle trace). The cycle then continues until the *S* response is again inverted and the *I* response is upright after 280 milliseconds (final trace). (Reproduced from E. Kupče and R. Freeman, *J.Magn.Reson.* A. **105**, 234 (1993) with the permission of Academic Press.)

build up at a rate determined by the appropriate coupling constant, so small couplings give relatively weak responses. Note the significantly increased number of cross-peaks as magnetization is transferred between all protons in the molecule, not merely those that are directly coupled.

11.7 Heteronuclear correlation

Correlation experiments can be performed between two different nuclear species, for example protons and an '*X* nucleus' where *X* might be carbon-13, or nitrogen-15. The basic mechanism for correlation is the same as in the COSY experiment, involving the creation of a differential population disturbance on the shared energy levels, but the symmetry of the problem is changed. As a result, magnetization transfer is unidirectional, $H \rightarrow X$ or $X \rightarrow H$. Another difference is the ability to decouple the spin–spin splittings in both frequency dimensions, thus collecting all the intensity of a cross-peak into a single resonance line, further simplifying the two-dimensional correlation spectrum.

If the transfer is in the direction $H \rightarrow X$, the sensitivity benefits from the high spin populations of protons, whereas transfer in the opposite direction $X \rightarrow H$ sacrifices this population advantage but exploits the intrinsically higher detection

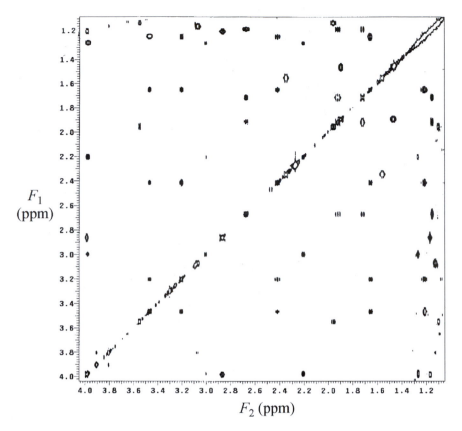

Figure 11.5 The 800 MHz two-dimensional total correlation (TOCSY) spectrum of erythromycin *A* recorded over the same frequency range as the COSY spectrum shown in Figure 11.3. All peaks are positive because this Hartmann–Hahn experiment causes net transfer of magnetization. Note the additional cross-peaks over and above those observed in the corresponding COSY spectrum, as magnetization is transferred throughout the molecule, not merely through direct couplings. (Spectrum courtesy of Toshiaki Nishida.)

sensitivity of proton NMR. The best techniques take advantage of both properties of the proton by performing a 'round-trip' transfer $H \rightarrow X$, followed by free precession at the X frequency to measure the chemical shift, and then a return transfer $X \rightarrow H$. For the case that X is carbon-13 the round-trip experiment is:

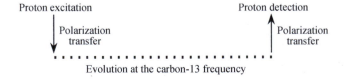

These are known as 'heteronuclear single-quantum correlation (HSQC)' experiments. The reason for the emphasis on 'single-quantum' will become evident in § 11.9.

If the X nucleus is present only in natural abundance (1.1 % for carbon-13 and 0.37 % for nitrogen-15) it becomes necessary to suppress the strong proton signals from the far more abundant molecules containing the non-magnetic carbon-12 or nitrogen-14 nuclei. Polarization transfer in the 'inverse' direction ($X \rightarrow H$) is executed in a difference mode so as to restrict the observed response to the transferred signal, cancelling the undesirable 'natural' signals at the proton sites.

Studies of biological macromolecules often employ samples labelled at specific sites with carbon-13 and nitrogen-15 nuclei. Not only does this improve sensitivity, but it also greatly simplifies the proton NMR spectra by restricting the observed responses to the chosen regions of the macromolecule. Alternatively, the isotopic enrichment may be global, the proton 'subspectra' being separated according to the chemical shift of the X nucleus. It is also feasible to perform round-trip transfers that involve paths via carbon-13 and nitrogen-15 at the same time, eliciting information about both these X nuclei simultaneously.

We see that all these two-dimensional correlation experiments are closely related, and follow the same general format. There is an initial evolution period, incremented in small time steps, which serves to encode the various nuclear precession frequencies. Then there is a fixed mixing period (measured in milliseconds) during which some form of population disturbance builds up. The mixing period may be negligible for COSY and HSQC experiments. Finally there is an acquisition period to allow the various NMR signals to be detected. The useful information is obtained from 'correlated' signals—those that originate at one chemical site but pass on information to spins at a different site, giving rise to cross-peaks in the two-dimensional spectrum. This act of 'passing the baton' may involve chemical exchange, cross-relaxation or spin–spin coupling. In this last case (COSY), the spin populations are disturbed in a differential manner, giving rise to a characteristic 'up–down' pattern in the cross-peaks. Mixing by this mechanism is achieved solely by radiofrequency pulses and is complete within a few microseconds.

The extension to three frequency dimensions is straightforward. We merely follow the relay race through a second baton change into the third stage. As an example, it is often quite useful to combine a COSY experiment with NOESY measurements to obtain both connectivity and proximity information in one fell swoop. We relabel the acquisition period t_3, and precede it with evolution periods t_1 and t_2, both of which are incremented independently in small steps.

Evolution (t_1) · · · · · · · · · | Mix | Evolution (t_2) · · · · · · · · · | Mix | Acquisition (t_3)

The result is a three-dimensional data array in the time domain, transforming into a three-dimensional spectrum in the frequency domain. The only real complications are the prolonged data gathering duration, the increased processing time, and the problem of devising a suitable three-dimensional display that allows frequencies to be accurately measured. The generally accepted solution to the display problem is to extract appropriate planes from the three-dimensional spectrum; then the familiar two-dimensional contour plots can be employed.

Three-dimensional Fourier transform experiments are also used in MRI, representing one of the standard ways to encode information about the three spatial dimensions (§ 12.8). Continuity between the three time dimensions is guaranteed—the precessing magnetization from a given voxel during t_1 simply changes its frequency during t_2 as a new gradient is applied along another axis, and changes it again during t_3 as a fresh gradient is imposed along a third axis. There are no mixing periods in this experiment; the linking intervals are just long enough to permit gradient switching and the decay of any induced eddy currents. Once again the key piece of information that is 'handed over' at the instant between the first and second evolution periods (or between the second evolution period and acquisition) is the phase angle accumulated through precession in the appropriate magnetic field gradient. This experiment 'correlates' distances along the x, y and z axes. Provided that motional effects are small enough to be neglected, there is no interference between signals from different voxels. No bumping or barging takes place in this particular relay race.

11.8 Polarization transfer (INEPT)

The polarization transfer stage mentioned in the previous section has acquired an importance in its own right. Termed 'insensitive nuclei enhanced by polarization transfer (INEPT)', this spin-off from the two-dimensional correlation experiment[10] is used as a building block for the construction of more elaborate schemes. The sequence of manipulations may be written:

$$\text{Protons: } 90°(X) - \tau - 180°(X) - \tau - 90°(Y)$$

$$\text{Carbon-13: } \underline{\hspace{2cm}} 180° \underline{\hspace{2cm}} 90° \text{ acquisition}$$

where the interval τ is chosen to be equal to $1/(4J)$ if we are dealing with a CH group. The corresponding vector diagram is set out in Figure 11.6. We label the two proton magnetization vectors α and β, reflecting the two possible spin states of carbon-13. In this scheme the 'evolution time' is no longer a variable but has a fixed value 2τ. Free precession for a period τ leaves the vectors α and β at right angles. At time τ a 180° radiofrequency pulse is applied, which refocuses the proton chemical shift at time 2τ. Simultaneously another 180° pulse is applied to the X-nucleus,

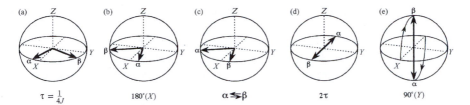

Figure 11.6 Vector diagram outlining the INEPT sequence for transferring polarization from protons to carbon-13. (a) Transverse proton magnetization precesses for a period $\tau = 1/(4J_{CH})$ as a result of chemical shift and spin–spin coupling, evolving into two component vectors, α and β, at right angles. (b) A proton radiofrequency pulse rotates these vectors through 180° about the $+X$ axis. (c) A 180° pulse applied at the carbon-13 frequency inverts the carbon-13 spin states, thus interchanging the α and β labels. (d) Free precession for a further period $\tau = 1/(4J_{CH})$ carries these vectors to the $\pm X$ axes. (e) A proton radiofrequency pulse rotates these vectors through 90° about the $+Y$ axis. This corresponds to equilibrium proton magnetization for one component (β) but a population inversion for the other (α). This population disturbance on the common energy levels enhances the carbon-13 responses in an up–down pattern.

which has the effect of interchanging the spin state labels α and β, ensuring that the spin–spin coupling continues to evolve (as in the spin echo modulation experiment described in § 9.7). After a further period of free precession τ, the two proton vectors reach the diametrically opposed condition, aligned along the $\pm X$ axes. Normally in the COSY scheme these would be the 'unused' magnetization components, but the next 90° proton pulse is applied about the $+Y$ axis (instead of the $+X$ axis) rotating the two vectors α and β into the $\pm Z$ axes. The vector α along the $-Z$ axis represents spin inversion and creates the maximum possible population disturbance on the shared energy levels, whereas the vector β along the $+Z$ axis corresponds to equilibrium and has no effect. Representing the populations schematically and allowing for the fact that proton frequencies are four times higher than carbon-13 frequencies, so that the relative intensities are also in the ratio 4:1, we have:

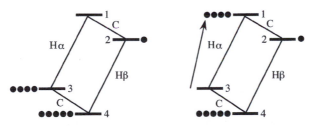

Equilibrium populations   Population disturbance

There is an enhanced effect on the carbon-13 lines that share these energy levels. When the final 90° pulse excites a carbon-13 response, one line is enhanced five-fold while the other increases threefold but is inverted. The *changes* in carbon-13 intensities are therefore four times as intense as the natural carbon-13 signals, with a characteristic 'up–down' pattern. This provides a welcome theoretical sensitivity advantage (fourfold for carbon-13 and tenfold for nitrogen-15).

A demonstration of the practical signal-to-noise improvement achieved by the INEPT technique is shown for the 125 MHz high-resolution carbon-13 spectra of pyridine in Figure 11.7. Two spectra are compared, both acquired with the same number of transients (128). The first is the 'conventional' proton-coupled spectrum with no enhancement, and it required 104 minutes of signal accumulation. The second is the INEPT spectrum which required only 46 minutes to collect the same number of transients. This is because the repetition rate of INEPT is governed only by proton relaxation, and the spin–lattice relaxation times of the protons ($T_1 = 6$ seconds) are shorter than those of carbon-13 ($T_1 = 14$ seconds). The INEPT spectrum shows the characteristic 'up–down' patterns, with a threefold intensity enhancement compared with the conventional spectrum. Although the respective spin population differences would suggest a theoretical improvement of a factor of four, the actual factor is smaller because the different CH couplings make it impossible to employ the optimum timing for all three sites in the INEPT sequence. However, the faster signal accumulation in the INEPT version corresponds to an additional sensitivity advantage of 1.5 (the square root of 104/46) so in this case INEPT offers an advantage of 4.5.

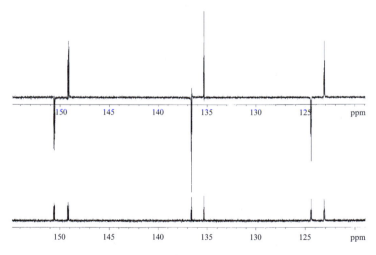

Figure 11.7 Enhancement of the natural-abundance proton-coupled carbon-13 spectrum of pyridine by the INEPT technique. The same number of scans was employed for the conventional spectrum (bottom) and the INEPT spectrum (top) but because spin–lattice relaxation of the protons was more than twice as fast as that of carbon-13, the INEPT measurements were completed in less than half the time. This advantage is in addition to the enhancement generated by the population effect, offering an overall improvement ratio of 4.5. (Spectra courtesy of Toshiaki Nishida.)

The timing required for optimum polarization transfer by the INEPT technique depends on the number of protons attached to the low-abundance species (for example, carbon-13). It can therefore distinguish between CH, CH_2 and CH_3 groups, and incidentally identify the remaining quaternary carbon sites because they exhibit negligible polarization transfer. There are now more refined techniques that perform this function more effectively. These form part of a family of experiments known as 'spectral editing' where the four different kinds of subspectra are identified according to the 'multiplicity' of the sites under investigation. This makes it unnecessary to record and analyse the spin-coupled version of the carbon-13 spectrum.

11.9 Multiple-quantum spectroscopy

Two-dimensional spectroscopy has other important applications not yet touched upon—schemes that do not fall neatly into the category of *correlation* experiments. Instead they exploit the evolution period by using it to monitor NMR processes that are not directly detectable in the spectrometer. The time-development of these 'invisible' magnetic resonance phenomena can be deduced by noting how they influence the phase of the signals observed during the normal acquisition period. This 'indirect detection' mode opens up some interesting applications.

Quantum mechanics implies the existence of fixed energy levels in atoms and molecules, and spectroscopy examines the transitions between these levels. This is why we observe a set of discrete sharp absorption lines in a spectrum rather than a continuum of frequencies. But not all possible transitions are 'allowed'; there are always some that are 'forbidden'. Spectroscopists formalize this in terms of 'selection rules' that govern which responses are normally observed in a given spectrum. For NMR, the selection rule states that the magnetic quantum number (m) can only change by one unit ($\Delta m = \pm 1$).

However, under certain conditions it is possible to violate the selection rules and make formally forbidden transitions observable. For example, in a coupled two-spin system (*IS*) where the coupling constant J_{IS} is comparable with the chemical shift difference δ_{IS}, the double-quantum transition ($\Delta m = +2$) can be observed if we significantly increase the radiofrequency power in a continuous-wave frequency-sweep experiment. A forbidden transition that is driven very hard becomes allowed. In this case it involves simultaneous flips of the I and S spins in the same sense. However, the corresponding zero-quantum transition ($\Delta m = 0$), where I and S flip in opposite senses, is not observable by this technique.

For want of a better name, we call these strange new entities multiple-quantum 'coherences'. They can be thought of as pairs of vectors locked into a configuration where they oppose or reinforce one another:

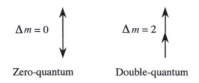

Zero-quantum   Double-quantum

This picture suggests that zero-quantum coherence would not induce a voltage in the receiver coil, but that, in certain circumstances, a response from double-quantum coherence might be detectable.

In two-dimensional spectroscopy a given multiple-quantum coherence is allowed to evolve during t_1, and then converted into an observable magnetization component detected during t_2 in the normal fashion. At the instant of conversion it 'passes on the baton' in the form of the accumulated precession phase. As t_1 is incremented, the time-development of this phase angle provides the information about the multiple-quantum frequency.

Consider the four energy levels appropriate to a weakly-coupled two-spin system (IS). Suppose that the S-spin doublet has been excited; creating precessing nuclear magnetization from states 1 and 3, and from states 2 and 4 (represented by wavy lines on the diagram). Now apply a frequency-selective 180° radiofrequency pulse that only affects one of the I-spin transitions, 1–2.

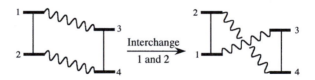

Single-quantum coherence   Zero- and double-quantum coherence

By interchanging these states, the 180° pulse creates zero-quantum coherence (between levels 1 and 3) and double-quantum coherence (between levels 2 and 4). These invisible coherences are allowed to evolve with time at their characteristic frequencies, $(\delta_I - \delta_S)$ and $(\delta_I + \delta_S)$, and are then reconverted into single-quantum coherence for detection. Note that these frequencies depend only on chemical shifts; spin–spin splittings are not involved. This is only one of several schemes for exciting multiple-quantum coherence.

By extension, a system of N-coupled spins can sustain N-quantum coherence. But because spin flips can be opposed in pairs, there can also be coherences of the order N-2, N-4, etc. Thus we can have five-spin three-quantum coherence, represented by four flips in one sense and one in the other:

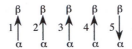

Five-spin triple-quantum coherence

When we examine the format of the HSQC round-trip polarization transfer scheme described in § 11.7, it is clear that at no time is the X response observed directly, it merely precesses during an evolution interval and then determines the initial phase of the final proton response. So it could just as well evolve in the form of multiple quantum coherence (MQC).

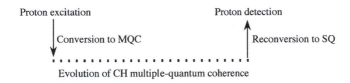

Evolution of CH multiple-quantum coherence

In this version the technique is called 'heteronuclear multiple quantum correl-ation 'HMQC)' and that is why the competing HSQC method emphasizes 'single quantum coherence'.

11.10 Molecular topology (INADEQUATE)

Multiple-quantum coherences have some unique properties that can be used to distinguish them from the familiar 'single-quantum' precessing magnetization that gives rise to conventional NMR responses. For example, N-quantum coherence is N times more sensitive to magnet inhomogeneity, applied field gradients, or radiofrequency phase shifts. This is what we might expect from the vector picture if these perturbations acted separately on each individual vector. Consequently, if we use two-dimensional spectroscopy to derive a zero-quantum spectrum from a system of coupled protons, it is virtually impervious to the inhomogeneity of the magnetic field. In principle, the resulting NMR responses exhibit natural line widths, determined by the spin–spin relaxation time. This remarkable compen-sation of the field inhomogeneity is only complete in homonuclear systems. For example, there is only partial compensation in the zero-quantum spectra involv-ing protons and carbon-13 because (in frequency units) the proton is four times more sensitive to magnetic fields.

These special properties have been exploited in several different ways. One interesting example is the experiment known as INADEQUATE (incredible nat-ural abundance double-quantum transfer experiment). Because carbon-13 is only

1% abundant in nature, the proportion of molecules having two particular carbon-13 spins directly adjacent is only about one in 10,000. Yet, it would be very useful to have spectra from just these coupled systems, rejecting the much more intense responses from singly-labelled molecules on the grounds that they cannot sustain C–C double-quantum coherence. By exciting carbon-13 double-quantum coherences and using their characteristic twofold sensitivity to radio-frequency phase shifts or applied magnetic field gradients, this very demanding filtration process can be achieved, and the resulting two-dimensional spectra give direct information about the connectivity of the carbon skeleton of an organic molecule. Each isolated pair of coupled carbon-13 nuclei gives rise to a four-line 'sub-spectrum' running in the F_2 frequency dimension, indicating that these two carbon atoms (I and S) are directly connected by a chemical bond.

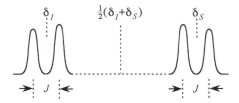

This subspectrum is completely independent of the others because, owing to the low isotopic abundance, each coupled carbon pair is isolated from all the rest by being in a different molecule. The subspectra are separated in the F_1 dimension according to their respective double-quantum frequencies $\delta_I + \delta_S$. Since the 'centre of gravity' of each four-line subspectrum lies at a frequency $\frac{1}{2}(\delta_I + \delta_S)$ in the F_2 dimension, and its F_1 ordinate is $\delta_I + \delta_S$, all the various subspectra are centred on the skew diagonal $F_1 = 2F_2$. This geometrical constraint helps in the identification of the responses when the signal-to-noise ratio is poor.

In this manner the INADEQUATE technique builds up the carbon connectivity one link at a time, the topology of the spectrum reflecting the topology of the carbon framework of the molecule. For example, an unbranched chain of carbon atoms might have an INADEQUATE spectrum like this:

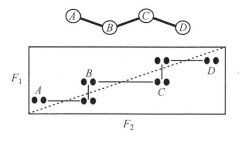

This is quite distinct from the corresponding spectrum from a branched chain:

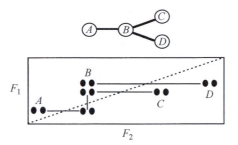

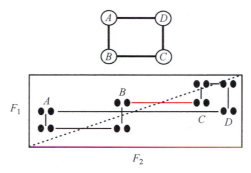

Ring formation has its own distinctive topology:

We can follow a chain of directly-bound carbon atoms until it terminates, or until a nitrogen or oxygen atom intervenes. This is a powerful and unambiguous structural tool.

Figure 11.8 is an illustration of the application of the INADEQUATE technique to the 50 MHz natural-abundance carbon-13 spectrum of a natural product, the *Ormosia* alkaloid panamine. Standard qualitative analysis indicates that the molecule contains three nitrogen atoms.

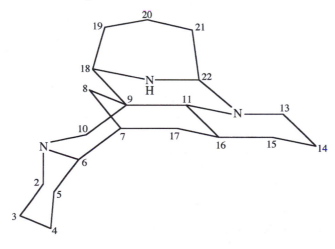

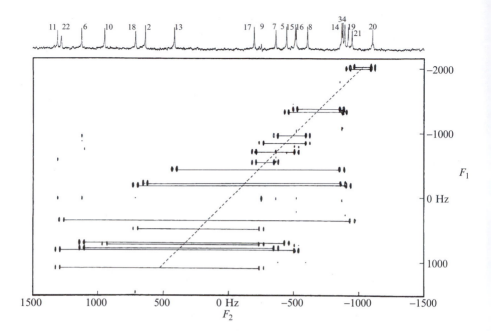

Figure 11.8 The 50 MHz carbon-13 INADEQUATE spectrum of panamine with the conventional spectrum running along the top margin. The response from the quaternary C-9 is very weak due to partial saturation attributable to slow spin–lattice relaxation. The characteristic four-line subspectra have been emphasised by the horizontal lines; each subspectrum establishes a direct connection between two carbon atoms. The subspectra are separated in the F_1 dimension according to the appropriate double-quantum frequencies, which means that the midpoints all fall on the dashed line $F_1 = 2F_2$. (Reproduced from T. H. Mareci and R. Freeman, *J. Magn. Reson.* **48**, 158 (1982) with the permission of Academic Press.)

The INADEQUATE spectrum[11] is made up of a series of four-line subspectra running in the horizontal (F_2) dimension, stacked one above the other according to the respective double-quantum frequencies in the F_1 dimension. The midpoint of each subspectrum lies on the dashed diagonal representing $F_1 = 2F_2$. Each of these four-line spectra indicates a direct correlation through a C–C bond, allowing us to assemble the carbon atoms into chains just like beads on a string. Because the chains are broken when there is an intervening nitrogen atom, the INADEQUATE results yield only a set of disconnected fragments of the overall molecular structure. However, the 'loose ends' are readily identified because the carbon atoms directly attached to nitrogen give rise to group of seven resonances with particularly low chemical shielding values, well separated from the rest. It is then a question of fitting the fragments together (using imaginary nitrogen links) to form a plausible whole. The connectivity information coupled with the assumption that all the rings are six-membered, allows the molecular skeleton (shown above) to be determined.

In MRS (Chapter 14) analogous multiple-quantum filtration experiments have proved their worth for extracting the NMR response of a desired compound that exists in a thick 'soup' containing many other biomolecules, often in much higher concentrations. One example is the use of zero-quantum filtration to derive a partial high-resolution spectrum (or a chemical shift image) showing only lactate signals, exploiting the fact that the lactate protons are coupled with a known coupling constant whereas the other constituents cannot sustain zero-quantum coherence.

11.11 Separation of NMR parameters

In some ways a high-resolution spectrum is *too* rich in information, sometimes presenting a veritable forest of resonance lines—a serious challenge to analysis. A drastic simplification can be achieved if the effects of chemical shifts (δ) can be separated from those of spin–spin coupling (J). Some applications can be solved on chemical shift evidence alone, others are more concerned with an accurate measurement of the coupling constants, while the majority rely on both parameters. The spin echo modulation phenomenon (§ 9.7) offers the key to such a separation of J and δ. The experiment employs a $180°$ pulse to refocus chemical shifts without affecting the spin–spin couplings, consequently the echo modulation frequencies provide an accurate measure of the coupling constants. Fourier transformation of the echo modulation displays this information in the form of spin–spin splittings. In its primitive form this experiment is not very practical because all the spin–spin splittings are superimposed and difficult to analyse, but by two-dimensional spectroscopy each splitting can be displayed on a different trace, set out in the second frequency dimension according to the relevant chemical shift. This is called a two-dimensional 'J-spectrum'.

In the case of two different nuclear species (protons and carbon-13, for example) a clean separation is readily achieved. Consider first the simple case of a sample of chloroform, containing one proton and one carbon-13 nucleus, with a spin–spin coupling J_{CH}. A carbon-13 spin echo is generated by the pulse sequence:

$$\text{Carbon-13:} \quad 90° - \tau - 180° - \tau - \text{Acquire}(t_2)$$

$$\text{Protons:} \quad \text{———} t_1 \text{———} \text{Decouple}$$

Note that $t_1 = 2\tau$ is the variable evolution period of a two-dimensional experiment. There is no echo modulation during t_1 and the carbon-13 chemical shift is refocused by the $180°$ pulse. Signal acquisition begins at time 2τ, at the peak of the spin echo. Fourier transformation of the second half of the echo (as a function of t_2) generates a conventional carbon-13 spectrum in the frequency dimension F_2. Proton decoupling during acquisition removes the CH splitting from this spectrum. In this form the experiment has a rather disappointing outcome—the two-dimensional spectrum consists of a singlet response at the carbon-13 chemical shift frequency in the F_2 dimension, and at zero frequency in the F_1 dimension.

All that has been gained is a rather narrower linewidth in the F_1 dimension due to the refocusing effect of the 180° pulse.

Now introduce a 180° proton pulse, synchronized with the carbon 180° pulse:

$$\text{Carbon-13:} \quad 90° — \tau —180° — \tau — \text{Acquire}(t_2)$$

$$\text{Protons:} \quad \text{———}180°\text{———Decouple}$$

As t_1 is incremented in small steps, this modulates the spin echo (§ 9.7), creating two frequency components, $\pm\frac{1}{2}J_{CH}$ Hz. Fourier transformation as a function of t_1 generates a doublet of splitting J_{CH}. Had there been two (equivalent) coupled protons (a methylene group) the spectrum in the F_1 dimension would be a 1:2:1 triplet, and if there were three coupled protons (a methyl group) it would be a 1:3:3:1 quartet.

So what has been achieved? A *conventional* carbon-13 spectrum can be very complex because the CH splittings are large (normally in the range 125–175 Hz) and adjacent spin multiplets can overlap in a very confusing manner. It is for this reason that these spectra are commonly run with broadband decoupling of the protons, sacrificing the coupling information but greatly simplifying the spectra. The two-dimensional experiment achieves the same simplicity in the F_2 dimension but retains the coupling information in the F_1 dimension, with the added advantage of better resolving power just where it is needed. Figure 11.9 shows a carbon-13

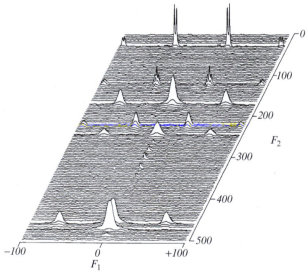

Figure 11.9 The two-dimensional J-spectrum of carbon-13 in a tricyclodecanone derivative. The responses are separated according to the carbon-13 chemical shifts in the F_2 dimension, while the F_1 dimension shows the individual CH splittings. These multiplets are basically singlets, doublets, triplets or quartets, reflecting the number of directly attached protons, but some long-range CH splittings are also observed. (Reproduced from M. H. Levitt and R. Freeman, *J. Magn. Reson.* **34**, 675 (1979) with the permission of Academic Press.)

two-dimensional J-spectrum of a tricyclodecanone derivative, displayed as stacked F_1 traces, with the chemical shift frequencies arrayed in the F_2 dimension.[12] This is the sense in which chemical shifts have been *separated* from spin–spin couplings.

A related experiment can be performed with a purely proton system, but then broadband decoupling during t_2 is not feasible. Spin–spin splittings are displayed in the F_1 dimension, but both chemical shifts *and* spin–spin splittings persist in the F_2 dimension. Consequently, each spin multiplet lies along a 45° diagonal of the proton two-dimensional J-spectrum. We may liken this to the operation of a Venetian blind—the conventional spectrum corresponds to a fully-closed blind, the two-dimensional proton–proton spectrum represents a half-open blind, whereas the corresponding (decoupled) proton–carbon spectrum is equivalent to a fully-open blind. Schematically, for a spectrum made up of a doublet, a triplet and a quartet:

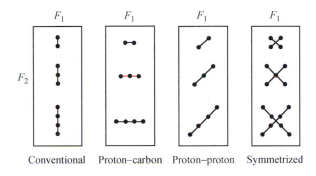

Conventional   Proton–carbon   Proton–proton   Symmetrized

We see at once that, even in the proton–proton case, a complete separation of J and δ could be achieved by projecting the two-dimensional J-spectrum at an angle of 45°, catching the spin multiplets in *enfilade*. Unfortunately, the peculiar line shapes in these proton spectra cause self-cancellation in such a projection. The problem can be circumvented by reflecting the two-dimensional spectrum about the axis $F_1 = 0$ and superimposing this on the original spectrum. Each multiplet then forms a symmetrical pattern and a symmetry filter can be used to separate them, even where there is a great deal of overlap.

Figure 11.10 shows the conventional high-resolution spectrum of the protons in dehydrotestosterone recorded at 400 MHz;[13] there is considerable overlap of spin multiplets, particularly for protons g and h which are separated by less than 0.01 ppm. Processing the 'reflected' two-dimensional J-spectrum with a symmetry filter gives the desired 'chemical shift spectrum' shown in the upper trace. Such 'stripped down' proton spectra can be very useful for analysing crowded spectra, or for matching to a library of characteristic chemical shifts.

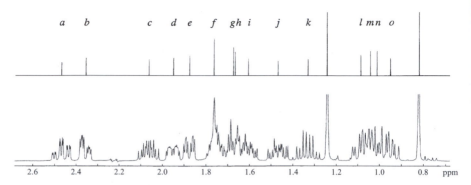

Figure 11.10 The 400 MHz high-resolution proton spectrum of dehydrotestosterone (lower trace), showing several overlapping spin multiplets. The strong (truncated) peaks at 0.82 and 1.24 ppm are from methyl groups. The top trace shows a 'chemical shift spectrum' derived from a symmetrized version of the two-dimensional J-spectrum, with the multiplets separated by means of a symmetry filter. The peaks g and h are separated by less than 0.01 ppm, while the response f is from two exactly degenerate resonances. This simplified form of a proton NMR spectrum is useful for assignment purposes and for creating a library of chemical shift information. (Reproduced from M. Woodley and R. Freeman, *J. Magn. Reson. A.* **109**, 103 (1994) with the permission of Academic Press.)

11.12 Diffusion-ordered spectroscopy (DOSY)

New applications of the general principle of two-dimensional spectroscopy continue to be introduced. High-resolution NMR suffers from serious limitations if the material under investigation is a mixture of several chemical compounds, as often happens in combinatorial chemistry (§ 16.2) and in the analysis of tissue extracts or biofluids (§ 15.1). In many such situations there is no time to use conventional chemical or physical methods to separate the various components. The DOSY technique[14] sets out to solve this problem by exploiting the different rates of molecular diffusion (§ 12.12), essentially performing the desired separation in the second frequency dimension of a two-dimensional experiment.

The pulsed field-gradient spin echo sequence introduced by Stejskal and Tanner[15] is one method for measuring the rate of molecular diffusion (§ 9.4). A short intense magnetic field gradient pulse first phase encodes the nuclear spins according to their positions, creating a regular helix of nuclear magnetization vectors along the direction of the imposed gradient (§ 12.5). For all stationary nuclear spins, the imposition of a hard 180° radiofrequency refocusing pulse followed by a second matched field gradient pulse of the same polarity 'unwinds' this phase-encoded helix, and generates a perfect spin echo at the end of the fixed interval Δ.

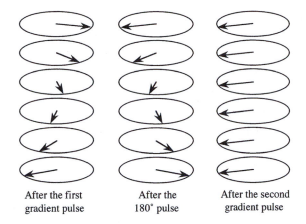

| After the first gradient pulse | After the 180° pulse | After the second gradient pulse |

However, any spins that have diffused during the Δ interval find themselves in the 'wrong' region of the second field gradient and are not properly refocused. This additional dephasing depends on the strength and duration of the two matched gradients and attenuates the spin-echo amplitude. The molecular diffusion coefficient can be extracted by fitting the echo peak heights as a function of gradient strength to the theoretical form. (This fitting procedure only works well when the signals from different components do not overlap in the chemical shift dimension, otherwise an intermediate value of the two diffusion coefficients is obtained.) A two-dimensional spectrum can then be constructed[16] where the diffusion coefficients determine the peak positions in the F_1 dimension, and the standard errors of the fitting process determine their widths. All the NMR responses from a given compound appear at the same ordinate in the diffusion dimension, and different compounds can be readily resolved in this dimension. One serious weakness of the DOSY technique is the distortion of the NMR lineshapes by eddy currents generated by the gradient pulses. Careful precautions have to be taken to minimize these effects by the use of bipolar gradient pulse pairs, stimulated echoes[17] or reference deconvolution.[18]

An example of diffusion-ordered spectroscopy is shown in Figure 11.11 for the 500 MHz proton spectrum of a perchloric acid extract from gerbil brain.[19] The pulse sequence of Gibbs and Johnson was used[17] with fifteen different spin echo spectra and a sixteen-step phase cycle in a ten-hour experiment. Diffusion coefficients and their standard errors were calculated for 116 separate peaks. Individual metabolites are well separated in the diffusion dimension and can be identified on the basis of their characteristic high-resolution NMR spectra. This 'virtual separation' technique compares well with the more conventional 'hyphenated' liquid chromatography-NMR method.

Multidimensional spectroscopy is not of course restricted to the applications described above. It is limited only by our ability to devise different ways to 'torture' the nuclei during the evolution period. In solid-state NMR, for example, where the observed spectrum is a function of the orientation of a single crystal

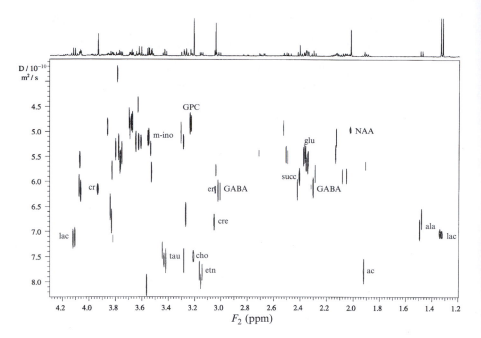

Figure 11.11 The 500 MHz DOSY spectrum of a complex mixture of metabolites extracted from gerbil brain with perchloric acid. The vertical axis corresponds to the diffusion constants extracted by fitting the spin echo decay curves as a function of field gradient strength. The full one-dimensional NMR spectrum is shown along the top margin. Selected metabolites have been assigned as follows: ac, acetate; ala, alanine; cho, choline; cr, creatine; cre, creatinine; etn, ethanolamine; GABA, γ-aminobutyric acid; gln, glutamine; glu, glutamate; gly, glycine; GPC, glycerophosphocholine; lac, lactate; m-ino, *myo*-inositol; NAA, N-acetyl aspartate; PC phosphocholine; succ, succinate; tau, taurine. (Reproduced from H. Barjat, G. A. Morris, S. Smart, A. G. Swanson and S. C. R. Williams *J. Magn. Reson. B.* **108**, 170 (1995) with the permission of Academic Press.)

with respect to the magnetic field (§ 10.1), it is possible to turn the sample progressively through small angles in the short interval between evolution and acquisition, allowing the complex trajectories of the various resonances in the spectrum to be followed as they cross and recross each other.

Further reading

A. Bax, *Two-Dimensional Nuclear Magnetic Resonance in Liquids*, Delft University Press, Delft, The Netherlands (1982).

N. Chandrakumar and S. Subramanian, *Modern Techniques in High-Resolution FT-NMR*, Springer-Verlag, New York (1987).

H. Friebolin, *Basic One- and Two-Dimensional NMR Spectroscopy*, VCH Publishers, New York (1993).

F. J. M. van de Ven, *Multidimensional NMR in Liquids: Basic Principles and Experimental Methods*, VCH Publishers, New York (1995).

S. Braun, H. O. Kalinowski and S. Berger, *100 and More Basic NMR Experiments*, VCH Publishers, New York (1996).

D. Canet, *Nuclear Magnetic Resonance: Concepts and Methods*, Wiley, Chichester (1996).

R. Freeman, *Spin Choreography*, Oxford University Press, Oxford (1997).

E. D. Becker, *High Resolution NMR: Theory and Chemical Applications*, Academic Press, San Diego, California (2000).

12

Magnetic resonance imaging

In 1972 magnetic resonance emerged from being a technique devoted almost entirely to chemistry to one that quickly became essentially a household word in medicine.[1] The initial excitement was boosted by the hope that it might serve as a foolproof diagnostic for cancerous tissue,[2] but it gradually became apparent that magnetic resonance had far wider implications as a method for obtaining images of human physiology, and even as the long-awaited window into how the brain functions. Soon the new tail (MRI) began to wag the old dog (NMR).

12.1 Basic principles

The key to obtaining images is the fact that the NMR frequency is strictly proportional to the strength of the magnetic field 'seen' by the nuclear spins. The nucleus acts as a very accurate 'clock' where the timekeeping is set by the magnetic field. If we focus attention on a single species, for example the protons in water, we would expect only a single sharp resonance response when the applied magnetic field is uniform across the sample. Now suppose we take five sample tubes containing water and place them in a row, and arrange that the strength of the applied magnetic field increases from one sample to the next. In other words, introduce a magnetic field *gradient* so that there are different field strengths $B_1, B_2, \ldots, B_5$ at the five locations. The NMR spectrum would consist of five separate signals, and if the tubes contain different quantities of water, the intensities of the responses would vary accordingly.

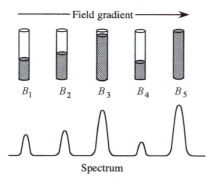

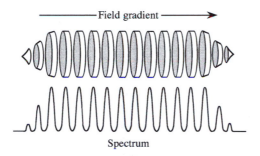

Now consider the case of an *extensive* sample—a salami might be an appropriate example. If we slice the salami and separate the slices, place them in the magnet and apply a field gradient along the long axis, we would again observe a separate NMR response from each slice.

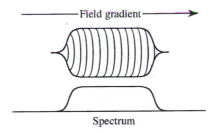

It is only a small step to see that if the slices were reassembled to form the original salami, we would observe a *continuous* NMR spectrum.

The intensity at any given point would be proportional to the number of spins with that particular resonance frequency—that is to say, all the spins within the appropriate slice. This is the *projection* of the total NMR signal intensity onto the gradient axis. This tells us nothing about the *shape* of the slices, and indeed nothing about the *distribution* of spins within a given slice, but it identifies the location of each slice with respect to the gradient direction.

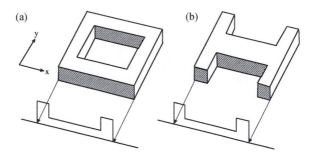

Figure 12.1 Assuming that these two solid shapes are uniformly filled with nuclear spins, the projections of their magnetic resonance signals onto the x axis would be identical. If we want to know more about their shapes, we have to measure projections in some other directions.

At this point we have rather begged the question of how the NMR spectrum is formed. In practice what is observed in the receiver is a jumble of different frequencies from nuclear spins the various slices—this composite signal is sometimes called an *interferogram*. The magnetic resonance information is in an inconvenient form for our purposes. We need to pick out the frequency components one at a time, and record the intensity of the NMR response carried at each frequency. These results must then be assembled in order of increasing frequency, to create a 'frequency-domain spectrum', essentially a graph of NMR intensity as a function of distance along the direction of the applied field gradient. This process of converting the raw time-domain interferogram into the frequency domain is called Fourier transformation (§ 3.7). It is implicit in almost all magnetic resonance imaging procedures.

We see that a single projection of spin density onto a given axis leaves considerable ambiguity about the nature of the sample. Consider, for example, an object in the form of a hollow square, containing a uniform distribution of protons (Figure 12.1). Projection of the proton spin density onto the x axis gives a profile that is identical to that from an object in the form of a solid letter 'H'. Indeed there are many other possible structures that would give the same projection, for the simple reason that all signals with the same x coordinate contribute to the same point on the projection—the y and z coordinates are unknown. To obtain an unambiguous image it is essential to view the object from some other directions, preferably the other Cartesian axes y and z.

To see how projections of the magnetic resonance response can be converted into a proton density map, we simplify the problem for the purposes of illustration, reducing it to two dimensions by considering a flat object of uniform thickness. Suppose the first measurement employs a magnetic field gradient that runs in the y direction, giving the projection of proton NMR intensity onto the y axis. We may choose a representative point on this intensity profile by selecting the appropriate NMR frequency, and the intensity measured at this point corresponds to the total proton response from the thin strip $A–A'$.

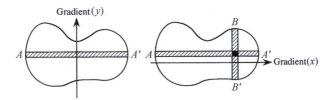

Then a second measurement is performed with the field gradient along the x axis, giving a profile of the proton intensity projected onto the x axis. A typical point on the profile represents the total intensity from the strip $B–B'$. Although the intersection of these two strips $A–A'$ and $B–B'$ defines the spatial coordinates of a particular voxel (the black square) it is rather less obvious how we establish the actual proton spin density of that voxel, since at this juncture we have only measured the total NMR intensities from the strips $A–A'$ and $B–B'$. We must find a way to link these two measurement together in order to solve the problem. A two-stage experiment is required, where the nuclear spins first evolve in a magnetic field gradient in the first direction (y) and then in a gradient applied at right angles (x). We say that behaviour of the nuclear spins during in the first time interval is *correlated* with the behaviour in the second time interval. This concept has already been examined in the context of two-dimensional NMR spectroscopy (§ 11.1) Information gleaned in one dimension is 'coded' according to the NMR response in the other dimension. For the moment let us take the essential encoding process for granted; it is considered in detail below (§ 12.5). With this key proviso we can map out the intensity of the magnetic resonance response at each and every point on a two-dimensional map. Usually there is no need to extend the treatment into a third spatial dimension because most MRI scans begin with a 'slice selection' stage (§ 12.3), so that, in effect, we are only dealing with a thin flat object.

12.2 Magnetic field gradients

In all applications of MRI the applied field gradients are extremely weak in comparison with the applied polarizing field, so we can completely disregard the tiny changes in nuclear spin populations, concentrating only on the variation in precession frequencies. The main magnetic field is applied in the z direction but field *gradients* can be imposed in any of the three directions in space x, y or z. To avoid confusion with the axes of the rotating reference frame (X, Y and Z) we shall retain lower-case letters (x, y and z) for the spatial coordinates. The Z and z axes will of course be the same. A gradient along any other arbitrary direction can be achieved by a suitable combination of these three orthogonal gradients.

Gradients are generated by currents in subsidiary coils around the sample. The magnetic field from a gradient coil runs from an extreme negative value to an equal extreme positive value, balanced about a point within the sample called the *isocentre*, where the additional fields from the gradient coils are all zero. If at all possible the applied field gradient should be a linear function of distance, otherwise the image will be distorted. When a superconducting solenoid is used for the main magnetic field, the gradient coils are wound on cylinders concentric with the main axis (z) of the magnet solenoid. The z gradient is generated by a 'Maxwell pair' of coils connected in opposition, while the x and y gradients are each produced by pairs of saddle coils (Figure 12.2).

At first sight it may not be obvious how the required gradients arise. The first essential point to note is that although the magnetic fields generated by the gradient coils alone are quite complex in shape, all that matters for magnetic resonance purposes are the components of these fields along the z direction. Focus attention on the overall field 'seen' by a given nuclear spin, the resultant of the intense main magnet field B_0 aligned in the z direction and the much weaker fields from the gradient coils. Any transverse (xy) components of the latter are so small in comparison with B_0 that the resultant field is still essentially directed along the z axis and is virtually unchanged in amplitude, whereas any z component of the gradient either adds to or subtracts from B_0 directly.

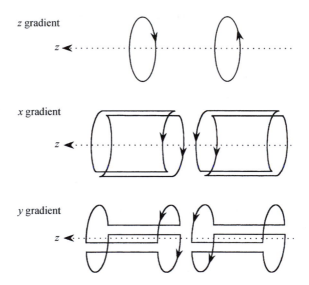

Figure 12.2 Coils used for creating z, x and y gradients in a superconducting solenoid imaging magnet where the main magnetic field is in the z direction. The arrows indicate electric current direction, and the leads are omitted for simplicity. For the z gradient, the opposed magnetic fields from the 'Maxwell pair' create a gradient that is approximately linear between the coils. In the 'Golay arrangement' for x and y gradients the main gradient contributions are from the currents in the innermost arcs (marked with arrows). For the x gradient, currents in the front and rear arcs generate magnetic fields in opposition, one enhancing the main magnetic field, the other reducing it. The y gradient Golay coils are identical except that they have been rotated 90° about the z axis. For clarity the three sets of coils are shown separately, but in practice all three are mounted on concentric cylinders.

It is easy to see that a single coil with its axis along the z direction generates a field that falls off as the distance from the plane of the coil. Two such coils aligned parallel and connected in opposition (the Maxwell pair) enhance this effect and create an z gradient that is approximately linear in the region enclosed by the coils. The optimum separation is given by the coil radius times the square root of three (1.732). This is the arrangement used to create the z gradient (Figure 12.2).

A similar opposed configuration is used to generate gradients transverse to the main magnetic field. One of the possible designs is the 'Golay pair'. In this arrangement two sets of saddle coils are used, and to a good approximation we can neglect all the electrical currents except those flowing in the innermost arcs (those indicated by the arrows). To produce the x gradient, the z component of the magnetic field generated by the rear sections of the saddle coils adds to the main magnetic field whereas the field from the front sections subtracts from the main magnetic field. In other words, the front and rear sections act in opposition and create a gradient in the x dimension. The operation to generate a y gradient is analogous; an identical Golay coil system is constructed, rotated by $90°$ about the z axis. Remember that the total field seen by the nuclear spins is *always directed along the z direction*; it is only its intensity that changes with the x, y and z coordinates.

Gradients are switched on and off at the appropriate times under computer control, and it is important to keep the rise and fall times as short as possible. In the intense main field of the magnet (B_0) the gradient coils vibrate as the gradient is switched, and act rather like loudspeakers, creating an uncomfortably noisy environment for the patient (§ 13.3). Furthermore, the act of switching induces eddy currents in nearby conductors, and these currents generate subsidiary magnetic fields that can persist for rather long times and interfere with the MRI measurement. One solution to this problem is a method called 'pre-emphasis' in which an initial negative gradient pulse cancels the eddy current contribution from the main (positive) gradient pulse. A better solution is to employ shielded gradient coils, where the magnetic field outside the main gradient coil is compensated by an opposite field from a subsidiary outer coil, thus minimizing the field reaching any nearby metallic conductors.

12.3 Slice selection

If we wish to examine the internal structure of an object, say an orange, we take a sharp knife and slice through the orange at a suitable point. Before the recent advances in medical technology, our knowledge of the internal structure of the human body had mostly relied on a similar procedure, hence the term *anatomy* (Greek: cutting up). Magnetic resonance imaging normally starts in a similar manner, by selecting a given slice for further examination, but in this case it is only a virtual slice—the patient has been spared the ordeal of a surgical intervention. The MRI slice has a certain thickness; enough to provide a sufficiently intense magnetic resonance signal, but not so thick that the tissues change significantly across the narrow dimension. Then we can anticipate construction of a two-dimensional map to reflect the structure of the tissues within the chosen slice.

Slice selection[3] involves the concept of a 'soft' radiofrequency pulse outlined in § 2.9. A soft pulse has low radiofrequency intensity and a correspondingly long duration. To take a practical example of slice selection, we might apply the field gradient along the main axis of the human body, from head to toe. Let us call this the z axis. Imagine the body divided into many parallel transverse slices; we select just one of these (for example, a slice across the chest) by adjusting the frequency of the selective pulse so that only these spins are at resonance.

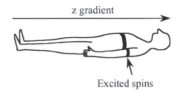

Excited spins

Spins outside this chosen slice are so far from the transmitter frequency that they experience negligible excitation. The thickness of the slice is determined by the effective bandwidth of the soft pulse and the strength of the applied gradient (a thin slice implies a long pulse duration or an intense magnetic field gradient).

So far we have said nothing about how the *profile* of the slice is defined. Viewed edgewise, the intensity profile should be uniform through the slice, falling off steeply at the edges. That is to say, the ideal profile would be a trapezium—almost a rectangle. Now a standard radiofrequency pulse excites a pattern of frequencies that is nowhere near rectangular—it has a central positive peak flanked by 'wiggles'. It approximates the Fourier transform of the pulse envelope—a sinc function.

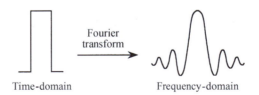

Time-domain   Frequency-domain

This is by no means an ideal excitation pattern—the edges are not very steep, the excitation is not uniform within the slice, and there could be overlap and interference with adjacent slices. What we would really like is the reverse relationship, where the time-domain envelope is a sinc function and the frequency-domain excitation pattern is approximately rectangular.

The usual remedy is to shape the time-domain envelope of the soft pulse according to a *modified* sinc function. To keep the pulse duration reasonably short, the wiggles are truncated at zero-crossing points of the sinc function; this gives a frequency-domain excitation profile that is very roughly trapezoidal with some residual oscillations:

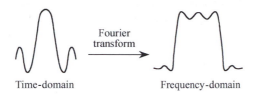

Time-domain   Fourier transform   Frequency-domain

Although this excitation profile is not ideal, the edges are reasonably steep, and there is only weak excitation of signals from adjacent slices.

If the transmitter frequency is set at resonance in the main magnetic field, then the selected slice is at the isocentre of the gradient coils, where the additional magnetic field is zero. The other slices are selected, one at a time, by suitably shifting the transmitter frequency. Once the excitation has been confined to a well-defined slice through the sample, we are ready to examine the variation in proton spin density in the two remaining dimensions (x and y) across this slice.

Couched in these terms, slice selection appears to be a relatively straightforward process, but there is a fundamental complication. It arises because the soft radiofrequency pulse causes an undesirable divergence of the nuclear magnetization vectors from different regions of the sample.[4] A hard radiofrequency pulse would pose no such problem—all the these vectors would be aligned along the $+Y$ axis immediately after the pulse. In contrast, a soft pulse causes a fanning-out of the phases of the nuclear spins depending on their offsets from exact resonance. We can think of this as arising because a soft pulse has a much longer duration than a hard pulse. The behaviour is a little complicated because the vectors representing different nuclear magnetization components rotate about tilted effective fields, but the net result is as if they had started to precess freely from a point near the centre of the soft pulse.

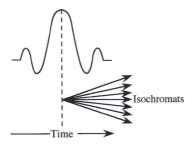

Isochromats

Time →

To a good approximation, the phase shift of nuclear spins within some small volume is directly proportional to the offset from resonance. Because the sample under investigation is made up of a continuum of nuclear spins, the corresponding magnetization vectors are soon spread out almost uniformly around a circle and the resultant is close to zero. Very little magnetic resonance signal is detected. The trick is to reverse the phase divergence by a gradient pulse of opposite sign and half the intensity of the slice-selection gradient.

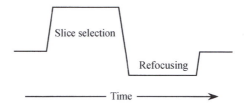

The factor half reflects the fact that the divergence starts near the centre of the soft pulse. Precession in the reversed gradient brings all the individual vectors back into alignment along the $+Y$ axis.

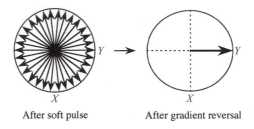

| After soft pulse | After gradient reversal |

This provides the full magnetic resonance response to the soft pulse.

After one slice has been examined, another can be excited without waiting for complete spin–lattice relaxation of the spins in the first slice, although it is preferable to employ an interleaving scheme so that consecutive slices are not adjacent. This permits multislice imaging (§ 12.8) which increases the rate of information-gathering and thus improves sensitivity.

12.4 The readout stage

Let us suppose that slice selection has been implemented by applying a field gradient along the z axis. (Remember that x, y and z represent the laboratory coordinates.) The next step is to determine the proton spin density within this two-dimensional sample as a function of the x and y coordinates, by applying magnetic field gradients along the x and y axes in turn. There are several different protocols for achieving this result; we outline here the simplest method, called 'two-dimensional Fourier imaging',[5, 6] later slightly modified and named the 'spin warp' method.[3]

In an applied x gradient we imagine the sample divided into strips running in the y direction.

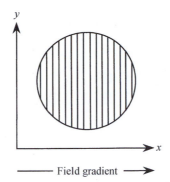

———— Field gradient ———→

All the nuclei within a given strip have the same precession frequency, but the remaining strips experience different values of the gradient and precess at different frequencies, forming an interference pattern. The convention is that the x gradient is applied during acquisition of the NMR response; it is therefore known as the 'readout' gradient.

12.5 Phase encoding

The readout stage provides a measure of the distribution of protons in the x dimension; now we have to examine the distribution in the y dimension. As mentioned above, it is not merely a question of repeating signal acquisition with a gradient imposed along the y axis, and then combining the two results. To see why this is so, consider the simple case of a phantom made up of two small tubes of water, both aligned in the z direction in an imaging magnet. The proton spin density in the xy plane might be represented by

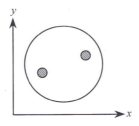

The time-domain NMR signal observed in the presence of a y gradient consists of two frequencies which beat together and decay with time, converted by Fourier transformation into a spectrum of two strong peaks. Similarly, the equivalent measurement made in the presence of an x gradient also generates two peaks (with a larger frequency separation in this case). If we simply combine these two measurements we obtain a *false* image consisting of four responses.

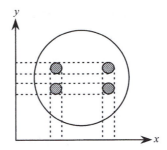

This is because the information obtained in the presence of the y gradient has not been *correlated* with that obtained in the x gradient.

In § 11.2 we used the analogy of a relay race to explain the concept of 'correlation' in the NMR context. Runners in the first leg of the race pass batons to members of the same team for the second stage. If one runner performs poorly in the initial stage he imposes a handicap on his teammate for the next stage. So it is with MRI. There are two independent time intervals—phase-encoding (t_1) with a gradient in the y direction, and readout (t_2) with a gradient in the x direction. The protons within a typical volume element (voxel) evolve during t_1 and retain information about their NMR frequency in the form of the accumulated precession phase. This determines the initial phase of these same nuclei as they begin to precess during readout, but has no effect at all on signals from other voxels if the spins remain in place throughout both t_1 and t_2. The observed signal is said to be 'phase encoded'. The extent of precession during t_1 is thus *correlated* with the precession frequency observed during t_2. This explains why the phantom consisting of two tubes of water excites two bright regions on the MR image, rather than four.

Phase encoding is not carried out in real time, but involves a sequence of independent measurements with stepwise incrementation of one of the evolution parameters. This can be achieved in two different ways. During the evolution period a field gradient is applied along the y axis, effectively dividing the sample into many parallel strips running in the x direction. All the nuclei within a given strip have the same precession frequency.

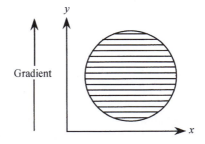

The rate at which nuclei in a typical strip accumulate precession phase is proportional to the strength and duration of the y gradient at that position. Consequently, there are two ways to perform the scan—if a *constant* gradient is used with progressive increments of the evolution time, it is called 'Fourier imaging'. If the evolution time is kept constant but the strength of the y gradient is incremented, this is known as spin warp imaging, as set out schematically below.

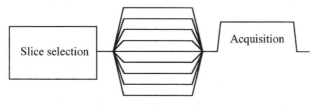

Phase-encoding gradient Readout gradient

Spin warp imaging is preferred because it avoids complications attributable to different degrees of spin–spin relaxation or other magnetization losses that would occur during a *variable* phase-encoding interval.

As described in § 3.5, there are some important rules governing the way in which magnetic resonance signals are sampled. In MRI this 'Nyquist criterion' sets an upper limit on the strengths of the magnetic field gradients that can be imposed. If these are too large, the precession frequencies of nuclear spins just beyond the edges of the desired field of view (measured in the rotating reference frame) are too high to be properly digitized. With the usual quadrature detection scheme these frequencies are 'aliased', that is to say, down-shifted in frequency by $2F$ where F is the sampling rate of the analog-to-digital converter. Aliasing can only be avoided if all the nuclear precession frequencies are constrained to fall within a 'Nyquist window' spanning the frequency range $-F$ to $+F$ Hz. If the applied field gradients are too strong to satisfy this requirement, any part of the image that would properly lie beyond one edge becomes aliased and appears inside the opposite edge, as illustrated in the 'giraffe cartoon' (Figure 3.6). Such a spurious displacement of some feature of a spin density map could prove disastrous in a clinical context. One remedy would be to increase the sampling rate, but this is not always feasible, particularly in the phase-encoding stage, for this would entail a long-duration MRI scan, proportional to the number of sampling operations. Fast sampling during readout is less serious, but is nevertheless limited by the practical shortcomings of the analog-to-digital converter.

Let us examine in more detail how aliasing comes about in the spin warp and Fourier imaging techniques. Consider first the Fourier imaging mode, where the gradient is held constant while the duration t_1 is incremented in small steps. Evolution in a magnetic field gradient imposed along the y axis builds up a phase 'handicap' for each strip of the sample, proportional to the duration of the evolution increment Δt_1, and this is the information that is passed on to the precessing spins during readout. A strip at the isocentre of the gradient coil will of course experience no phase handicap at all. For all other strips, the imposed y gradient induces a clockwise or anticlockwise rotation of the precession phase, depending on whether that particular strip lies above or below the isocentre. To avoid aliasing, it is essential that this phase accumulation be kept within the limits of $\pm 180°$ for all strips in the sample and for each and every increment of the evolution time Δt_1. We can simplify the picture by considering the very first increment, where the magnetization vectors from all regions of the sample start off with exactly the same phase. After precession during Δt_1 the accumulated phase shifts (positive and negative) are greatest for the strips at the top and bottom of the field-of-view where the gradient field is strongest (Figure 12.3). The Nyquist condition requires that these phase shifts should not exceed $\pm 180°$ at these extreme locations, otherwise aliasing will occur because of the periodic nature of the phase angle. For example, a phase angle of $+190°$ is indistinguishable from one of $-170°$, so a magnetic resonance response from a strip just above the top of the window would appear to originate from a false location just above the bottom of the window. This imposes an upper limit on the step size Δt_1 and, as a direct consequence, on the extent of the field of view in the y dimension. A wider field of view can be achieved by increasing the sampling rate (smaller increments) but if we limit ourselves to the same total scan duration, the spatial definition is degraded—the same number of pixels are spread over a larger distance in the y dimension.

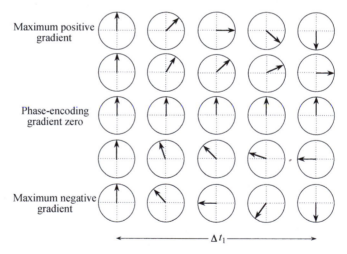

Figure 12.3 Aliasing in the phase-encoding dimension in Fourier imaging. Five representative magnetization vectors (left) from voxels in different regions of an applied magnetic field gradient evolve during the interval Δt_1, building up phase shifts that depend on their locations in the y dimension. The increment Δt_1 must be sufficiently short that the maximum precession angle never exceeds $\pm 180°$ (top right and bottom right). Otherwise aliasing occurs because, for example, the angle $+190°$ is indistinguishable from $-170°$. This is the Nyquist condition; if it is violated, parts of the image appear at a false locations.

A compromise must be made between fine detail and the overall extent of the image. Analogous restrictions apply to the spin warp technique. The evolution time t_1 is now fixed, while the y dimension is explored by incrementing the strength of the imposed y gradient. Because the maximum permissible phase shift is $\pm180°$ this sets an upper limit on the size of the gradient increments.

When the experimental data are processed, the phase-encoded information is examined in the appropriate sequence, starting with the largest negative y gradient and stepping through systematically to the largest positive y gradient. Now a phase angle that increases linearly with time is essentially a frequency, albeit defined here in a stepwise manner. Consequently, each horizontal strip of the sample has been labelled according to its intrinsic nuclear precession *frequency*, proportional to the height of that particular strip in the y dimension.

Two stages of Fourier transformation serve to separate the frequency components arising from individual voxels. Consequently, with phase encoding in a gradually incremented y gradient, followed by frequency encoding in a fixed x gradient during readout, the coordinates of any given voxel are uniquely defined, while its intrinsic intensity determines the brightness of that region of the image.

12.6 The concept of k-space

We see from the previous sections that a typical imaging sequence is made up of three successive stages:

1. slice selection in a constant z gradient
2. phase encoding in a stepped y gradient
3. readout in a constant x gradient.

The raw experimental data are stored in what is known as 'k-space'. Strictly three dimensions are involved, although we are principally concerned with the axes k_x and k_y, having taken slice selection in the z direction for granted. In the Fourier imaging method, k_y is a time axis, as is k_x. In the more common spin-warp protocol, k_y represents gradient amplitude for a *fixed* phase-encoding interval. The experimental response is sampled in real time along the k_x axis, but the k_y information is acquired in a succession of separate measurements. Two-dimensional Fourier transformation of data in k-space converts to proton spin density in *image space*, just as data gathered in two time dimensions in high-resolution NMR transforms into a spectrum in two frequency dimensions (§ 11.2). The appearance of a k-space map bears no obvious relationship to the desired magnetic resonance image, although all the required information is present in the raw experimental data. Each individual data point in k-space contributes information to all the pixels in image space, just as each point on an NMR free induction decay contributes to the entire high-resolution NMR spectrum.

We could of course regard k-space merely as a two-dimensional array of numbers, soon to be transformed by a computer into an image, but it is quite instructive to establish the *order* in which the experimental data points in k-space are acquired. Exactly how the data gathering is organized to explore k-space has some important practical consequences for the quality of the final image. This is called a *trajectory* in k-space. In the usual MRI sequences there is no other option than to acquire the readout (k_x) information as a function of real time, which corresponds to a horizontal trace through k-space, but the phase-encoding gradients can be imposed in any desired order. The overall k-space trajectory might simply be a set of horizontal traces stacked one above the other, reminiscent of the way in which a television picture is constructed:

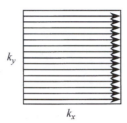

In high-resolution NMR spectroscopy, there is sometimes an artefact near the beginning of the free induction decay, caused, for example, by a temporary receiver overload from the intense transmitter pulse. It is a general property of the Fourier transform that an amplitude artefact near the origin of the time-domain signal transforms into a low-frequency sine wave running across the entire spectrum in the frequency domain. In high-resolution NMR this problem is called the 'rolling baseline'. Conversely, an amplitude spike late in the time-domain response transforms into a high-frequency sine wave. In MRI the origin is the centre of the k-space diagram, and data points near the centre transform into low-frequency components of the spin density map, determining the gross (low-resolution) shape of the image, whereas points nearer the periphery of k-space transform into high-frequency components, determining the fine structure of the image. We can hardly dispense with data near the centre of k-space, but eventually we can stop gathering data in the outer reaches, once sufficient image resolution has been achieved. This is important, for it sets upper limits on the required strength of the applied field gradients and on the duration of data gathering.

But why is the k-space trajectory so important? It turns out that the various imaging protocols each follow a characteristic trajectory, and this determines the nature of artefacts that can appear in the final image. Consider for a moment a technique employed in the computer-aided tomography (CT) scanner which records the absorption of X-rays in a set of different directions equally spaced around a circle. However complex the internal structure, these multiple views provide sufficient information to define an accurate two-dimensional image; no features are hidden. The results are processed by a reconstruction algorithm which computes the unique X-ray map that is consistent with all the different views.

In the analogous MRI projection–reconstruction procedure,[1] spin density is projected not *along* these skew axes but *onto* them (line projections). The measurement is repeated many times while stepping the *direction* of the magnetic field gradient in the xy plane. This implies a polar (as opposed to Cartesian) diagram.

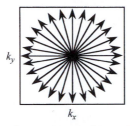

The procedure necessitates simultaneous switching of the amplitudes of the x and y gradients, carefully planned (according to sine and cosine tables) so that the resultant gradient changes direction but remains of constant amplitude. The method has the advantage that signals are gathered in real time—there is no need to wait for a phase-encoding step, making it useful for rapidly decaying signals from samples with a short spin–spin relaxation time T_2. The raw data are converted by a projection–reconstruction algorithm that calculates the only possible image consistent with all the line projections. This procedure concentrates data sampling near the origin of k-space (where all the arrows are bunched together). One consequence is a slight improvement in sensitivity over Fourier imaging because the local signal-to-noise ratio is highest near the origin. However, projection–reconstruction images suffer blurring from imperfections in the applied gradients, whereas the widely-used spin warp method shows only minor *distortions* from the same perturbations. The projection–reconstruction technique is indirect and rather sensitive to magnetic field inhomogeneities, so for most applications it has been superseded by more robust methods.

Another useful trajectory in k-space was devised to avoid rapid switching of the field gradients. An electric current that follows a sine wave is applied to the x gradient coil, with a simultaneous cosine waveform of the same amplitude and frequency applied to the y gradient coil. As the two currents are gradually increased from zero, the k-space trajectory spirals outwards from the centre until a suitable area has been covered.

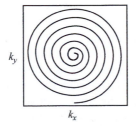

At no time do the gradient currents need to change rapidly, so the induced eddy currents are minimal. We shall come across another important k-space trajectory in the next section.

12.7 Echo planar imaging

Imaging over a two-dimensional slice is normally a time-consuming operation because two orthogonal field gradients (the phase-encoding and readout gradients) must be explored independently. Acquisition during the readout gradient is no problem; it is complete within a fraction of a second, but acquisition as a function of the phase-encoding gradient necessitates N consecutive measurements, each involving a recycling delay (TR) for spin–lattice relaxation, followed by a new excitation pulse. Such measurements can be rather protracted. Yet for many MRI applications it is important to obtain a 'snapshot' image. In this photographic analogy, we need a very short 'exposure'. This implies speeding up the imaging sequence so as to obtain in one shot all the information that was traditionally acquired over a much longer time in N separate measurements. In this manner it becomes possible to image those regions of the anatomy that are subject to motion, voluntary or involuntary, essentially 'freezing' the movement to eliminate motional artefacts. Fast imaging is important when we have to deal with 'uncooperative' patients (for example, infants), it permits measurements while a patient holds his breath, and it improves throughout and thereby reduces the cost per examination.

An obvious extension of this concept is to obtain a *time-dependent* set of images—the equivalent of a movie rather than a still photograph. For example, studies of the activation of specific regions of the human brain by functional MRI (Chapter 17) often involve a physical stimulus followed by a rapid observation of the consequent changes in a localized region of the image. We are interested in seeing which regions of the brain 'light up' as a result of the stimulus, and how they develop with time. Another application would be to view the motion of a beating heart, requiring several images per cycle (synchronized with the heartbeat).

One such rapid imaging technique has been called 'echo planar imaging'.[7] It relies on the fact that the vectors representing spin isochromats are returned to their initial orientations at the time of a gradient-recalled echo (§ 9.2), and they are then ready to undergo many further cycles of dispersal and refocusing throughout an extended train of echoes. Only a single radiofrequency excitation pulse is employed, and the entire measurement is completed before the signal has decayed significantly through spin–spin relaxation. (There is of course the technical problem of ensuring that the field gradients can be switched sufficiently rapidly, a property made easier by the use of shielded gradient coils which minimize eddy currents.) Whereas the traditional imaging sequence explores k-space one horizontal trace at a time, echo planar imaging can complete the entire raster in a single acquisition. A typical echo planar measurement can be accomplished in about a tenth of a second.

In echo planar imaging, exploration of the k_y dimension is implemented by imposing small 'blips' in the y gradient in the intervals between spin echoes. These small increments have a cumulative effect on the phase of the nuclear precession, shifting each successive horizontal scan a small step in the k_y dimension, thus completing a k-space trajectory that is very similar to that employed for scanning the image on a television screen (Figure 12.4). The read gradients alternate in sign, so the horizontal scans alternate in direction. This procedure[8] is known as 'BEST' (blipped echo planar single-pulse technique). The complete sequence is set out in Figure 12.5. Note that no time is wasted, signal acquisition takes place throughout the entire sequence.

Because there is a practical limit on the total time a patient can remain inside an imaging magnet and we must be sure to use this time to the best effect. After slice selection with a soft radiofrequency pulse we have to allow a relatively long recycle time (TR) for spin–lattice relaxation (§ 4.1) before these nuclear spins can be excited again. But this restriction does not apply to the remainder of the sample, where the nuclear spins remain polarized. So it is quite feasible to excite a second slice elsewhere in the sample while the nuclear spins in the first slice are still recovering through spin–lattice relaxation. The time required to acquire the magnetic resonance signal from a single slice by the echo planar method might be of the order of one-tenth of a second, whereas the recycle time TR needs to be of the order of one second, so there is scope for improvement in the rate of data gathering. Because there can be a certain amount of 'cross-talk' between adjacent

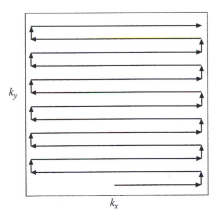

k_y

k_x

Figure 12.4 Trajectory in k-space corresponding to the echo planar imaging scheme. The 'read gradients' alternate in sense, corresponding to traces in the positive and negative k_x dimension, while the short phase encoding gradients ('blips') cause the cumulative displacement in the positive k_y dimension.

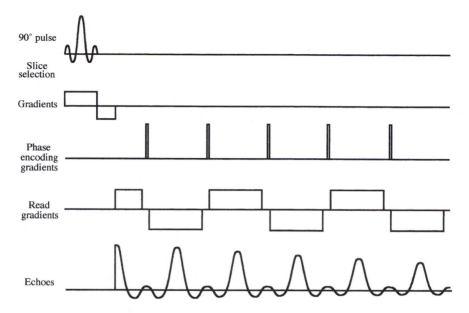

Figure 12.5 Sequence for echo planar imaging. The soft 90° pulse and its associated pair of gradients select magnetic resonance signals from the chosen slice. The remaining gradients explore this slice by creating the *k*-space trajectory shown in Figure 12.4. Acquisition of all the spin echoes provides imaging information from the entire slice in a single shot. This is far faster than conventional imaging protocols.

slices, it is preferable to arrange the multi-slice sequence such that successive slices are well separated in space, for example by an interleaving procedure. In this manner an entire set of different slice-selection operations can be performed, increasing the sensitivity without significantly extending the total length of the MRI scan. In practice the 'nesting' of the slice selection, phase-encoding and read-out operations is subject to permutations designed to obtain an image in the shortest possible time.

12.8 Imaging in three dimensions

Instead of examining many slices one at a time, we can also implement true three-dimensional imaging in which nuclear spins from the entire sample volume are excited simultaneously. The initial radiofrequency pulse is non-selective (a 'hard' rather than 'soft' pulse) and acts in the absence of applied field gradients. The innovation is to introduce another period of phase encoding with an incremented gradient applied in the z dimension, followed by the usual phase encoding in the k_y dimension and then frequency encoding during readout. One implementation can be written:

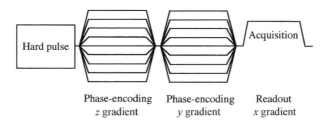

Phase-encoding   Phase-encoding   Readout
z gradient y gradient x gradient

This is necessarily a longer scan for it involves M times N separate signal acquisitions where M and N are the number of phase encoding steps in the z and y dimensions, but it offers high intrinsic sensitivity because the signal is derived from the entire volume rather than from a single slice. Furthermore, the image slices are contiguous and can be very thin without danger of the kind of interference that can occur in slice-selection methods. It is possible to operate with voxels that are tiny cubes with the same spatial resolution in all three dimensions, making it simpler to compute the proton density map in any arbitrary plane (axial, coronal, sagittal or oblique). In practice, time constraints usually impose a lower spatial resolution in the two phase-encoding directions, elongating the voxels in these dimensions. The Nyquist condition for phase-encoding must be satisfied in both the z and y dimensions.

12.9 Contrast

So far it has been implied that a magnetic resonance image is simply a map of the proton spin density within the sample. We are mainly concerned with mobile protons. If the protons are stationary (as in solid material such as bone) they have long spin–lattice relaxation times and very short spin–spin relaxation times, and their responses are therefore weak and broad, contributing very little to the proton density map. But even for mobile protons, the image is not fixed once and for all, it can be *manipulated* at will. One of the great advantages of MRI over the CT scanner is that discrimination between various soft tissues can be greatly improved by varying the operating conditions. In other words, we can enhance the contrast of the image to favour a particular clinical feature, in a manner similar to varying the contrast of a television picture. The most common distinguishing parameters are the spin–lattice relaxation time (T_1) and the spin–spin relaxation time (T_2) (Table 12.1). Spin density is still a major factor in determining image brightness, but this is now modified by relaxation effects, providing a higher degree of discrimination between tissues. But because spin density determines the maximum signal obtainable, contrast is achieved at the expense of some loss of sensitivity.

Suppose a particular feature has a longer-than-average spin–lattice relaxation time T_1 (§ 4.1). Cerebrospinal fluid (CSF) is a good example; a typical spin–lattice

Table 12.1 The time parameters used in magnetic resonance

T_1: the spin–lattice relaxation time.

T_2: the spin-spin relaxation time.

T_2^*: the decay time constant due to instrumental effects.

TR: the recycle time between successive excitations.

TE: the time interval between excitation and the peak of the spin echo.

TI: the time interval between population inversion and signal acquisition.

---

relaxation time (T_1) would be between 2 and 4 seconds, depending on field strength, compared with about 0.4 second for the white matter in the brain. If consecutive measurements are separated by a recycle time $TR = 0.4$ second, a steady-state regime is established in which the recovery of the proton spin populations in CSF is far less complete than that of protons in white matter. We could say that the CSF protons are preferentially saturated so that the corresponding CSF signal is weaker, showing up as dark regions on the T_1-weighted image. This saturation technique was first used in high-resolution NMR spectroscopy.[9] In MRI applications the actual proton spin density has not been altered, but the relative intensities of the partially saturated signals are altered, enhancing image contrast.

Contrast enhancement by T_1 weighting is widely used in MRI studies, often implemented by the preferential saturation technique where the faster-relaxing regions appear brighter on the image. High-resolution images can be obtained, as evidenced by the close-up view of the human eye shown in Figure 12.6, where the pixel size is only 0.31 × 0.31 mm. A radiofrequency surface coil was used. This T_1-weighted image clearly shows the lens, the optic nerve and the muscles that lie behind the orbit. The retro-orbital fat is bright because it has a short spin–lattice relaxation time, whereas the aqueous humour is dark because it has a long spin–lattice relaxation time.

An alternative approach to this preferential saturation technique is to apply a 180° 'inversion pulse' a short time TI prior to the main imaging sequence. In this mode the recycle time TR must be long compared with the relevant spin–lattice relaxation times so that the system is close to Boltzmann equilibrium at the start of each new pulse sequence. The 180° prepulse inverts the nuclear spin populations at all the proton sites, and they return to equilibrium along an exponential curve of time constant T_1. If TI is short compared with the appropriate spin–lattice relaxation time, the observed signal is negative; when TI is about 0.7 T_1 the signal passes through a null, and at longer settings of TI the signal becomes positive again. Consequently, this 'inversion-recovery' method can achieve a very high level of discrimination between tissues with different spin–lattice relaxation times. For example, it is possible to operate under conditions where the signal from fat is at the null condition while the tissues of interest still give inverted signals (§ 4.1).

Recent relaxation of the American Food and Drug Administration (FDA) regulations now permits imaging measurements at a magnetic field of 3 tesla, where the quality of the images is superior. Figure 12.7 shows a high-contrast T_1-weighted axial image of the brain in which the contrast between gray and white matter is very high. This can be clinically important in a number of diseases, for example epilepsy.

Although MRI is billed as a non-invasive technique, there can be occasions when it is advantageous to inject some chemical agent into the patient to enhance the contrast of the image. Paramagnetic ions are an example because, even at low concentration, they accelerate spin–lattice relaxation by providing intense local magnetic fields that fluctuate near the Larmor frequency. Often the uptake of these 'contrast agents' is specific to a particular tissue type or pathology. The most commonly used relaxation agent is the gadolinium Gd^{3+} ion chelated with diethylenetriamine penta-acetic acid (DTPA), but iron compounds have also been used. Inversion-recovery is probably the most sensitive sequence for exploiting these contrast agents.

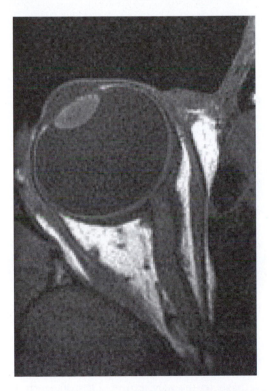

Figure 12.6 A close-up of a 1.5 tesla axial T_1-weighted image of the eye showing the lens, the optic nerve, and the retro-orbital muscles and fat. A 3-inch diameter surface coil was used. The slice thickness was 2 mm and the pixel size was 0.31 × 0.31 mm, which accounts for the high definition. (Image courtesy of Dr Peter Barker, Johns Hopkins University School of Medicine).

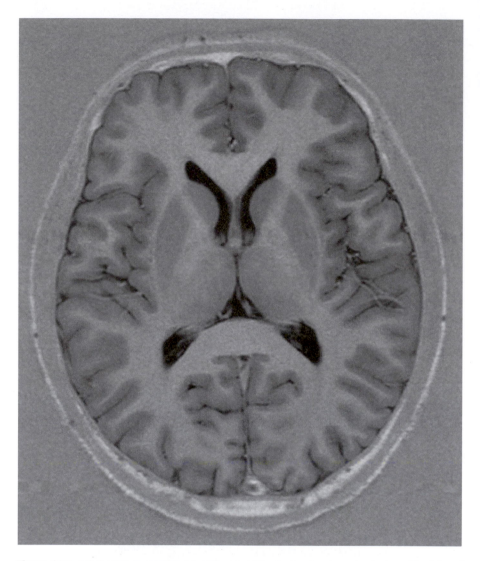

Figure 12.7 A 3.0 tesla T_1-weighted axial image of the brain of a normal volunteer. The interval between spin inversion and signal detection (*TI*) is 400 milliseconds. The field-of-view is 230 × 180 mm, with a slice thickness of 4 mm. Note the high contrast between gray and white matter, based on differences in spin–lattice relaxation. (Image courtesy of Dr Peter Barker, Johns Hopkins University School of Medicine).

Now suppose we have set the recycle time *TR* sufficiently long in comparison with all the spin–lattice relaxation times that all types of protons are close to Boltzmann equilibrium at the time of each new excitation pulse, so all spin populations are roughly the same. We now have a second important parameter at our disposal, the time *TE* between excitation and detection of the first spin echo (Chapter 9). The strength of the spin echo signal depends on how much phase coherence has been lost through spin–spin relaxation during the interval *TE*, as the local magnetic fields from nearby spins upset the precise timekeeping of the nuclear 'clock'. A representative spin–spin relaxation time (T_2) for cerebrospinal fluid is of the order of a second, whereas that of brain white matter is about 90 milliseconds. If we set $TE = 90$ milliseconds, the proton spin echo signal from white matter decreases to roughly 37 % of its initial value, whereas that from CSF diminishes by a negligible amount and consequently appears much brighter on the T_2-weighted image. Contrast has been enhanced, but in the opposite sense to that achieved in the T_1-weighted image mentioned above. Figure 12.8 shows a coronal T_2-weighted image of the brain.

We see that although the instrumental parameters *TR* and *TE* both affect relative signal intensity, judicious choice of one of these variables can ensure that the image contrast is determined principally by T_1 or by T_2. It is not usually a good idea to try to exploit both relaxation mechanisms unless the straightforward contrast methods fail.

12.10 Motion artefacts

In an ideal world, MRS would be practised on a patient where the organs of interest were perfectly motionless. It is more productive to perform MRI scans on patients who are still alive, so we must cope with respiration, heartbeat, blood flow, peristalsis and other involuntary movements. Most imaging protocols are based on the gradient-recalled spin echo, and this is particularly sensitive to changes in the intrinsic precession frequency of a given voxel as it moves from one part of the gradient to another. The result may be loss of signal intensity, blurring or misregistration of the image, or the formation of 'ghost' images. A ghost is a replica of some genuine feature of the image at a displaced position, usually with much lower intensity. Ghost artefacts are displaced in the phase-encoding dimension. They arise from a spurious phase modulation caused by pulsatile blood flow or some periodic translational motion of the spins, for example, movement of the chest wall during respiration. The phenomenon is related to the appearance of spinning sideband responses (§ 6.2) in high-resolution NMR spectroscopy, and as with spinning sidebands, there can be multiple ghosting.

There are several ways to compensate motion artefacts, or at least minimize their impact. Take the case of respiratory motion during imaging of the abdomen, where ghosting is caused by the periodic displacements. The most obvious remedy is to complete the entire imaging sequence while the patient holds his breath. Another method is to synchronize the data gathering with the respiratory cycle, using a pressure transducer to generate a trigger signal, and choosing to acquire data when there is least movement.

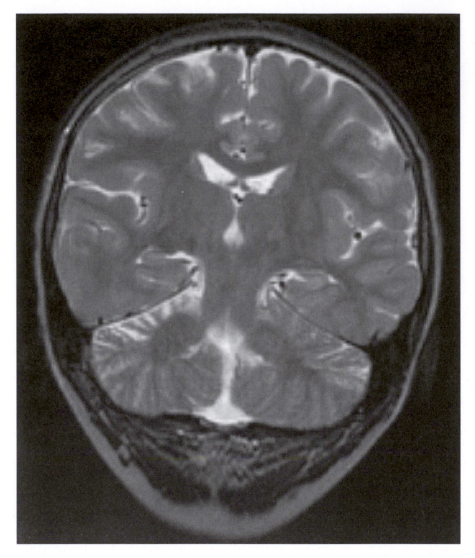

Figure 12.8 A 1.5 tesla T_2-weighted image of the brain obtained by the spin echo technique. This is a coronal section taken towards the back of the head. (Image courtesy of Dr Peter Barker, Johns Hopkins University School of Medicine).

A more sophisticated application acquires images of the beating heart, using an electrocardiogram (ECG) signal for synchronization. An image can be acquired at a fixed interval after the ECG trigger pulse, when the heart has a particular configuration. By varying this delay, a sequence of different images can be obtained, and a video loop can be improvised showing the configuration of the heart at different points of the cardiac cycle. There are obvious problems if the heart rate is irregular. An alternative approach (called retrospective gating) abandons the idea of direct synchronization of data gathering, but uses the trigger pulse as a time-reference to record and store in the computer the instant in the cardiac cycle when each measurement was carried out. This is followed by reorganization of the experimental data to form a sequence of images as a function of the delay after the trigger pulse.

Blood flow can degrade the quality of a magnetic resonance image as a result of two different types of flow phenomena—inflow effects, where the nuclear spins within the volume under investigation are replaced by fresh spins that have undergone a different preparation, and phase effects, where motion through a field gradient spreads out the nuclear precession phases. Both factors are usually at play at the same time. Flow in the readout direction causes a phase dispersal and loss of signal intensity, but the effect can be compensated by a scheme outlined in the next section, where we shall see how the effects of blood flow can be put to good use in a technique known as magnetic resonance angiography, generating 'bright blood' or 'dark blood' images according to the conditions.

Another flow artefact is misregistration, caused by motion in the plane of the image slice. It arises because the spins in a given voxel move during the appreciable time lag between the application of the phase-encoding and readout gradients. If the blood flow has a component in the phase-encoding direction (the y axis), the MRI response corresponds to the y ordinate these spins occupied when they were phase-encoded—not to their y ordinate during readout. The corresponding response from the flowing blood appears to have been slightly displaced in the y dimension of the image.

12.11 Magnetic resonance angiography

The study of blood flow in arteries is known as angiography and has been conventionally investigated by X-rays methods using iodinated contrast agents. Magnetic resonance angiography was discovered by accident. The gradient-recalled echo technique generates undesirable artefacts when there is appreciable motion along the gradient direction. A prime culprit is blood flow. In an attempt to minimize these effects by applying compensating gradients, it was noticed that the images of the blood vessels were enhanced in intensity. This was how the new field of magnetic resonance angiography was born.

First, a few comments about the nature of a flowing liquid. The motion of blood inside a blood vessel can be *laminar*, where the velocity profile across the diameter of the vessel is approximately parabolic, *turbulent* where the profile is irregular, or *pulsatile*, where the velocity varies in a cyclic manner. In general, the faster-flowing blood shows up brightest in the angiogram because these nuclear spins are less subject to saturation. Schemes that highlight the normal laminar flow of blood show a loss in intensity if the ordered flow becomes turbulent due to pathological conditions such as stenoses (narrowing) of the arteries. Occasionally the normal laminar flow can be disrupted into localized vortex flow, for example, at the bifurcation of the carotid artery, and this also reduces the brightness of this region of the image.

There are two techniques that can be used to study blood flow—'time-of-flight' and 'phase contrast' methods, and we consider them in turn. It is many years since I was at high school, but I still have a vivid memory of our gymnastic classes. They were always followed by a ritual visit to the cold showers. These were situated in a short corridor where the shower heads were arranged to spray the entire cross-section, so there was no obvious escape from the very cold water. Fortunately, the flow rate was low, and the accepted practice was to run as quickly as possible through the corridor; anyone who foolishly stood still got *saturated* with freezing water, and was treated with derision.

Time-of-flight angiography is very similar in principle. Within the chosen imaging slice the nuclei are subjected to a rapid sequence of small flip-angle radiofrequency pulses. Because the recycle time TR is short compared with T_1, stationary tissue reaches a steady state of almost complete saturation and generates little magnetic resonance signal. On the other hand, blood flowing into the slice contains spins initially at equilibrium, and if the flow rate is high enough, they experience rather few radiofrequency pulses before leaving the slice; consequently they are only mildly saturated. The result is a 'bright-blood' image where the blood vessels stand out against a dark background from the surrounding tissues. Note the importance of using a small pulse flip angle (our custom of 'running the gauntlet' through the showers would not have worked if the shower heads had worked at full volume).

A related 'dark-blood' technique employs presaturation of the nuclei upstream from the imaging slice. The surrounding tissue generates its normal magnetic resonance response but nuclei in the flowing blood are saturated and produce very little magnetic resonance response. Alternatively the upstream nuclear spins can be prepared by a population inversion followed by a short delay. Since this method is sensitive to the flow direction, it is useful for distinguishing arterial and venous flow. In one rather crude implementation, nuclear spins in the blood flowing through arteries to the brain are saturated by means of a subsidiary radiofrequency coil wound around the neck of the patient.

Unlike X-ray angiography, these MRI time-of-flight measurements do not normally require contrast agents, but if injected relaxation agents such as the gadolinium chelate mentioned in § 12.9 *are* employed, the sensitivity is greatly increased, allowing the duration of the MRI scan to be reduced to a few seconds, which permits temporary suspension of respiration by the patient in order to avoid other motional artefacts.

Phase-contrast angiography is based on an entirely different principle. As outlined in § 9.2, the gradient-recalled echo technique presupposes that the nuclear spins remain stationary throughout the sequence. If there is some concerted flow in the direction of the field gradient, the phase divergence that builds up during the first field gradient pulse is *overcompensated* by the second field gradient pulse because these spins have now moved into a stronger region of the gradient. This leads to a net loss of signal intensity at the first echo. Flow along the gradient direction leads to a *progressive* speeding up or slowing down of the nuclear precession frequencies. However, it is possible to devise a gradient-recalled echo scheme that refocuses not only the stationary spins but also those flowing at a constant velocity. It is based on the fact (initially discovered in high-resolution NMR spectroscopy) that phase errors are compensated on even-numbered echoes (§ 9.8) if a symmetric time-reversed sequence of gradient pulses is used.

We can appreciate how this comes about by considering a vector model in which a typical stationary voxel is represented by the vector S and a typical voxel of flowing spins by the vector F (Figure 12.9). Without prejudice to the argument we can assume that the direction of blood flow is such it carries the flowing spins into a stronger part of the magnetic field gradient (so S and F can also stand for the slow and fast vectors). The precession frequency of the flowing spins continuously accelerates and the phase evolution follows a curved function of time. However, we can simplify the discussion by considering the *mean* rates of precession in each of the four intervals; they are in the ratio $+1: -2: -3: +4$ as the vector F moves successively into more and more intense regions of the imposed

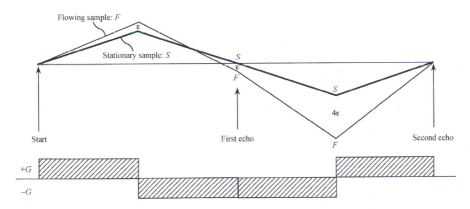

Figure 12.9 Phase evolution diagram demonstrating refocusing on even-numbered echoes. When blood flows through an applied magnetic field gradient there is a progressive change in its precession frequency and the resulting phase shift interferes with the formation of the first gradient-recalled echo. Although the 'well-behaved' stationary isochromat S is refocused at both the first and second echoes, the flowing 'rogue' isochromat F moves into more and more intense local magnetic fields, increasing its mean rate of precession in the ratio $+1: -2: -3: +4$ in the four successive intervals. The alternation in the sense of the applied gradients refocuses the phase error at the time of the second echo. For simplicity, the curvature of the phase evolution graph for the flowing nuclear spins is not shown.

gradients. Figure 12.9 illustrates the precession phases at the end of each interval. We see at once that the vector S representing stationary spins refocuses at the time of both the first and second echoes, as expected. In the first interval the vector F rotates anticlockwise faster than S and accumulates a phase lead of ϵ. The mean rate of precession of F is doubled during the second interval and causes clockwise rotation, so at the time of the first echo F still leads S by a phase angle ϵ. This clockwise rotation accelerates during the third interval and F builds up a phase lead of 4ϵ. During the fourth interval the vector F continues to accelerate, but by rotating anticlockwise, it catches up with the stationary vector S and both are exactly in focus at the time of the second echo. By extension, we see that both stationary and flowing spins contribute fully to all even-numbered echoes. More complex gradient sequences can be devised to compensate for higher-order effects, for example, accelerating or pulsatile flow.

This compensation scheme permits the acquisition of a reference image that is not affected by the blood flow. This reference image is then subtracted from images acquired without flow compensation, leaving a differential display showing only the flowing blood. The experimental parameters for the non-compensated image are adjusted for the maximum flow rate (which gives the brightest regions in the difference image) while slower-moving blood appears less bright. The reason for this precaution is that the primary observable is a phase angle, and there is a critical flow rate beyond which the phase deviation exceeds $360°$. Because a phase angle of, say, $365°$ is indistinguishable from a phase angle of $5°$, aliasing occurs (§ 12.5), causing fast flow rates to appear to be much slower.

As outlined above, phase contrast angiography monitors the component of blood flow in the direction of the applied field gradient. However, when the measurement is repeated with gradients along the other two Cartesian axes, we have all the information necessary to calculate the flow in any desired direction. This serves to remind us of an important physiological fact—the vascular system is seldom confined to a single imaging slice but extends in all three dimensions of space. This complicates the determination of flow rates unless they happen to be parallel to one of the field gradient directions. Flow at right angles to the field gradient would render this section of the vasculature invisible.

A scheme called 'maximum intensity projection' is employed to tackle this difficulty. If we assemble two-dimensional angiogram slices one behind the other we have essentially a three-dimensional image. We can then choose a viewing direction, and for each parallel 'ray' in this direction the computer selects the brightest pixel and projects it onto a viewing plane normal to the ray (Figure 12.10). In this way the most intense signal is recorded and no part of the vasculature is overlooked, as it might well have been if we had examined only one slice and the flow direction happened to be normal to that slice. The calculation of the maximum intensity projection may then be repeated for different viewing directions and the resulting set of images used to create a video loop in which the three-dimensional angiogram appears to rotate on the screen. This is probably the

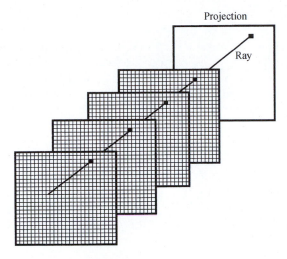

Figure 12.10 Magnetic resonance angiography risks losing track of blood vessels that do not lie in one of the imaging planes. The 'maximum intensity projection' avoids this problem by collecting the strongest magnetic resonance response along each 'ray'. The final projection highlights all the blood vessels so that no part of the angiogram is missed.

most revealing mode of display for a complex three-dimensional structure. While some quantitative intensity information has been sacrificed in the maximum intensity projection, the important point is that it leaves no false gaps in the angiogram. Figure 12.11 shows a maximum intensity projection angiogram of the brain of a patient who has suffered a stroke. There is a stenosis (narrowing) of the left middle cerebral artery (on the right-hand side of the image, indicated by the arrow).

12.12 Diffusion

There is another form of motion that affects spin echo formation—the random movement of the molecules. Each individual molecule in a liquid makes small jumps in random directions due to thermal agitation, an effect called Brownian motion, which can just be made visible under a microscope by sprinkling a fine powder on the surface of the liquid. This haphazard motion of the molecules is quite different from the *concerted* motion treated so far—one step forward is likely to be partly cancelled by the next step in another direction. It is rather like comparing the staggering trajectory of a particularly drunk individual with the purposeful gait of a pursuing policemen. Theoretical treatments of molecular diffusion treat it as a 'random walk' where, for simplicity, the step-length is assumed to be constant.

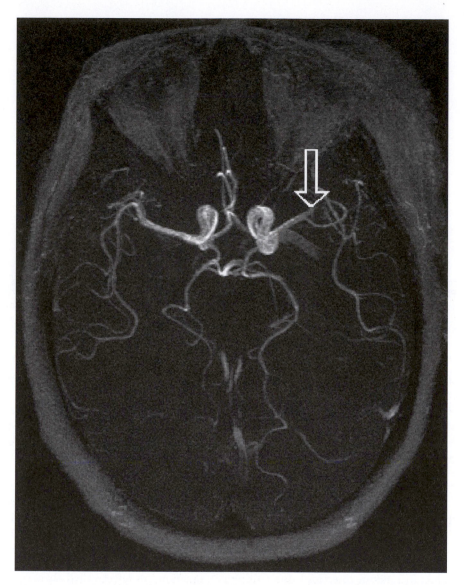

Figure 12.11 Magnetic resonance angiogram of the brain of a stroke patient with a stenosis (narrowing) of the left middle cerebral artery (indicated by the arrow). The 'maximum intensity projection' is shown. In MRI the left side of the patient is always represented by the right side of the image. (Image courtesy of Dr Peter Barker, Johns Hopkins University School of Medicine).

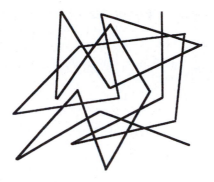

For magnetic resonance applications the net displacement is calculated in just one dimension, the direction of an imposed field gradient. The overall displacement after many jumps increases quite slowly in comparison with bulk motion such as blood flow. Diffusion should be carefully distinguished from *perfusion*, which is treated in Chapter 17.

Diffusion distances are rather small—water molecules normally move only about 20 microns (millionths of a metre) in a tenth of a second. Since this distance is comparable to the dimensions of a typical cell (where the diffusion might be expected to be restricted in some manner) diffusion measurements offer the possibility of probing cell pathology. Diffusion is irreversible and it interferes with the formation of echoes. The rate of diffusion can be measured by exploiting this effect. As described in § 11.12, we apply a pair of gradient pulses of equal duration and amplitude, separated by a fixed interval Δ, with a 180° refocusing pulse at the midpoint of the Δ interval. To be properly refocused by the second gradient pulse, a typical nuclear spin would have to experience a magnetic field *exactly equal* to the field of the first gradient pulse. Diffusion into a slightly different position interferes with this process. The consequent change in precession phase is proportional to the diffusion coefficient, an intrinsic property of the liquid. The experimental observable is a reduction in the intensity of the echo.

In investigations of diffusion, an obvious precaution is to minimize other motional influences that might mask the effect, for example, by employing the flow-compensated sequence described in § 12.10. Much of the clinical research on diffusion has focused on the brain, where cardiac and respiratory motional effects are minimal. The gradient-recalled echo technique probes the diffusion in the direction of the gradient, which may be applied along the x, y and z directions in turn. In this manner diffusion in the white-matter tracts of the brain has been shown to be anisotropic, that is to say, it is faster along the direction of the tracts than it is transverse to them.

Incorporation of a matched pair of gradient pulses into a standard imaging sequence produces a 'diffusion-weighted' image. At first sight this would appear to be counter-productive, reducing the global brightness of the image. But it was discovered that certain types of pathology *restored* the brightness in specific regions of the image by *restricting* the normal diffusion. The case of cerebral ischemia has proved to be the most exciting because changes in the diffusion-weighted image are observed very early after the onset of a stroke, long before T_1- or T_2-weighted images (§ 12.9) show perceptible changes. It is surmised that this may be a result of cell swelling.

12.13 Magnetic resonance microscopy

The exciting new imaging technology described above is not of course limited to scanning the human body. It is often very useful to examine the internal structure of an inanimate object, a small animal or a plant, without having to section it first. Often the samples are physically much smaller than those appropriate to medical imaging, consequently, for the same electric currents, the pulsed magnetic field gradients can be more intense, permitting much higher spatial resolution. However, the resolution is eventually limited by the rate of spin–spin relaxation, and can be degraded by molecular diffusion (§ 12.12) or discontinuities in magnetic suscepti-bility (§ 6.2). In favorable cases it can approach a few micrometres. However, compared with a conventional optical microscope, the resolution of magnetic res-onance microscopy still leaves a lot to be desired and the cost is far higher. The technique comes into its own for applications where the non-invasive feature is crucial, or where the usual NMR tricks can be exploited to achieve an image with high contrast (§ 12.9). Much of materials science is concerned with heterogeneous samples where we would like to learn more about the microstructure.

Translational motion of molecules adversely affects the quality of the image because the movement of nuclear spins through an applied field gradient spreads out the individual precession phases and interferes with the formation of spin echoes. However, as we have seen in (§ 12.11), such effects can be put to good use to monitor molecular motion, be it random or coherent. If the extent of molecular motion differs from one voxel to the next, the pulsed-gradient echo techniques can be used to derive spatial maps that represent velocity information rather than mere intensity. This may reflect macroscopic flow (as in a capillary) or restricted diffusion (as in a biological cell). Molecular motion is interrupted by boundaries within the structure, for example, droplets of oil in a food sample or water within a cell. Many interesting materials involve the motion of fluids through interconnected pores and capillaries, sometimes randomly arranged and sometimes in an approximately regular lattice. In principle all these different motions are susceptible to investigation by magnetic resonance microscopy.

NMR microscopy operates on the same principles as the MRI scanner, but the equipment is more likely to be a high-resolution NMR spectrometer with a narrow-bore superconducting solenoid rather than a modified MRI system. The most critical feature is the set of coils used to generate intense pulsed magnetic field gradients. Gradients are needed in all three spatial dimensions, and they

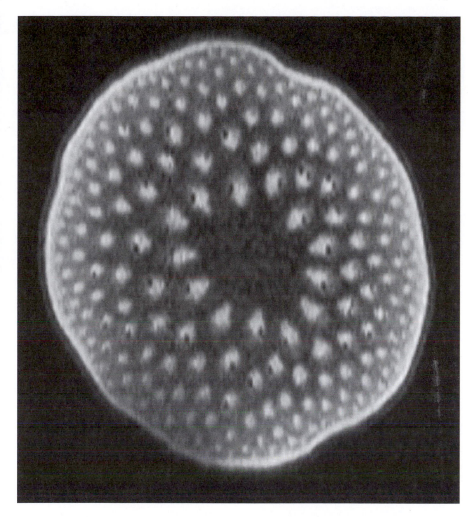

Figure 12.12 Image of an asparagus stalk obtained by NMR microscopy using the spin warp technique. The spatial resolution is 40 microns and the image was obtained in 8 minutes. (Photograph courtesy of Professor Laurie Hall, Laboratory of Medicinal Chemistry, Cambridge).

should be one or two orders of magnitude stronger than those used for medical imaging, necessitating very high stability and reproducibility for precise echo refocusing. Usually these coils are actively shielded to minimize eddy current effects.

We may be tempted to regard manufactured objects, plants or food products as eminently disposable and therefore amenable to investigation by sectioning and conventional microscopy. But this is not always the case; it may be necessary to monitor a sequence of related objects continuously without destroying them. More importantly, the ability to manipulate the contrast of magnetic resonance images according to the relaxation properties or molecular diffusion, makes this form of microscopy particularly attractive in food science and plant physiology. An illustrative example is shown in Figure 12.12, which is a spin warp image of an asparagus stalk with a resolution of 40 microns, showing the detailed internal structure.

Soft matter presents a novel problem in physics, particularly for the response of soft materials to deformation, shear and flow, the science of rheology.[10] NMR can help elucidate the dynamics and alignment of molecules, and when coupled with applied field gradients, NMR microscopy allows these properties to be spatially localized. This has important applications in the study of many polymeric substances. On the macroscopic scale, fluid mechanics can be investigated by monitoring the spatial distribution of the velocity of nuclear spins in an applied magnetic field gradient.

Further reading

P. G. Morris, *Nuclear Magnetic Resonance Imaging in Medicine and Biology*, Oxford University Press, Oxford (1986).

P. T. Callaghan, *Principles of Nuclear Magnetic Resonance Microscopy*, Clarendon Press, Oxford (1991).

M. K. Stehling, R. Turner and P. Mansfield, 'Echo-Planar Imaging: Magnetic Resonance in a Fraction of a Second' *Science*, **254**, 43 (1991).

D. G. Gadian, *NMR and its Applications to Living Systems*, 2nd ed., Oxford University Press, Oxford (1995).

E. D. Becker, C. L. Fisk and C. L. Khetrapal, *Encyclopedia of Nuclear Magnetic Resonance*, Vol. 1: *Historical Perspectives*, Wiley, New York (1996).

M. A. Brown and R. C. Semelka, *MRI Basic Principles and Applications*, 2nd ed., Wiley, New York (1999).

E. M. Haacke, R. W. Brown, M. R. Thompson and R. Venkatesan, *Magnetic Resonance Imaging: Physical Principles and Sequence Design*, Wiley, New York (1999).

13

How safe is magnetic resonance imaging?

Many clinical procedures involve a certain degree of risk to the patient; the justification being that, without them, the consequences to health would be far more serious. The use of X-rays is one well-known example, involving penetration by potentially dangerous ionizing radiation. While MRI is far safer than X-ray methods, it is unusual in that it involves some new kinds of potential hazard— exposure to strong, constant magnetic fields, magnetic field gradients, time-varying magnetic fields, and radiofrequency irradiation. Until relatively recently there was no reason to immerse humans in intense magnetic fields, and there was very little empirical evidence about possible health hazards. Even less information was available on the effects of magnetic field gradients or on time-dependent magnetic fields. On the other hand, the heating effect of radiofrequency and microwave fields is well documented, and they have been used for physiotherapy and in hyperthermia for cancer treatment. Recently, concern has grown about the possible hazard from low-frequency radiation from electric power lines and the radiofrequency radiation emitted by mobile telephones.

There is therefore every reason to investigate the possible adverse effects on a patient undergoing an MRI or MRS examination. There are many *potential* mechanisms whereby radiofrequency irradiation or strong magnetic fields could interact unfavorably with the physiology or biochemistry of the patient, so it is not possible to dismiss the dangers out of hand. Furthermore, it is important to be able to reassure a patient faced with an MRI scan that this large and rather daunting machine poses no risk to his health. There has been some conflicting evidence from different laboratories concerning the potential hazards of MRI, but on the whole it paints a reassuring picture. No one should be deterred from a magnetic resonance scan when it is required for diagnostic reasons.

13.1 The magnetic field

We are all continuously subjected to the very weak Earth's magnetic field, which amounts to roughly 0.5 gauss, depending on location on the Earth. This is a very weak field; we can get a feel for its strength by noting that it can just move the magnetized needle of a compass, provided that it has a reasonably free suspension. The SI (Système International) unit of magnetic field is the tesla, which is equal to 10,000 gauss. Consequently, the magnetic fields used in MRI are four to five orders of magnitude more intense than the Earth's field. The standard used in routine clinical imaging is a magnetic field of 1.5 tesla, and more than 100 million individuals have been examined at this field strength. Experimental work on thousands of human volunteers has been carried out at fields of 3 and 4 tesla, and some recent investigations have employed 8 tesla magnets. The drive towards higher fields is motivated by the increased sensitivity that can be obtained, but this advantage must be offset against the increased cost of a whole-body magnet at high field. In the USA, the Food and Drug Administration has recently changed the regulations to allow clinical imaging at magnetic fields of 3 tesla. (Note that magnets for high-resolution NMR spectroscopy employ fields as high as 23 tesla, but it is easier to generate a high field when the solenoid has a very narrow bore, typically about 50 millimetres.)

The first and most obvious hazard is the strong force acting on ferromagnetic objects in the fringe field of an MRI magnet. Because there is such a large field gradient in this region just outside the magnet itself, iron or steel objects are drawn, often quite violently, from the 'stray' field in the laboratory towards the intense field inside the magnet. It is easy to overlook the danger of some steel tool slipping from the grasp of a technician and flying into the magnet bore. Most people are unaccustomed to the idea of an intense magnetic field; after all, there is nothing they can actually *see*, so there is a tendency to overlook these dangers. With the intense fields that are used in high-resolution NMR laboratories there have been countless tales of gas cylinders or sheets of steel being violently pulled against the superconducting solenoid and damaging the magnet itself. On a more mundane level, credit cards and mechanical wristwatches can easily be ruined if they come too close to the magnet.

A more serious health hazard arises while the patient is being moved through the peripheral field into the magnet bore if he has an implanted device such as an aneurysm clip. Proper screening procedures should reduce such unfortunate incidents to the absolute minimum. Cardiac pacemakers are of particular concern because they normally contain ferromagnetic components and could experience appreciable torques when moved into the main magnetic field. Such patients are almost always excluded from examination by MRI, and in general they are not allowed to enter magnetic resonance laboratories at all. On a less serious note, any internal ferromagnetic device (for example, an orthodontic brace) can so distort the main magnetic field that it renders the image unreliable or even un-usable.

But what is the effect of the steady, intense, uniform magnetic field once the patient is in place? In principle there could be biological consequences if the magnetic field has an appreciable effect on the motion of ions (atoms or mol-ecules that carry an electric charge), but this seems unlikely. A more significant interaction arises from the property known as diamagnetic susceptibility (§ 6.2)— a measure of the ease with which the applied magnetic field penetrates a particu-lar material. The diamagnetic susceptibility of a cell or a cluster of molecules may not be the same in all directions—there is some 'anisotropy'. The intense applied magnetic field then exerts a torque acting to align these units in the direction of the field, but this tendency is rather weak and is opposed by the chaotic thermal motion in a liquid. The partial alignment phenomenon is well documented at the very intense magnetic fields employed in modern high-resolution NMR spectrom-eters, and has been used to study internuclear distances in protein molecules partially oriented in a solution of bicelles (§ 10.6). However, at the far weaker fields currently employed in MRI, the degree of alignment should be very much smaller and most probably negligible in the clinical context.

The MRI technique necessarily involves the application of magnetic field *gradi-ents* superimposed on the uniform field of the magnet. In principle, field gradients can induce relative motion between regions of different magnetic susceptibilities. To take an extreme case, in laboratory experiments *in vitro* very intense field gradients have been used to achieve a physical separation of deoxygenated blood (deoxyhemoglobin is paramagnetic) from normal blood. Even more startling is the 'Moses effect' in which water is enclosed in a horizontal tube and subjected to a very intense magnetic field gradient. The gradient acts on the difference in magnetic susceptibilities of air and water and splits the water into two parts with a void in between, reminiscent of the Biblical account of the parting of the Red Sea. Fortunately such high gradient strengths are not employed in clinical MRI; furthermore any concerted motion, for example blood flow, would inhibit the effect.

There is one interesting and surprising report of an apparent effect of a mag-netic field gradient on the behaviour of rats.[1] A field gradient as high as 13 tesla per metre was generated in the fringe field of a small 4 tesla magnet in one arm of a T-shaped maze, with a mock magnet in the other arm. Presented with this choice, the rats showed a strong aversion (greater than 90 %) to entering the leg of the maze containing the magnet. This suggests some form of nerve stimulation, but the detailed mechanism remains unclear, although there are other species that are known to exploit the Earth's magnetism for orientation purposes.

13.2 Free radical reactions

The human body is known to contain small quantities of some extremely reactive species called free radicals, the result of splitting a stable molecule into two parts. Free radicals are extremely reactive and rather indiscriminate in their choice of target so they are potentially harmful, although the body possesses some defence mechanisms against free radical attack. Under certain conditions, free radicals can initiate chemical reactions that are dependent on the strength of the applied magnetic field. It is just conceivable that in MRI, the main magnetic field might influence the direction of a particular free radical reaction, inducing chemical changes that pose a hazard to the health of the patient. An attack on the DNA (deoxyribonucleic acid) molecule would be particularly serious.

Experimental evidence for the effect of a strong magnetic field on free-radical reactions comes from high-resolution NMR spectroscopy, where the phenomenon of 'chemically-induced nuclear polarization' is well known. Most of the studies involve photochemical excitation. In a stable molecule the two electrons that form a chemical bond are paired, that is to say they have opposite orientations with respect to the direction of the field. This is known as a 'singlet state'. Absorption of light can break the chemical bond, splitting the molecule into two free radicals. Instead of recombining at once, they may become separated and wander about, repeatedly colliding with solvent molecules. They do not part company entirely but remain trapped in a 'cage' of solvent molecules for quite long periods, undergoing many collisions before they come together again.

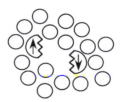

We now extend the interpretation of a 'singlet state' to this pair of radicals. Even though separated by an appreciable distance, the two trapped radicals remain in this singlet state unless there is some further magnetic perturbation. At some later time they may collide again and recombine to form the original molecule; a process known as 'geminate recombination'. On the other hand, during the trapping period, a singlet-to-triplet conversion may occur:

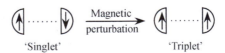

The probability of such a change depends on the interaction (the 'hyperfine coupling') between the electron spin and any magnetic nucleus in the radicals, on the strength of the applied magnetic field, and on the time for which the radical pair remains trapped in the solvent cage. When two free radicals in a triplet state collide, they cannot form a chemical bond. These 'impotent' radicals eventually escape from the solvent cage and attack some other chemical entity, forming a *different* product. In this manner the course of a chemical reaction can be tipped in one of two possible directions, generating 'cage' or 'escape' products, depending, among other things, on the strength of the magnetic field. In high-resolution NMR, this phenomenon can easily be monitored by observing some anomalous intensities in the resulting spectrum.

Now, apart from the effect of sunlight on the skin, it is unlikely that photochemistry is involved during an MRI examination, but the human body contains millions of free radicals, and we cannot entirely rule out a similar field-dependent steering of a chemical reaction when a patient is immersed in a strong magnetic field. No human physiological effects of chemically induced nuclear polarization have been established to date, but a remote possibility certainly exists, and the consequences could be quite subtle.

13.3 Time-varying magnetic fields

Magnets for MRI examinations are now almost exclusively superconducting solenoids, where the energizing coils are maintained at a very low temperature by a liquid helium bath surrounded by a second container filled with liquid nitrogen (§ 2.2). An intense electrical current continually flows in these coils. There is a danger, admittedly very small, that such a magnet might 'quench', that is to say, lose its superconductivity in a catastrophic event. The main magnetic field collapses from a very high value to near zero over a period of the order of ten seconds. The intense electric current flows through windings that have now become resistive, creating a large amount of heat which boils off the cryogenic liquids over a period of about half a minute, releasing large quantities of helium and nitrogen gases. The magnitude of this problem increases with the strength of the magnetic field and the physical size of the superconducting magnet. If a quench should occur while a patient is inside the solenoid, he would be subjected to a rapidly changing intense magnetic field and this might be dangerous. Precautions must also be taken to evacuate the large amounts of helium and nitrogen gases released during the quench to avoid any possible danger of asphyxiation.

There is one well-known physiological effect of the intense field of the MRI magnet—patients can experience vertigo, and sometimes nausea, as a result of rapid head movements. This seems to be caused by eddy current effects in the canals of the middle ear, misinterpreted by the brain, and causing confusion with the visual signals that provide information about motion of the head. The obvious remedy is to limit head motion by physical restraints, or to persuade the patient to make only slow movements of the head while in the magnet.

Spatial encoding in MRI necessarily involves pulsed field gradients (§ 12.2). It is the time-dependence of these gradients that constitutes a potential hazard. The most obvious manifestation is the loud noise generated by the gradient switching. A gradient coil carrying a switched electric current in an intense field acts in a similar manner to a loud speaker. The patient can hear the complex sequences of gradient switching used for the MRI investigations. The sound level is minimized by embedding the coils in a plastic material that limits their motion, but it is nevertheless appreciable and can routinely reach as high as 70–80 decibels, even higher for some gradient switching sequences. Even when ear protection is used, this noise can be quite disconcerting to the patient.

'Faraday induction' describes the generation of an electrical current in a conductor placed in a time-varying magnetic field. There are several possible conductive paths within the human body but they are very difficult to quantify. Two different direct physiological effects have been reported—flashes of light, and some perceived nerve stimulation. The visual sensation has been known for a long time and is sometimes called a 'magnetophosphene'. It is believed to be caused by tiny electrical currents induced in the retina by the pulsed field gradients. Frequencies below 100 Hz are implicated. The effect does not persist after the exposure to the pulsed gradients, and is not thought to be hazardous to health.

Since the time of Galvani it has been known that muscles can be stimulated by an electrical current. The eddy currents induced by pulsed magnetic field gradients certainly cause some nerve stimulation. For example, volunteers reported nerve sensations when their forearms were exposed to gradients changing at a rate of about 200 tesla per second. There has been some concern that switched field gradients might cause cardiac muscle stimulation, or even induce ventricular fibrillation. However, the threshold for such an excitation has been calculated to require rates of change of magnetic field that are an order of magnitude higher than those which cause nerve stimulation, so the latter acts as an early-warning safeguard with respect to any possible hazard to the heart. The recommended upper limit for the rate of change of magnetic field is 20 tesla per second.

There are several other sources of concern about the potential dangers of pulsed field gradients. Particular attention has been focused on the development of the embryo and the fetus, but the evidence from chick embryo experiments is equivocal. Note that there are some imaging protocols that avoid rapid gradient switching by using sinusoidal magnetic field modulation designed to trace out a spiral trajectory in k-space (§ 12.6)

13.4 Radiofrequency heating

It is well known that radiofrequencies or microwaves can heat the body, and local radiofrequency heating has been used in physiotherapy for many years, and in cancer treatment by hyperthermia. (At one point in the Second World War, hospital diathermy units were pressed into service to jam enemy low-frequency radar.) Theoretical calculations of the temperature rise induced by radiofrequency radiation are complicated, since the thermoregulatory effects of blood flow and perspiration are difficult to quantify, but a *specific absorption rate* (SAR) of 4 watts/kg of body weight (averaged over the whole body) is found to cause a core body temperature rise of the order of 1°C. This is taken to be an acceptable upper limit. There may be an associated slight increase in heart rate as the blood flow to the skin is increased to assist cooling through perspiration. These considerations apply to whole body imaging, but note that the use of surface coils (§ 14.3), which have very non-uniform radiofrequency fields, could be more hazardous because they induce quite localized heating effects. At higher frequencies, conductivity effects begin to act as a shield to penetration by the radiofrequency field. In the context of metallic conductors, electrical engineers call this the 'skin effect', which is confusing for a clinician.

Care should therefore be exercised in MRI to limit the specific absorption rate of radiofrequency energy and the duration of the patient's exposure. Organs that lack cooling by perfusion, such as the eyes, or organs that normally operate at a lower temperature, such as the testes, are particularly sensitive to any imposed radiofrequency heating. Research at 1.5 tesla[1] indicated only minor increases in corneal temperature with no hazard to ocular tissue. Another investigation[2] found that the scrotal skin temperature rise in human patients was below the threshold for affecting the testicular function. On the other hand, experiments on rats using prolonged high exposure to radiofrequencies resulted in transient infertility. Particular attention should be paid to patients with a health condition (hypertension or cardiovascular disease) or those on medication. Some concern has been directed to the possible hazards of radiofrequency heating to human embryonic development.

In high-resolution NMR spectroscopy analogous problems of radiofrequency heating are encountered during broadband decoupling experiments (§ 8.5) and some MRS experiments employ decoupling (Chapter 14). For most situations the efficiency of decoupling increases with radiofrequency power, and in high-resolution NMR there is an ever-present danger that delicate samples (such as proteins) can be modified or destroyed. Because radiofrequency heating takes place throughout the active sample volume, an external stream of cold air or nitrogen is not particularly effective as a cooling method, just as perspiration has its limitations for cooling the human body. In MRS, decoupling is probably the most serious heating effect, because the radiofrequency power is relatively high and it is applied continuously, whereas most pulse sequences involve intermittent irradiation. The thermal effect is likely to be highest in experiments that involve carbon-13 decoupling because the irradiation has to cover the wide range of carbon chemical shifts. The problem increases if the magnetic field is increased to 4 tesla or even 8 tesla, since the chemical shift range increases in proportion. The remedy is to employ more efficient decoupling techniques, for example, adiabatic frequency-sweep decoupling (§ 8.5). These methods achieve decoupling over a wide band of frequencies with far less heating.

13.5 Conclusions

Of the three physical phenomena outlined above, radiofrequency heating appears to be the most serious potential health hazard. Regulatory guidelines suggest a maximum core body temperature rise of 1°C, corresponding to a specific absorption rate of radiofrequency energy of about 4 watts/kg of body weight. Higher specific absorption rates may be tolerated for shorter durations, provided that the temperature increase remains below 1°C. Pulsed magnetic field gradients constitute the next most serious hazard. Intense gradients and high switching rates can cause visual artefacts and painful nerve stimulation, but appear unlikely to prove dangerous to the heart function. Finally, the constant intense field of the magnet appears to be the most innocuous factor of the three, provided that care is taken with respect to implants, and the use of iron or steel objects in the MRI laboratory.

There have been literally hundreds of animal and human studies seeking to detect adverse effects of clinical MRI. The *vast majority* report no significant effect on blood flow, blood pressure, heart rate, bone marrow, carcinogenic effects, respiratory function, sperm, egg, ovarian or embryo development, growth rate, genetic damage, behaviour, memory or cognitive function. These widespread negative findings tend to focus attention on a very small number of positive indications. Studies on rats[3] indicated inhibition of morphine-induced analgesia. Mice with tumours kept in a magnetic field of 2.35 tesla showed an apparently increased immune response, demonstrated by longer latency and smaller tumours.[4] Many other claims for real effects have not been substantiated by later research.

The positive findings for humans during routine MRI scans suggest that the principal potential hazards are slight peripheral nerve stimulation, possible temporary hearing loss due to loud noises from gradient switching, slight nausea and vertigo attributable to head movement, and isolated cases of patient burns, possibly due to metallic implants. All of these appear to be avoidable, and none seem to pose a serious threat to the well-being of the patient. Clearly MRI involves some small degree of risk, but the medical benefits far outweigh the hazards.

Further reading

P. Mansfield and I. L. Pykett, Biological and Medical Imaging by NMR, *J. Magn. Reson.* **29**, 355 (1978).

P. G. Morris, *Nuclear Magnetic Resonance Imaging in Medicine and Biology*, Clarendon Press, Oxford (1986).

R. Magin and B. Persson (eds.), *Biological Effects and Safety Aspects of Nuclear Magnetic Resonance Imaging and Spectroscopy*, New York Academy of Sciences 285 (1991).

A. Kangarlu and P-M. L. Robitaille, *Biological Effects and Health Implications in Magnetic Resonance Imaging, Concepts in Magnetic Resonance*, **12**, 321 (2000).

Website: www.mrisafety.com

14

Magnetic resonance spectroscopy

The most useful and immediate impact of magnetic resonance in medicine has undoubtedly been the ability to display images of living systems (MRI) but some scientists are more excited about an alternative avenue of research—the non-invasive study of biochemistry within the human body. This is now generally referred to as MRS, or sometimes *in vivo* spectroscopy. The basic principle is very simple—focus attention on a restricted volume within a particular organ of the body and then study the high-resolution NMR spectrum from that site. The way in which that spectrum changes with variations in metabolism, disease, or drug treatment affords an unprecedented insight into human biochemistry. Unlike MRI, *in vivo* spectroscopy appears to offer the possibility of suggesting biochemical treatments for disease rather than merely a diagnosis of pathology. Progress in MRS has however been slower than in MRI, probably because the technical problems have been more severe. Magnetic resonance imaging quickly achieved widespread acceptance because it promised better pictures than the well-established X-ray methods; *in vivo* spectroscopy had no true forerunner at all.

14.1 NMR spectra *in vivo*

High resolution NMR works very well when the sample is homogeneous, reasonably pure, and is small enough to be enclosed in a simple radiofrequency coil. The technique is less successful when the sample is grossly heterogeneous, very large, and is made up of many different chemical compounds. For these reasons the early investigations of the biochemistry within the human body by proton NMR achieved only limited success. The biomolecules involved are very large, with very complex proton NMR spectra, and they exist in a rich soup containing hundreds of different substances, some in very low concentrations. The sample is heterogeneous, and access to the internal organs of interest is difficult. Although good progress was made in the study of isolated body fluids *in vitro* (Chapter 15), high resolution NMR *in vivo* was found to be much more demanding. Yet the prospect of studying human biochemistry by a non-invasive method is very attractive indeed.

14.2 Phosphorus spectra

The first breakthrough occurred with the discovery that *in vivo* spectra of phosphorus-31 comprise only a relatively small number of different resonances, and the individual lines are reasonably well-resolved, giving rather simple 'fingerprints' of the range of metabolites involved.[1] The interpretation of these phosphorus spectra is therefore rather straightforward (Figure 14.1). The chemical shifts are quite large and their variation between samples rather small, so the resonance peaks can be assigned by comparison with reference spectra. In most situations one can see strong responses from inorganic phosphate (Pi), phosphocreatine (PCr) and the three resonances from adenosine triphosphate (ATP). The early studies concentrated on the relative intensities of these metabolites, and to a lesser extent on the displacement of the frequency of the inorganic phosphate signal as the chemical exchange equilibrium is altered by the generation of lactic acid (§ 7.8). Only the signals from mobile components give narrow resonance responses; the largely immobilized membrane phospholipids normally have only broad responses that merely distort the baseline of the phosphorus spectrum.

The phosphorus-31 nucleus is 100% abundant in nature and its gyromagnetic ratio is roughly 40% of that of the proton, but because MRS involves metabolites at rather low concentrations, the high-resolution NMR spectra are quite noisy. This has encouraged the use of higher magnetic fields than those currently employed for MRI. Proton broadband decoupling slightly improves both sensitivity and resolution of phosphorus spectra but care must be taken to minimize radiofrequency heating effects from the decoupler (§ 13.4) Initially these phosphorus-31 investigations were performed *in vitro* because no one relished the idea of surgically inserting a radiofrequency coil inside the human body. This was all changed with the introduction of the *surface coil* (§ 3.2), a flat radiofrequency coil placed on the surface of the patient or animal.[2]

14.3 Surface coils

Two factors are important in determining the NMR signal detected from nuclear spins at a particular point in space. One is the intensity of the radiofrequency

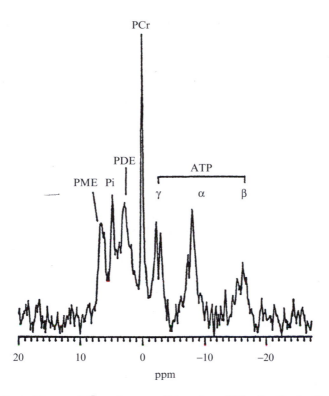

Figure 14.1 Magnetic resonance spectroscopy of phosphorus-31 in a localized region of the brain, showing peaks from phosphomonoester (PME), inorganic phosphate (Pi), phosphodiester (PDE), phosphocreatine (PCr) and three chemically shifted peaks from adenosine triphosphate (ATP). (Spectrum courtesy of Brian Ross).

field generated by the coil at that particular location, and the other is the coupling of the excited nuclear spins back to the coil. If we are using a single coil rather than a crossed coil arrangement (§ 3.2) these 'transmit' and 'receive' functions follow the same geometrical dependence. As would be expected, a radiofrequency solenoid generates an intense radiofrequency field (and strong coupling) in the enclosed volume, and a diminishing field (and coupling) above and below the coil windings.

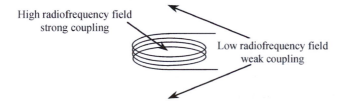

A 'flat' coil, with a high ratio of diameter to length, nevertheless excites and picks up detectable NMR signals from regions above and below the plane of the coil. When such a coil is placed on the surface of the body, the detection efficiency is rather low because much of the radiofrequency field is 'wasted' on the immediate surface layer which is of little interest, or the opposite side of the coil where there is no sample at all. Adequate phosphorus MRS signals can nevertheless be detected at a depth of the order of the coil radius.

At first these investigations concentrated on observing signals from the muscles in the limbs, but soon they were extended to the heart, kidneys, and liver—in fact any part of the anatomy with sufficient coupling to an external radiofrequency coil. The field of view is determined principally by the radius of the surface coil. Special pulse sequences can be designed to vary the depth at which the maximum signal response is detected, or to minimize the signal from subcutaneous fat. Flexible surface coils have been designed that wrap around any convex feature to give a snug fit. It is even possible to design an array of small surface coils that operate in unison to examine an extended feature, such as the spine (Figure 3.1(d)). But when all is said and done, the surface coil is a rough-and-ready method of spatial localization. Its main advantages are its simplicity and flexibility.

In investigations of localized spectroscopy using a surface coil, the active volume of the sample is poorly defined; it is rather like gazing into a pond and trying to estimate how many fish there are—our perception falls off quite slowly with depth and with radial distance from the eye, so the count can never be more than a very rough approximation. Consequently, the *absolute* intensities of the responses in MRS *in vivo* have little significance. On the other hand, the *relative* intensities can be very useful. Usually there is little scope for inserting a separate reference material of known concentration, so recourse is made to the ratios of the intensities of certain chosen resonance lines, for example, the ratio of the phosphocreatine response to that of inorganic phosphate for phosphorus spectra.

A surface coil is not always the most efficient device for MRI or for detecting NMR signals *in vivo*. Specialized radiofrequency coils have been developed to *enclose* the head or a limb, exploiting the high detection sensitivity for MRS signals from the region inside the windings. Complex structures, such as the 'birdcage coil' have been constructed to ensure that the radiofrequency field inside the coil is as uniform as possible (§ 3.2). They are widely used for MRI scans of the head, for example. The disadvantage of such large coils for MRS is that localization has to be achieved by specialized pulse sequences (§ 14.5).

Animal studies make possible a more drastic approach. Cardiac metabolism in the rat has been investigated by excising the beating rat heart and suitably perfusing it while enclosed inside a purpose-built solenoid coil. Measurements can be made in the high magnetic field (and narrow bore) of a superconducting magnet intended for high-resolution NMR spectroscopy. The coil filling factor is high and the signal-to-noise ratio for phosphorus-31 quite adequate for the purpose. The high-resolution spectra can be monitored to study the pathology of the cardiac function.

While MRI is now an established 'routine' clinical practice, MRS remains much more exploratory. The measurements are made on volunteers and are therefore not subject to the restrictive ethical protocols of MRI. For this reason it is possible to work at higher magnet field strengths (for example 4.7 tesla) where the detection sensitivity is higher and the chemical shift range proportionately expanded. Unfortunately a whole-body magnet at 4.7 tesla is very large and expensive, and the stray field extends an appreciable distance outside the main coil windings, so precautions must be taken to prevent passers-by entering this fringe field where a heart pacemaker might be adversely affected. Many investigations have to 'make do' with the 1.5 tesla magnets built for imaging purposes.

14.4 Other nuclear species

As the technology evolved, and with the advent of higher-field magnets, the intrinsic sensitivity of MRS improved, and high-resolution *proton* spectra became amenable to study. Proton spectra are far richer in information than phosphorus spectra, provided that the resonances of interest are well-resolved and can be reliably assigned to the chemical compounds involved. Proton studies benefit from higher metabolite concentrations and more favorable relaxation parameters than phosphorus-31, and much of the interest has now shifted towards proton MRS, particularly of the brain. Apart from the enormous intrinsic interest in brain pathology, the cerebrum has the advantage of being immune to the motion artefacts that can affect magnetic resonance studies of many other organs of the human body. Today, proton MRS has largely superseded phosphorus-31 spectroscopy.

Special techniques, for example selective presaturation, are employed to suppress the intense proton signal from water which could otherwise interfere with the signals of interest (§ 3.6). In the brain, the strongest metabolite signals are generated by N-acetyl aspartate (NAA), creatine and phosphocreatine, choline, and myo-inositol (mI). Creatine and phosphocreatine give a composite peak that is sometimes used as an intensity reference. Glutamine and glutamate give overlapping responses unless high fields are used. The signal from lactate is usually below the detection threshold but its intensity can increase significantly in ischemia, brain tumours and other abnormalities. Occasionally that alien substance ethanol can be detected in brain spectra.

Although surface coils can be used to investigate metabolites in the brain, better spatial specificity is achieved by one of the localization schemes described below (§ 14.5) where the magnetic resonance response is elicited from a single voxel. To obtain an acceptable signal-to-noise ratio this voxel is often quite large, for example, a cube of side 2 cm; reducing this to a 1 cm cube would excite eight times fewer spins and degrade the signal-to-noise ratio by a similar factor.

Let us examine here just one illustrative application of proton MRS. Intensity ratio measurements of brain metabolites appear to indicate a diagnostic role for

MRS in monitoring the progression of Alzheimer's disease and for following its response to drug treatment. To quantify the intensities of the proton resonances, the strong peak at 3.03 ppm, representing phosphocreatine plus creatine (Cr), is usually chosen as the standard because this has the most stable concentration, although it does change in certain pathologies. One useful parameter is the ratio of N-acetyl aspartate (NAA) to creatine measured for a set of normal adults. This ratio is typically about 1.4, but can be 10 to 20% higher for children and 10 to 20% lower for elderly patients. Another parameter is the ratio of myo-inositol (mI) to creatine which has a typical value of 0.6 and is not significantly dependent on age. The volume of interest for the spectroscopic study is chosen from an MRI brain scan, concentrating on an occipito-parietal white matter region or on an occipital grey matter location. In order to present the MRS results in a form suited to diagnosis (or ruling out) Alzheimer's disease, a 'nomogram' can be plotted where the horizontal axis is the ratio NAA/Cr and the vertical axis the ratio mI/Cr (Figure 14.2). The points on this scatter-plot for normal elderly patients fall in the lower right-hand corner, whereas those from patients suffering from Alzheimer's disease fall in the upper left-hand corner, corresponding to reduced NAA and increased mI. Although there is not an entirely clear-cut distinction between these two possible diagnoses, proton MRS provides a relatively simple and rapid test for this distressing medical condition.

As the technology has improved, other nuclear species have been employed for localized MRS. Proton-decoupled carbon-13 and nitrogen-15 nuclei provide well-resolved spectra because the chemical shifts are large. The low intrinsic sensitivity of these nuclei can be offset by signal enhancement by the nuclear Overhauser effect

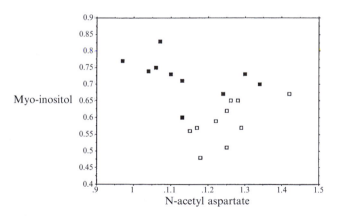

Figure 14.2 A scatter-plot in which the intensity of the myo-inositol peak from the proton NMR spectrum of the brain is plotted against the intensity of the N-acetyl aspartate peak, both normalized to the intensity of the creatine peak. Results from normal patients (open squares) can usually be distinguished from those of patients suffering from Alzheimer's disease (filled squares). (Diagram courtesy of Brian Ross).

(§ 4.3) and more importantly by infusion of isotopically enriched compounds such as carbon-13-labelled glucose or nitrogen-15-labelled ammonium acetate. Isotopic enrichment has the important practical advantage that the very weak background responses from naturally-abundant carbon-13 or nitrogen-15 nuclei can then be safely disregarded.

Even in natural abundance, carbon-13 spectroscopy can be successfully applied to studies of metabolism *in vivo*. A practical example is provided by a recent investigation by Blüml[3] of Canavan disease, a rare inborn brain disorder due to a deficiency of aspartoacylase, resulting in demyelination with megalocephaly, blindness, spasticity, and death within the first few years of life. The proton-decoupled carbon-13 spectrum from a selected region of the brain of a Canavan disease patient (Figure 14.3) shows elevated levels of NAA (+50%) and mI and a striking reduction in glutamate (to 46%) when compared with a control spectrum (not shown). This may be a result of the sequestration of aspartate in NAA and the reduction of free aspartate (synthesized from glutamate). Clearly natural-abundance carbon-13 spectroscopy has much to offer.

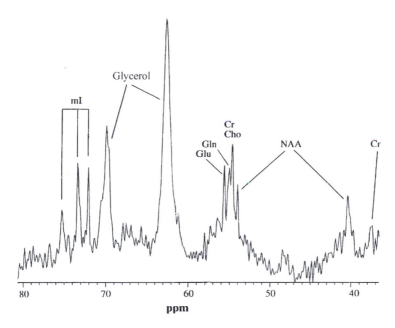

Figure 14.3 Part of the 1.5 tesla proton-decoupled carbon-13 spectrum from the brain of a young patient with Canavan disease. Compared with a normal control spectrum (not shown), the levels of myo-inositol (mI) and N-acetyl aspartate (NAA) are increased, whereas glutamate (Glu) is markedly decreased. The remaining metabolite signals are from glutamine (Gln), creatine (Cr) and choline (Cho). (Reproduced from S. Blüml, *J. Magn. Reson.* **136**, 219 (1999) by permission of Academic Press.)

14.5 Localization techniques

When the radiofrequency coil completely encloses the sample of interest, (for example, the head) some alternative method of localization is required, otherwise we would see a composite signal arising from all material within the enclosed volume of the coil, having little diagnostic value. We need to focus attention on a particular region, so this is often called the 'single voxel' method. This is achieved by designing a pulse sequence that suppresses all signals except those from the designated volume of interest.

These spatial localization techniques employ frequency-selective radiofrequency pulses (§ 2.9) acting in applied magnetic field gradients, and they define the volume of interest as the intersection of three orthogonal slices through the sample. The first stage is the well-known slice-selection operation used in most imaging protocols (§ 12.3). Suppose this slice is in the xy plane. After a second stage of slice selection (in the yz plane) the only remaining response is from a thin strip running in the y dimension (Figure 14.4). The third stage of slice selection (in the xz plane) picks out the signal from a short section of this long strip and rejects the rest. The intersection of the three orthogonal slices has thus defined a small 'box' where the NMR signals are reinforced; in all other regions the signals are cancelled. This box has the shape of a cube if the frequency selectivity is the same in all three dimensions, and it can be moved at will by choosing the appropriate frequencies for the three selective pulses.

We can appreciate that this is a much more precise method of spatial localization than the use of a surface coil, allowing attention to be focused on the most interesting region of the organ in question, with quite sharp transitions to near-

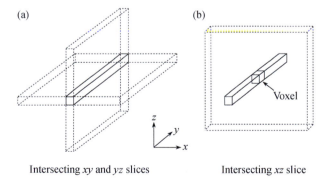

(a)   (b)

Voxel

Intersecting xy and yz slices   Intersecting xz slice

Figure 14.4 The principle of spatial localization by the 'single voxel' technique. (a) Slice selection in a z gradient followed by slice selection in an x gradient suppresses all signals except those within a thin strip running in the y dimension, at the intersection of xy and yz slices. (b) Subsequent slice selection in a y gradient further restricts the signal to a small 'box' where the xz slice intersects the y strip. The three orthogonal slices can be moved independently to position the active voxel at any desired location.

zero signal outside the designated volume of interest. This volume can be expanded so as to enclose a larger number of nuclear spins if sensitivity is at a premium, or made smaller to achieve higher spatial resolution. For example, the relatively low intrinsic sensitivity of phosphorus MRS of the brain typically requires a minimum voxel size of $3 \times 3 \times 3$ cm, whereas a high-resolution proton spectrum can be obtained with a voxel size of the order of $1 \times 1 \times 1$ cm. Three commonly-used sequences, ISIS, PRESS and STEAM, are outlined here; we start with a description of the ISIS technique on the grounds that it is the most simple conceptually.

14.6 ISIS (Image-selected *in vivo* spectroscopy)

This method exploits a well-known magnetic resonance trick—taking the difference between the responses from two successive scans, one of which has been perturbed in a selective fashion. The ISIS technique[4] employs a radiofrequency pulse that prepares the system by inverting the nuclear spin populations in just one restricted region. It is a frequency-selective 180° pulse operating in an applied magnetic field gradient. Most of the nuclei in the sample are too far from resonance to be influenced by the 180° pulse; only those very close to exact resonance are inverted (§ 12.3). The first scan employs the usual 'hard' radiofrequency pulse to excite the NMR response from the entire sample, whereas in the second scan, excitation is preceded by a selective population inversion pulse. The difference between these two signals represents the response from this selected region while all other signals cancel because they are identical in both scans.

The selective pulse is shaped so as to give an approximately rectangular profile in the frequency domain. In the time domain its envelope is usually a sinc function truncated at the second zero-crossing points (§ 12.3). Let us suppose that a magnetic field gradient has been applied along the x direction. We can imagine the sample divided into a set of parallel slices normal to the x axis, each slice being labelled with its characteristic NMR frequency, determined by the value of the magnetic field generated by the x gradient at that position. By choosing the frequency of the selective 180° pulse we can invert the spin population in any one of these slices.

The ISIS sequence is set out in Figure 14.5. To achieve localization in all three spatial dimensions, a threefold extension of the basic 'on/off' sequence is required, with three selective 180° pulses and magnetic field gradients applied successively along the x, y and z directions during the preparation period. After a short interval to allow any eddy currents to decay, the usual hard 90° read pulse is applied. Eight scans are recorded, employing all eight possible on/off combinations of the three selective pulses followed by the appropriate addition and subtraction of the acquired signals.

The advantage of the ISIS technique is its relative insensitivity to signal loss through relaxation, because during the preparation stage it acts on the nuclear spin populations (which can only recover by the relatively slow process of

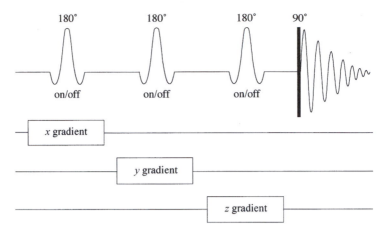

Figure 14.5 The ISIS sequence for spatial localization. A frequency-selective ('soft') 180° radio-frequency pulse applied in a magnetic field gradient inverts the nuclear spin populations in a particular slice through the sample. By difference spectroscopy only the inverted spins contribute to the observed signal. Three successive slice selection operations in the *x*, *y* and *z* dimensions limit the response to nuclear spins within a small 'box' defined by the intersection of the three orthogonal slices. The coordinates of this box can be changed by selecting the appropriate frequencies of the soft pulses.

spin–lattice relaxation) rather than on precessing nuclear magnetization (which decays by the faster spin–spin relaxation). The PRESS method outlined below does not enjoy this advantage. On the other hand, ISIS offers no opportunity to optimize the homogeneity of the main magnetic field while observing the localized signal, because the latter is never observed directly but is only obtained by subtraction. Furthermore, the method assumes that the nuclei remain in place throughout the eight-step cycle, any motion of the nuclear spins through the applied magnetic field gradients would seriously interfere with the subtraction process. For these reasons ISIS has proved to be more useful in phosphorus MRS (where motion is not so critical because the signal is derived from a voxel that forms part of a larger organ with similar properties. Proton studies are more demanding.

14.7 PRESS (Point-resolved spectroscopy)

The PRESS technique[5] also employs the concept of a selective radiofrequency pulse acting in an applied magnetic field gradient, but in this case the first pulse serves to excite the nuclear spins, while the second and third are 180° refocusing pulses designed to form spin echoes (Figure 14.6). Suppose the initial (90°) excitation pulse is applied in the presence of a magnetic field gradient in the *x* direction. Nuclear spins lying within a *yz* slice close to resonance are excited, but all other spins in the sample remain at equilibrium and play no further part (Figure 14.7(a)).

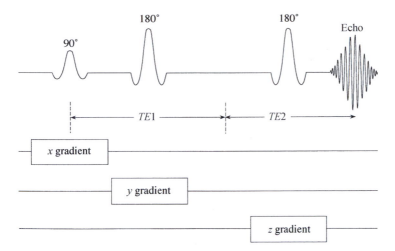

Figure 14.6 The PRESS sequence for spatial localization. The first 90° selective radiofrequency pulse (applied in an x gradient) excites NMR signals from a slice in the yz plane. The next selective 180° radiofrequency pulse (applied in a y gradient) serves to generate a spin echo, restricting it to spins located in a thin strip running in the z dimension. The final selective pulse (applied in a z gradient) generates a second echo from spins confined within a small 'box'.

The next stage of the sequence employs a selective 180° pulse applied in y gradient, forming a spin echo at time TE1. This selects the NMR response from a narrow strip of the sample running in the z direction. Note that in general this strip is parallel to, but not coincident with the z axis; it is offset by an amount determined by the frequency of the selective radiofrequency pulse. The final stage employs a second 180° pulse applied in a z gradient to reduce this strip to a small 'box' of nuclear spins (Figure 14.7(c)). We see that the general principle resembles that of the ISIS sequence—the intersection of three orthogonal planes defines the voxel that is excited.

So how does the echo phenomenon achieve spatial localization? After the initial slice selection, the x gradient is removed and replaced by a y gradient. Within the excitation slice there is now a linear distribution of resonance frequencies, nuclei near one edge of the slice precessing fast compared with those at the centre, while those at the opposite edge precess correspondingly more slowly. When we consider the total signal from the yz slice as a whole, it decays with time as the individual spins get out of phase with one another. We divide the slice into narrow strips running in the z dimension and assign each a small vector to represent the strength of its nuclear magnetization. Initially all these vectors would be aligned along the Y axis of the rotating frame (Figure 14.8(a)). Precession in the applied field gradient has the effect of twisting this distribution of vectors into a helix with essentially zero resultant along the Y axis (Figure 14.8(b)).

Now the selective 180° pulse is applied. Let us suppose for simplicity that it has been suitably shaped so that its frequency profile is rectangular—only nuclear

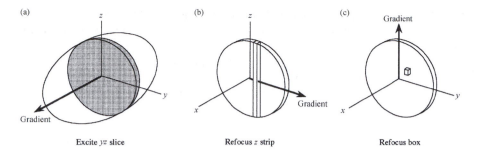

Figure 14.7 Principle of the PRESS technique. (a) The excitation stage in an x gradient defines a slice in the yz plane. (b) Refocusing in a y gradient restricts the spin echo signal to a thin strip running in the z dimension. (c) Refocusing in a z gradient restricts the second spin echo to a small 'box' defined by the intersection of the three orthogonal slices.

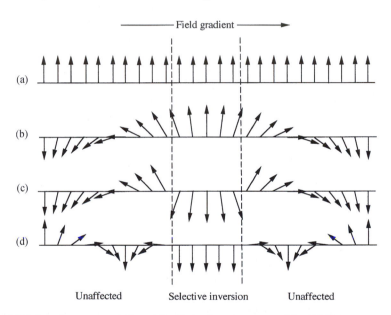

Figure 14.8 A vector representation of the first refocusing stage of the PRESS sequence. (a) All magnetization vectors are initially aligned along the Y axis of the rotating reference frame. (b) The applied field gradient disperses these vectors into a helix with no net resultant. (c) Selective refocusing rotates vectors in the chosen strip by 180° about the X axis. (d) Only these vectors are focused; the rest continue to precess in the same direction and are dispersed along an even tighter helix.

spins close to resonance are inverted, all the rest remain unaffected. We must now consider separately the motion of nuclear spins affected by the refocusing pulse (resonant spins) and those outside its effective range. As in the Carr–Purcell method (§ 9.3), the resonant vectors are rotated through 180° about the X axis (reversing their Y components), while the remainder remain unchanged (Figure 14.8(c)). After the 180° refocusing pulse, the applied y gradient remains in operation, so all the individual vectors continue to precess in the same directions as before. We see that within the chosen thin strip these vectors gradually come into alignment to form a (negative) spin echo (Figure 14.8(d)). All the rest continue precessing as before, twisting into an even tighter helix which induces no net magnetic resonance response.

The time at which a spin echo occurs is usually called 'TE'. Here we have called it $TE1$ because we are about to generate a second spin echo. At time $TE1$ the magnetic field gradient in the y direction is replaced by a gradient in the z direction. The precession frequencies within the selected strip are now spread out along the length of the strip, and, after an interval of free precession, another helix of vectors is created. The second selective 180° pulse refocuses isochromats in only one short region of the strip, generating a second spin echo at time $TE1 + TE2$. This echo represents the NMR signal from a magic 'box' which contains only those spins lying close to resonance for all three radiofrequency pulses. All other nuclear spins give zero resultant signal; either they were not excited initially or they were not refocused by the second or third pulses of the sequence. Exactly as in the ISIS technique, the chosen 'box' may be moved to any location within the sample simply by choosing the frequencies of the three selective pulses. The size of the box is determined by the frequency selectivity of the pulses and the strengths of the applied gradients.

The PRESS technique does not rely on taking differences between the responses from two successive scans, permitting it to be used to optimize the homogeneity of the magnetic field within the chosen box by adjusting the currents in the field correction coils to give maximum response. This is a distinct advantage compared with the ISIS technique. On the other hand, PRESS relies on nuclear magnetization that continues to precess throughout the entire period $TE1 + TE2$, so there is a significant loss through spin–spin relaxation. For this reason PRESS is more suited to proton studies than to phosphorus NMR.

Proton MRS is dogged by the ubiquitous water signal that is so intense that it risks 'swamping' the signals of real interest. For this reason the PRESS technique is usually preceded by a water suppression sequence, often a selective 90° saturation pulse at the water frequency, followed by a 'spoiler' gradient to disperse the transverse components of the water signal. All other resonance remain unaffected.

14.8 STEAM (Stimulated echo acquisition mode)

The stimulated echo has been treated in detail in § 9.6. It has found wide application in the STEAM technique[6] used for localized spectroscopy, where the relative insensitivity to losses through spin–spin relaxation affords a distinct advantage. The STEAM pulse sequence is set out in Figure 14.9. It consists of three frequency-selective 90° radiofrequency pulses that act in magnetic field gradients applied in the x, y and z directions. We saw in § 9.5 that the first two 90° pulses actually refocus only half of the available NMR signal at time *TE*. The famous 'figure-of-eight' distribution of spin isochromats of the Hahn echo can be resolved into 50% transverse magnetization and 50% longitudinal magnetization. The latter component is aligned along the $\pm Z$ axes, stored in two equal parts—a group of isochromats along $+Z$ representing spins at equilibrium, and another group along $-Z$ representing spins that have suffered a population inversion. These two groups may also be characterized by their average precession frequencies which remain the same during the two intervals $\frac{1}{2}$ *TE*. The former are the 'fast' vectors, while the latter are the 'slow' vectors. When the third 90° pulse is applied, these two sets of vectors are brought into the *XY* plane where they are once again free to precess at their characteristic frequencies. The fast group catches up with the slow group at time *TE* + *TM*, forming the 'stimulated echo' along the $-Y$ axis. It has the same sense as the Hahn echo, and if spin–lattice relaxation losses can be neglected, the Hahn echo and the stimulated echo have equal magnitudes.

In analogy with the PRESS scheme described above, the STEAM sequence applies the three frequency-selective pulses in the presence of successive *x*, *y* and *z* gradients, selecting first a slice of the sample in the *yz* plane, then a strip in the *z* direction, and finally a small box—the volume of interest. The frequencies of the selective pulses determine the *x*, *y* and *z* coordinates of this volume of interest; the pulse durations and the strengths of the applied gradients determine the dimensions of the voxel. A high degree of spatial localization implies a relatively low sensitivity for detection.

The key feature of the stimulated echo is the 'time out' interval *TM*, during which all the important information is stored as spin populations, and spin–spin

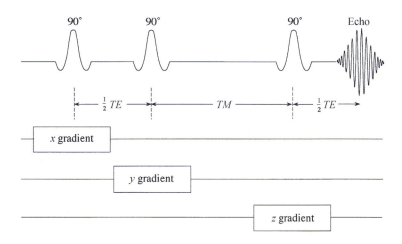

Figure 14.9 The STEAM sequence for spatial localization using three stages of slice selection. As in the Hahn spin echo sequence, the first two selective 90° radiofrequency pulses return some of the nuclear spins to the $\pm Z$ axes of the rotating frame, but only those in a thin strip running in the z dimension. After a period *TM* the third selective 90° pulse generates a 'stimulated echo', but only for nuclear spins in a small 'box' defined by the intersection of the three orthogonal slices.

relaxation has no effect. For many samples of biochemical significance the spin–lattice relaxation time (T_1) is considerably longer than the spin–spin relaxation time T_2. Consequently, for many purposes, we may neglect relaxation losses during the interval *TM*. This makes the STEAM technique preferable to the PRESS scheme for metabolites with relatively fast spin–spin relaxation. However, reliance on the stimulated echo sacrifices half of the available signal.

14.9 Chemical shift imaging

It was tacitly assumed in the imaging chapter that only the proton resonance of water was involved in MRI. In practice this is only an approximation, for the human body also contains appreciable amounts of fatty tissue which gives rise to a second, chemically shifted response (roughly 3.4 ppm from water). The standard MRI sequences cannot distinguish this frequency shift from that imposed by a field gradient. In effect there are two images, one from fat and one from water, displaced from one another in the direction of the applied field gradients. The two images merge only if the imaging gradients are made sufficiently intense that these fields become much stronger than the chemical shift difference, so that the 3.4 ppm frequency displacement between the fat and water signals is hidden inside a single voxel. This unfortunate chemical shift 'artefact' is most evident at the boundaries of the adipose tissue where it can render that region of the image either brighter or darker than it should be.

This phenomenon can be turned to good advantage by deliberately separating the image from one chosen chemical species and suppressing the rest. Called 'chemical shift imaging' or 'spectroscopic imaging'[7] it provides a halfway house between MRS and MRI. It works best at a high applied magnetic field because this spreads out the chemical shifts, making separation easier. The procedure involves slice selection, phase encoding, and frequency encoding, followed by acquisition of the free induction decay in the absence of field gradients. Separation of the signal from the chosen chemical species is achieved by a further stage of Fourier transformation. In a sense, the chemical shifts appear in a fourth frequency dimension. For this reason the measurements are necessarily protracted, but yield a large amount of useful information—in principle one could derive separate maps showing the spatial distribution of all the chosen metabolites within any slice through the sample.

The main limitation is sensitivity. Often we are interested in a minor constituent (at a concentration as low as millimolar) with inherently poor signal-to-noise ratio, so the voxel size has to be large, typically about one centimetre cube, and spatial resolution is reluctantly sacrificed. But the rewards are impressive. For example, a chemical shift image showing only the disposition of choline can be recorded and then superimposed on a conventional proton image of the brain, providing an invaluable insight into brain chemistry. The process of separation can sometimes be improved by specific 'spectral editing' techniques. For example, a 'lactate image' can be obtained by filtration through zero-quantum coherence (§ 11.9), exploiting the fact that lactate consists of spin-coupled protons with a known coupling constant. This discriminates the lactate response from much stronger overlapping lipid signals.

A practical clinical example of proton chemical shift imaging is shown in Figure 14.10. This patient has a disease called 'acute disseminating encephalo-myelitis' that has produced bilateral lesions in the brain. The MRI scan indicates a selected voxel within one lesion (the black box) which gives rise to the abnormal

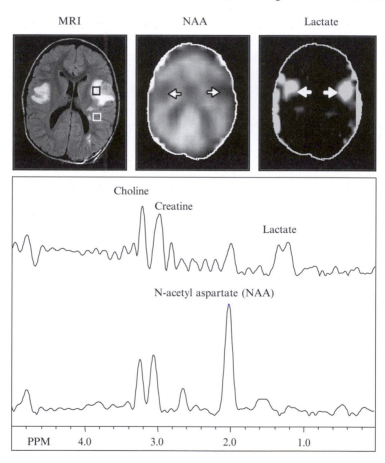

Figure 14.10 MRI scan and chemical shift images for N-acetyl aspartate (NAA) and lactate from the brain of a patient with acute disseminating encephalomyelitis. The lower trace shows the proton NMR spectrum from a voxel in the normal region of the brain (the white box) with a strong signal from NAA but no lactate signal. The upper trace is the spectrum from a voxel located within the lesion (the black box) showing a diminished signal from NAA and an enhanced signal from lactate. (Images and spectra courtesy of Peter Barker.)

proton spectrum (upper trace) where the lactate signal is enhanced and the N-acetylaspartate (NAA) signal is reduced. A voxel in a normal part of the brain (the white box) shows a proton spectrum with a strong NAA signal and no lactate signal (lower trace). Chemical shift images are shown for NAA and lactate, with arrows to indicate the abnormal regions.

Sensitivity constraints restrict most chemical shift imaging applications to nuclei of high natural isotopic abundance (protons or phosphorus) but carbon-13 enriched compounds can be employed in situations where the agent is injected. We may then neglect the carbon signals from all other compounds because they are almost two orders of magnitude weaker. Alternatively, since a carbon nucleus has a large spin–spin coupling to a directly attached proton, the spin echo modulation phenomenon (§ 9.7) can be exploited to detect only those protons adjacent to carbon-13, rejecting all other proton signals. This has been put to good use in the study of brain metabolites.

Further reading

D. G. Gadian, *NMR and its Applications to Living Systems*, Oxford Science Publications, Oxford University Press, Oxford (1995).

M. A. Brown and R. C. Semelka, *MRI: Basic Principles and Applications*, 2nd ed., Wiley-Liss, New York (1999).

E. R. Danielsen and B. D. Ross, *Magnetic Resonance Spectroscopy: Diagnosis of Neurological Diseases*, Marcel Decker, New York (1999).

15

High-resolution NMR of body fluids

Even before the advent of MRI, high-resolution NMR spectroscopists were already exploring applications to human biochemistry. Some of these involved the analysis of human body fluids, which, in many cases, are readily accessible. NMR spectroscopy became yet another high-technology weapon in a well-stocked armoury of clinical tests. A parallel line of research led to the introduction of *in vivo* MRS (Chapter 14). However, the study of biofluids has the advantage over MRS in that the samples are normally isotropic liquids, and far more homogeneous than the organs or tissues of the human body. This makes them more amenable to high-resolution NMR spectroscopy.

15.1 Chemistry and medicine meet

The study of human body fluids is one area where the medical and chemical aspects of magnetic resonance overlap comprehensively. No attempt is made to form an image or to focus on a particular region, instead the method examines internal biochemistry by recording the *in vitro* high-resolution NMR spectra of blood, plasma, bile, urine, milk, saliva, sweat, cerebrospinal fluid, aqueous humour, gastric or pancreatic juices, synovial, amniotic, seminal or prostatic fluids. In most cases, these body fluids can be examined with little alteration—merely the addition of a minimal amount of heavy water for the purpose of field regulation through the deuterium NMR signal (§ 6.2).

Proton NMR spectra have proved the most useful in this context, because sensitivity is an important factor. High-field spectrometers are the most appropriate as they provide good dispersion of the chemical shifts and high sensitivity. One of the main instrumental problems stems from the very intense signal of water. Shortcomings of the analog-to-digital converter (§ 3.6) restrict the attainable dynamic range of the proton spectra so that signals from very weak metabolites are improperly digitized and disappear below the noise level. An effective water suppression technique is therefore essential; there is a vast literature on this subject. Selective presaturation of the water resonance seems to be the most generally favoured technique, achieving suppression factors of the order of 1000. The alternative is to freeze-dry the sample and then reconstitute it in heavy water; in addition this allows the concentration of the sample to be artificially increased.

These spectra have a high information content because the number of components is very large. There is an enormous range of concentrations involved; the detection threshold is of the order of one-tenth of a micromole for some metabolites in the highest-field NMR spectrometers. Low-intensity contributions to the spectrum are so numerous that they are often dismissed as 'chemical noise' that largely outweighs the electronic noise of the instrument itself. Often it is this chemical noise that restricts the achievable sensitivity.

Some biofluids have an almost constant composition, some are affected by diurnal, dietary and hormonal variations, while others, for example urine, are very variable and therefore more difficult to analyse. The spectra may be even more complex for samples where there is compartmentation, partial molecular alignment, or binding of small molecules to macromolecules. The broad lines from macromolecules may be suppressed by spin echo methods, exploiting their fast spin–spin relaxation (§ 4.5). All these factors combine to ensure that a *complete* assignment of the NMR spectrum of a human body fluid is hardly ever possible, but this still leaves a great deal of extremely useful information.

The power of the method lies in the fact that changes in composition of biofluids reflect the influence of toxicity, disease, or drug therapy. A large number of metabolites can be detected simultaneously by a technique that does not itself perturb the relative concentrations. Normally there is a high-resolution spectrum from a control sample available for comparison. Identification of the spectrum of a given metabolite can usually be achieved by addition of a small amount of the pure compound, noting which resonances increase in intensity. Where ambiguities in assignment arise, it is often possible to separate the component spectra in a second frequency dimension (see Chapter 11).

15.2 Blood plasma

Take the case of human blood as an illustrative example. The physical properties of whole blood render it rather unsuitable for direct examination by high-resolution NMR. Some of the interesting spectral information is masked by a broad envelope arising from the presence of paramagnetic molecules derived from haemoglobin, and several macromolecules with broad responses. Furthermore, the spectra may have poor reproducibility owing to erythrocyte sedimentation. The usual procedure is to separate the plasma by centrifuging whole blood, freezing and storing at $-40°$, then thawing again just before the NMR investigation. Usually a small percentage of heavy water is added to provide a deuterium signal for field regulation.

The conventional proton NMR spectra of blood plasma are complex, with many broad overlapping components, but they can be simplified by employing a spin echo method (§ 9.3). This has the effect of delaying the acquisition of the signal (typically for a time of the order of 100 milliseconds), allowing the rapidly-decaying components from macromolecules to be attenuated, but leaving the slowly-decaying components that give rise to sharp NMR responses of the mobile species (§ 4.5). The problem of complexity of conventional blood plasma spectra can be addressed by two-dimensional spectroscopy, for example, techniques such as correlation spectroscopy (COSY) or total correlation spectroscopy (TOCSY), where the information is spread out into the second frequency dimension and where the connectivity through spin–spin coupling is also put to good use (§ 11.5).

There are hundreds of low molecular weight metabolites in blood plasma that can be detected and assigned in a high-field NMR spectrometer. Some of the more intense responses arise from galactose, alanine, glycerol, threonine, glucose, taurine, myo-inositol, choline, histidine, phenylalanine, tyrosine, creatinine, creatine, formate, asparagine, trimethylamine, dimethylamine, aspartate, methylamine, citrate, pyruvate, glutamine, acetoacetate, methionine, glutamate, acetone, proline, acetate, alanine, arginine, lysine, lactate, fucose, 3-hydroxybutyrate, valine, isoleucine, leucine and cholesterol. In addition there are several highly-ordered structures and macromolecules that give rise to broad baseline responses. Some of the interesting metabolites may become undetectable because of binding to a large molecule of low mobility; for example, an appreciable proportion of lactate appears to be 'invisible' for this reason.

As an illustrative example, a partial 750 MHz high-resolution NMR spectrum of human blood plasma[1] is shown in Figure 15.1. The broad contributions from protein and lipoprotein signals have been greatly reduced by employing the Carr–Purcell spin echo sequence (§ 9.3), starting acquisition after a delay of 88 milliseconds to allow appreciable attenuation of these signals by spin–spin relaxation. Resolution enhancement (§ 6.4) has been used to bring out more detail in the central region of the spectrum. Many of the metabolites are identified in Figure 15.1.

This kind of NMR information about the concentration levels of small molecules in blood plasma can be used to monitor metabolic disorders, because disease upsets the control mechanisms that maintain metabolites within their normal concentration ranges. For example, diabetic patients that are not being treated with insulin show increased levels of hydroxybutyrate, acetoacetate, acetone and glucose in their plasma spectra. Furthermore, it is possible to monitor the improvements achieved by changes in diet or by insulin therapy by observing the decrease in intensity of the fatty acid signals.

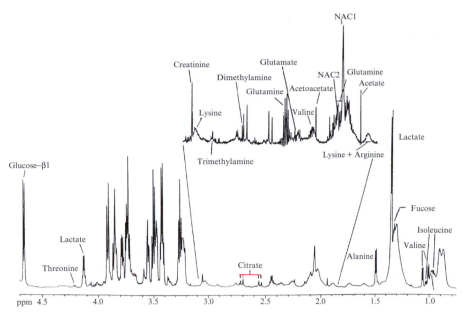

Figure 15.1 Part of the 750 MHz high-resolution proton NMR spectrum of a typical sample of human blood plasma. Broad contributions from proteins and lipids have been minimized by the Carr–Purcell spin echo technique (§ 9.3). Resolution enhancement has been applied to the central region (inset, slightly expanded). NAC1 and NAC2 refer to acetyl signals from a glycoprotein. The congested region between 3.2 and 4.0 ppm contains signals from glycerol, glucose and aminoacid CH protons. (Adapted from J. K. Nicholson et al., *Anal Chem.* **67**, 793 (1995) with permission of the American Chemical Society.)

The long-sought-after Holy Grail would be a definitive test for malignancy by NMR methods. There was a flurry of interest in a proposed test for cancer based on linewidth changes in the high-resolution proton NMR spectrum of blood plasma.[2] It was reported that plasma from patients with malignant tumours showed slightly narrower linewidths for certain proton responses compared with plasma from healthy patients, with intermediate results for patients with benign tumours. The reproducibility of this 'test' was challenged and largely discredited by later investigations, although some cancer patients certainly have unusual NMR spectra in the critical frequency regions. The results are complicated by overlap effects at the resonance frequencies in question. It is possible that future technological improvements may permit a more reliable test to be devised.

15.3 Toxicity

One may lump all foreign substances, toxic or not, into the general term *xenobiotics*. In almost all cases they upset the balance of concentrations of biofluid metabolites in some manner, thus changing the NMR spectrum. In favorable cases these changes characterize the site and mechanism of the xenobiotic action, although the metabolic pathways may be complex and the interpretation quite subtle. One way around this complexity is to treat the NMR information by computer-based pattern recognition techniques, without any attempt at assignment.[3] We can think of the high-resolution NMR spectrum as a multidimensional object where each separate element may change as a result of the toxic insult. Instead of trying to interpret the NMR spectra directly, we are merely looking for the changes in a complicated multiparameter 'fingerprint'.

One such approach is *principal component analysis*, a method that calculates weighted linear combinations of the raw NMR variables (frequencies and intensities) to give new parameters called *principal components*. The latter have the two important properties—they are uncorrelated and they are ordered according to their information content. Thus we may focus attention on the first two or three principal components and ignore the rest. Only this very condensed information is used in the interpretation stage.

An illustrative example comes from a study of toxicity in rats by monitoring metabolite concentrations in the urine. Figure 15.2 shows 600 MHz high-resolution proton spectra of rat urine.[3] The first point to notice is that the spectra from two different control rats are similar but by no means identical, reflecting the known variability of urine samples. When the rats are treated with the toxic compound hydrazine, the urine spectrum shows intense new peaks, primarily from creatine and 2-aminoadipic acid. This tells us something about the sites and mechanism of the toxic process. When the levels of the different metabolites are measured and the results processed by principal component analysis, a graph is constructed showing the first principal component plotted against the second for a series of different toxins. In this illustrative example the points on this scatter-plot form two well-defined clusters—one for toxins that attack the renal cortex, the other for toxins affecting the testes or liver.[4] A more sophisticated cluster analysis is able to differentiate toxins on the basis of the actual site of the lesion within the kidney.

15.4 Disease

As would be expected, the composition of many biofluids changes significantly where disease is present. An important illustrative example is the detection of inborn errors of metabolism in neonatal infants. Here the speed of high-resolution NMR is important because the patient's condition can deteriorate rapidly unless suitable therapy is provided. Taking a urine sample is a quick and non-invasive method for monitoring a wide spectrum of metabolic disorders and it is unlikely that any serious abnormality would be overlooked because so many different metabolites are measured in one shot. Metabolic abnormalities in infants can generate unusually high concentrations of certain compounds in the urine, for example

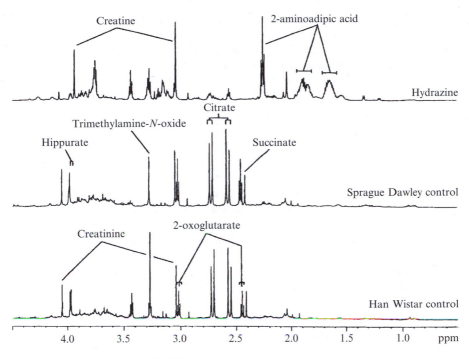

Figure 15.2 High-resolution 600 MHz proton spectra of rat urine, showing the intense new peaks that appear several hours after treatment with the toxic substance hydrazine (top trace). Note the small but significant differences between the spectra of the untreated control rats. (Adapted from J. K. Nicholson, et al., *Xenobiotica*, **29**, 1181 (1999) with permission of Taylor and Francis Ltd http://www.tandf.co.uk/journals.)

trimethylglycine, a feature that might be overlooked in a conventional clinical analysis.

Cerebrospinal fluid (CSF) is a clear, non-viscous liquid that surrounds the spinal cord and supports and protects the brain. It can carry substances from the brain into the blood stream and may transport drugs to the brain. Changes in the composition of CSF provide evidence of damage to the central nervous system. Cerebrospinal fluid normally has a low protein content, making it suitable for simple pulse-acquire NMR spectroscopy, although the spectrum may be contaminated by broad protein responses if there has been serious damage to the brain or an acute infection.

Cerebrospinal fluid is only extracted from a healthy subject when there is good reason, because it involves the delicate invasive technique of lumbar puncture. However, post-mortem samples are a different matter. Samples may be freeze-dried and then reconstituted with a tenfold increase in concentration, thus lowering the NMR detection threshold for minor constituents of the fluid. Many diseases have been studied by this means, one of the more interesting being the distressing condition known as Alzheimer's disease. Post-mortem samples of CSF from diseased and control groups showed significant differences in the high-resolution spectra, the key being the much reduced level of citrate in the Alzheimer's patients, possibly attributable to reduced levels of pyruvate dehydrogenase in the cortex.[5]

15.5 Drug metabolism

Drug metabolites are conventionally studied by introduction of radioactive tracer versions of the drug, but this raises obvious ethical questions about safety for studies on humans. The alternative is to employ chromatographic techniques, but these rely, at least in part, on the ability to predict the course of the metabolism, and it is possible that unexpected metabolites could be overlooked by these methods. High-resolution NMR avoids these difficulties, provided that the metabolite signals are sufficiently intense. The drug itself normally generates a spectrum of many lines, thus constituting a well-defined 'fingerprint', while its related metabolites are also easily recognized.

One advantage of the high-resolution NMR approach is that isotopically enriched drugs can be employed—carbon-13, for example, can be enriched almost 100-fold compared with its natural abundance, and there is no question of radioactivity. Quite complex substances can be partially enriched biogenetically, by feeding suitable organisms with acetate or carbon dioxide enriched in carbon-13. Isotopic enrichment of a drug has the effect of 'highlighting' its mode of operation by making the relevant parts of the carbon-13 spectrum abnormally intense. Carbon-13 acts as a benign 'marker' and drug action of the carbon-13 enriched molecule is in no way different from that of the normal carbon-12 molecule. Similar considerations also apply to enrichment with nitrogen-15.

The power of the NMR method can be enhanced by coupling it to a high-performance liquid chromatograph, where the HPLC eluent flows through the NMR probe continuously. This hyphenated arrangement permits the separation of the spectra of metabolites in a new 'dimension'—the retention time of the chromatography column. An even more sophisticated version[6] bleeds off a small proportion of the eluent (typically 5 %) into an ion-trap mass spectrometer, thus providing complementary evidence for the molecular structures. A related approach separates NMR subspectra as a function of their differing rates of random molecular diffusion (§ 11.12). This 'diffusion-ordered spectroscopy (DOSY)' is particularly valuable for studies of blood plasma where there is a wide range of molecular weights and hence a wide spread of molecular velocities.

The biofluid of choice for monitoring drug metabolism would be urine, since blood plasma samples contain far lower drug concentrations, and the metabolites may bind to proteins and 'disappear' from the spectrum through excessive line broadening. Unfortunately, the sensitivity of the NMR method often proves inadequate for the detection of drugs prescribed in low doses, or where the structure

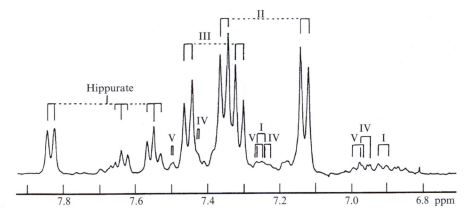

Figure 15.3 Part of the 500 MHz high-resolution NMR spectrum of a human urine sample collected four hours after ingestion of one gram of the analgesic paracetamol (I: N-acetyl-4-aminophenol). The NMR responses of the major metabolites are indicated. II: 4-glucuronosido-acetanilide; III: N-acetyl-4-aminophenolsulphate; IV: N-acetyl-2-(N-acetyl-1-cysteinyl)-4-aminophenol; V: N-acetyl-2-(1-cysteinyl)-4-aminophenol. (Adapted from J. K. Nicholson and I. D. Wilson, *Progress in NMR Spectroscopy*, **21**, 449 (1989) with the permission of Pergamon Press.)

is complex, or there are many different metabolic pathways. Detection of drug overdoses is a different matter, because the concentrations are so much higher. For example, the commonly-used analgesic, paracetamol (N-acetyl-4-aminophenol), is often used in suicide attempts. Its metabolism and excretion in urine for normal therapeutic doses has been well documented.[7] The NMR spectrum of this drug is simple, there are only five major metabolites and they can be detected with a very high reliability. However there are some overlap problems, which are evident in the 500 MHz partial proton NMR spectrum (Figure 15.3) of human urine collected four hours after ingestion of one gram of paracetamol.[8] If necessary, the overlap question can be resolved by two-dimensional correlation spectroscopy (COSY) described in § 11.5, because this picks out the patterns of connectivity. Unfortunately, COSY experiments are time-consuming and not really suitable for routine clinical studies.

Further reading

J. K. Nicholson and I. D Wilson, *Progress in NMR Spectroscopy*, **21**, 449 (1989).

J. C. Lindon, J. K. Nicholson and J. R. Everett, *Annual Reports on NMR Spectroscopy*, G. A. Webb, ed. Academic Press, London (1999).

J. C. Lindon, J. K. Nicholson, E. Holmes and J. R. Everett, *Concepts in Magnetic Resonance*, **12**, 289 (2000).

16

The search for new drugs

The origins of pharmaceutical chemistry are lost in the mists of time, but Chinese traditional medicine certainly stands out as an example of impressive progress through a great deal of hard work over thousands of years. This essentially trial-and-error method has had its successes and, no doubt, some dangerous failures. The basic problem is that natural substances tend to be found in complex mixtures, and at that epoch there were no sure means to determine the active ingredient and probably no way to isolate it. Even today, we still have only an incomplete understanding of human and microbial biochemistry. Many western drugs have been discovered essentially by accident, probably the best-known example being that of penicillin. Some turn out to be useful, but not at all for the purpose for which they were intended (Viagra).

Organic chemists made an important step forward, first by showing how it was possible to isolate and purify the active ingredient in a natural product, how to determine its molecular structure, and then how to modify that structure to retain the sought-after therapeutic function with the minimum of undesirable side effects—aspirin is a case in point. Instrumental techniques, such as X-ray crystal-lography, infrared spectroscopy, mass spectrometry and high-resolution NMR, rendered structure determination relatively straightforward, allowing the molecular features responsible for drug action to be identified. This was the golden age of medicinal chemistry.

16.1 Screening procedures

But the complexity of human biochemistry remains a stumbling block. New drugs are slow to be discovered. It is usually quite impossible to predict theoretically the molecular structure of a substance that would be effective for a particular disease. The needs of the medical profession (and the appetite of the pharmaceutical industry) are not satisfied, and biochemists are forced to fall back on trial-and-error methods yet again. These involve the 'screening' of a very large number (sometimes called a 'library') of chemical substances in a search for possible drug activity, choosing the most promising candidates, and then examining these in more detail with regard to efficacy and absence of side effects. If a substance is only eliminated late in the screening procedure this makes the search very expensive, so the aim is to drop most candidates at an early stage. The danger is that, just occasionally, a potentially useful drug can be overlooked.

This is not quite as mindless an exercise as it might first appear. The chemist has a wealth of ideas about the structures of possible drugs but lacks the time to perfect the necessary synthetic procedures. Instead of sitting down and trying to devise the best route to the synthesis of a desired product, the synthetic chemist now takes an automated approach, referred to as 'combinatorial chemistry'. This is a powerful method for generating large numbers of structurally diverse compounds.[1]

One approach employs solid-phase synthesis—polymer beads (for example, a styrene-divinylbenzene gel) are anchored to an organic reactant by a variable length molecular 'tether'. In a suitable medium (such as cyclohexane or dioxane) the polymer beads swell, generating spaces where 'solid-phase reactions' are facilitated.[2,3] The gel-phase sample is a slurry, neither a solid nor a true liquid, and direct NMR measurements are complicated by line broadening caused by the heterogeneity of the sample and differences in magnetic susceptibility (§ 6.2). This is more serious for protons than for nuclei with a wide chemical shift range, like carbon-13, fluorine-19 or phosphorus-31. Magic angle spinning (§ 10.2) can generate high-resolution spectra by removing the effects of internal magnetic susceptibility differences and dipole–dipole interactions (§ 10.1). The magic angle spinning probe is derived from those used for solid-state NMR, but spinning rates are lower (1 to 3 kHz) and particular care is taken with all materials in the non-spinning part of the probe in order to minimize local discontinuities in magnetic susceptibility. These devices can achieve linewidths of only a few Hz. An alternative approach employs chemical methods to separate the desired product from the resin beads, and then acquires a conventional high-resolution NMR in the liquid phase. In favorable circumstances, cleavage of the substrate from a *single* bead as small as 90 micrometres in diameter can yield enough material to record an acceptable high-resolution NMR spectrum.[4]

A second approach employs solution-phase reactions.[1] Suitable reagents, for example cyclic anhydrides and primary amines, are mixed under a series of different conditions and a small quantity of each product is collected. Automatic NMR sample changers, controlling a sequence of conventional 5 mm spinning-sample tubes, can be used to investigate the high-resolution NMR spectra of the large number of products generated by combinatorial methods. However, this operation is not immune to mechanical problems, such as sample tube breakage or failure to spin the sample. A neutral bystander can derive a certain perverse amusement from the sight of a robotic device doggedly dropping two or more sample tubes into the same probe at the same time. Each time a sample is changed the system must automatically reacquire a signal for locking the magnetic field, and then readjust the field inhomogeneity.

In practice, a higher throughput can be achieved by automated flow-injection systems adapted from existing hyphenated liquid chromatography-NMR methodology.[5] Typically the individual samples, each having a slightly different structure, would be collected on a plastic 'microtitre' plate containing 96 small open 'wells'. The NMR probe is modified to accommodate an automated flow system instead of individual sample tubes. Normally the flow is discontinuous; a predetermined small 'slug' of the analyte is pumped from one of the wells on the microtitre plate into the flow probe, and the NMR spectrum acquired while the slug remains stationary, so that good sensitivity and resolution are achieved. Then the flow is restarted, flushing out this sample with pure solvent before the next slug of analyte arrives (Figure 16.1). A compromise is reached between the throughput rate and the permitted degree of contamination from the previous sample. Cost considerations favour protonated rather than deuterated solvents, and standard solvent suppression techniques (§ 3.6) are used. As the physical properties of the successive samples tend to be very similar throughout the run, retuning of the receiver coil and readjustment of the field homogeneity are usually not required; the entire process runs without operator intervention. High-resolution spectra are generated at a typical rate of one every two to five minutes.

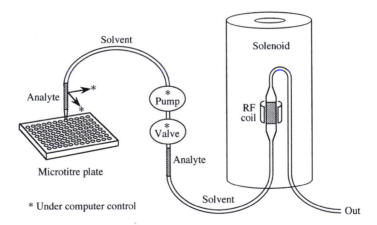

Figure 16.1 Schematic diagram of a flow-injection NMR spectrometer adapted for screening a series of samples prepared by combinatorial chemistry. A robotic device selects a 'slug' of analyte from the microtitre plate, and this is pumped into the flow cell. In order to achieve high resolution and good sensitivity the flow is temporarily interrupted while the transient NMR signal is being detected. The analyte is then flushed out by pure solvent to make way for the next sample in the pipeline. Not drawn to scale.

Samples generated by combinatorial chemistry, like those of human body fluids (§ 15.1), are often complex mixtures and may require some form of separation into their basic components. High performance liquid chromatography (HPLC) is one approach, and many investigations now rely on a flow system where the eluent from the HPLC column is fed into an NMR flow-injection probe, similar to the scheme sketched in Figure 16.1. The inherently low sensitivity of these hyphenated techniques should improve considerably with the development of miniaturized radiofrequency probes and cryogenic receiver coils. Diffusion-ordered spectroscopy (DOSY) can also be applied to the same problem, separating the NMR spectra of the components of a mixture in a second frequency dimension (§ 11.12).

The high rate of acquisition of NMR spectra from combinatorial chemistry can cause a bottleneck at the interpretation stage that follows. It is advantageous to have software programs that identify the products by comparing their spectra with a library of known chemical shifts and (possibly) coupling constants. The fit need not be exact; indeed the method requires only a binary decision—whether a particular spectrum represents a promising product or not. Data reduction offers an alternative approach. Each experimental NMR spectrum is stripped down into a much simpler form, for example a display of proton chemical shifts without spin multiplet structure (§ 11.11), or a set of integrals of the NMR intensities in predetermined regions of the spectrum. The reduced spectra of mixtures can be handled as linear combinations of the reduced spectra of the pure components, held in a library. This is an application where the conventional NMR spectrum is far too rich in information for the purpose of choosing the 'best' product from a large set of related compounds.

It seems a pity that the economics of this mode of drug discovery have forced the medicinal chemist to abdicate his classical creative role—inventing a model for drug action, imagining a likely molecular structure for a potential drug and then devising a suitable synthesis. This only emphasizes the importance of obtaining a far deeper understanding of human biochemistry, in the hope that, one day, each disease will be treated with its own specific 'magic bullet' based on rational drug design, with trial-and-error methods only used for fine-tuning the final drug.

16.2 Design strategies

Fortunately there are still many scientists pursuing the goal of rational drug design. This line of biochemical research has acquired the name 'molecular recognition' and it focuses on the interaction of a small ligand molecule (the potential drug) with a target receptor (usually a protein). The idea is to study the association of the ligand at a particular binding site on the protein, using X-ray crystallography or high-resolution NMR methods to evaluate of the three-dimensional structure of the complex. The NMR results provide structural constraints which, when combined with molecular dynamics calculations, establish the structure. The presumption is that once we understand the specificity of the drug-receptor interaction, we might be able to establish a logical strategy to design the most effective drug.

One key parameter is the affinity of the drug for the protein. Weak binding allows the small ligand molecule to jump on and off the protein very rapidly, corresponding to the limit of fast chemical exchange (§ 7.8). A nuclear spin on the ligand exhibits only a single NMR response at the weighted mean of the 'free' and 'bound' chemical shifts. In this fast exchange case the 'averaged' ligand signals are broadened because they have contributions to their line widths from the bound state where the ligand motion is greatly restricted.

On the other hand, strong binding of the ligand to the protein corresponds to the case of slow chemical exchange (§ 7.8). The ligand spends so much time in either the free or the bound state before an exchange event occurs that we see two separate NMR responses. If an excess of the ligand is used, saturation transfer experiments (§ 7.8) may be useful for assigning the bound signals, provided that the exchange is sufficiently rapid in comparison with spin–spin relaxation. The changes in NMR intensity are most evident when displayed in a difference mode where the selectively saturated spectrum is subtracted from a non-saturated control spectrum. This method of detecting binding is simple to implement in a screening experiment and can give detectable results for as little as one-millionth of a mole of protein.

A related magnetization transfer approach uses the 'transferred nuclear Overhauser effect' to enhance signals on the ligand bound to the protein. This works best under fast exchange conditions, but can also operate under the slow exchange conditions described above. In screening experiments, the transferred nuclear Overhauser enhancement can be used to pinpoint the active component in a mixture of several potential drug molecules.

Suppose a potential drug candidate has been discovered that binds to a particular site on the protein. The information about the location of the binding site and the binding affinity may then be used to suggest improved ligand molecules, and these can then be synthesized and tested by NMR methods of the kind outlined above. Even weak binding can be detected by observing the perturbations of the proton and nitrogen-15 chemical shifts of the protein. Once a suitable candidate has been identified, an excess of the ligand is used to fully occupy the binding site so that further experiments can be run to try to discover a second ligand that binds to an adjacent site on the protein. If this search is successful, the first and second ligands are then chemically joined by an appropriate synthesis with a view to creating a new composite molecule that binds at both sites and has an enhanced affinity for the protein. This type of research exploits the power of the screening method and at the same time reinstates the authority of the biochemist.[6]

16.3 Molecular recognition

These ideas can be illustrated by the extensive research carried out on a particularly well-defined system involving drugs used in the treatment of certain childhood leukaemias and bacterial infections.[7] The 'target' is a cellular enzyme (a small protein) called dihydrofolate reductase which catalyses the conversion of folate and dihydrofolate to tetrahydrofolate. The latter product is an important precursor in the biosynthesis of purines and pyrimidines. Among the possible 'antifolate' drugs are methotrexate (anti-cancer), trimethoprim (anti-bacterial) and pyrimethamine (anti-malarial), and they act by inhibiting the action of the enzyme in invasive cells. For example, trimethoprim selectively inhibits the enzyme in bacterial cells by up to four orders of magnitude more than that in normal mammalian cells. This work on inhibitors of purine and pyrimidine metabolism was highlighted by the award of the 1988 Nobel Prize for physiology and medicine.

X-ray crystallography and NMR spectroscopy have been used to establish the structures of many of the complexes of dihydrofolate reductase, providing the basic groundwork for molecular modelling calculations on related complexes. However, NMR has the advantage that it can study molecular structures in the physiologically relevant aqueous state, and these could differ from the solid-state structures. NMR is also well suited to the investigation of the specificity and dynamics of the protein-ligand interaction. Assignment of the NMR spectra of these complexes employs multidimensional spectroscopy (§ 11.7) of dihydrofolate reductase uniformly labelled with carbon-13 and nitrogen-15, bound to ligands either with or without specific isotopic labelling. The proton spectra can be 'edited' according to the isotopic labelling, providing the essential assignments needed to interpret cross-relaxation measurements obtained by the NOESY technique (§ 11.4). The resulting changes in signal intensities can be interpreted in terms of distances between protons on the ligand and protons on the protein, establishing intimate details of the structure of the binding site.

Apart from the obvious medical significance of studying the action of drugs used to treat cancer, malaria or bacterial infections, these investigations of the binding of dihydrofolate reductase to small molecules serve as a useful model for drug-receptor interactions in general. Not only is it possible to investigate specific interactions between the enzymes and their substrates and inhibitors, but one can also study the multiple conformations of these complexes, and measure the rates of chemical exchange. This new science of molecular recognition should eventually form a rational basis for drug design.

Further reading

'Special Issue on Intelligent Drug Design', *Nature* (Supplement), **384**, 1 (1996).

M. J. Shapiro and J. S. Gounarides, 'NMR Methods Utilized in Combinatorial Chemistry Research', *Progress in NMR Spectroscopy*, **35**, 153 (1999).

17

Functional imaging of the brain

Historically, our knowledge about the structure of the brain and the function of its various regions was largely obtained by autopsy after the death of patients who had suffered a stroke or who had sustained brain damage as a result of an accident. Of course animal experiments have provided many important insights into brain structure and function, but human behaviour and human capabilities in language, abstract thinking, mathematics, etc. cannot be studied in animals. For human beings, magnetic resonance has provided one of the first truly non-invasive methods for exploring the brain.[1-3] Functional magnetic resonance imaging of the brain (fMRI) aims to pinpoint those regions of the brain that 'light up' as a consequence of some physical or mental stimulus—often visual, auditory, or tactile.

In the simplest implementation of functional imaging, two successive maps of the brain are acquired; the first detects the effect of the stimulus and the second acts as a control so that a 'difference image' can be displayed. NMR intensities in the key regions of this difference map are temporarily enhanced by the stimulus and are often displayed as bright yellow or orange pixels superimposed on a conventional grey-scale map of the brain. Usually these bright features appear in the regions of grey matter in the brain rather than in the white matter. The bright pixels can be as small as 0.5×0.5 mm, so the stimulated regions can be precisely located.

At first sight these observations seem to suggest a simple phenomenon, but the deeper one delves into the mechanism the more complicated it appears to be. In fact the processes that change the local MRI signal intensities in the brain image are complex and time-dependent. To some extent they are also influenced by the intensity of the applied magnetic field used in the experiment—usually 1.5 tesla, but as high as 4 tesla or even 7 tesla in some recent experimental investigations. Further evidence for complexity is the surprising observation that if the time-domain resolution of the experiment is high enough, the NMR signal intensity initially goes *negative* before changing sign to become positive again at later times. To begin to understand these strange phenomena we first need to outline some of the physiology of the vasculature of the brain.

17.1 Blood flow

In articles about magnetic resonance imaging of the human brain, we shall see many references to the term 'perfusion'. Perfusion is the process by which blood delivers oxygen and nutrients to tissue at the capillary level, and also carries away by-products. Oxygenated blood arrives through an artery, which divides into several narrower arterioles, which in turn split up into much smaller diameter capillaries where the perfusion takes place. In the capillaries, some of the oxygen leaves the blood and is utilized by the surrounding tissue. The partially deoxygen-ated blood is carried away in the capillaries which then merge into venules (or venuoles) which in turn join together to form the veins. The mean diameter of capillaries is approximately 5 microns (millionths of a metre), whereas the venules have diameters up to 20 microns, and the veins are 500 microns or larger. Capil-laries in the brain are fairly uniformly distributed and are separated from one another by distances of the order of 50 microns. Perfusion represents a macro-scopic movement of blood and the motion is therefore considerably faster than the process of *diffusion* (§ 9.4) which proceeds by random displacements on a molecular scale.

The rate of perfusion of blood is an important measure of the viability of the tissue involved, offering a key clinical diagnostic of both disease and also brain activity. Cerebral blood flow on the macroscopic scale can be monitored by a 'tagging' technique where the spin states of the nuclei are used as an innocuous label. For example, in a rather crude experiment a second radiofrequency coil around the neck of the patient can be used to invert the spin populations of the protons in the blood flowing to the brain. When these inverted spins reach the brain, they partly cancels the normal NMR response, reducing the detected signal intensity, giving a 'dark blood' image from the flowing blood. The intensity loss can be related to the blood flow rate.

This type of macrovascular flow is not really germane to our discussion; it is more important for our purpose to measure the effect of *changes* in blood flow in the *capillaries* as a result of brain activity. Two successive brain images are meas-ured—one corresponding to the 'stimulus' and the other to the 'control'. In the presence of an applied magnetic field gradient (typically in the axial direction) nuclear spin populations are inverted by a frequency-selective 180° radiofrequency pulse that affects a chosen slice through the brain (§ 12.3). In the absence of any blood flow, these inverted spins would recover quite slowly by spin–lattice relaxation (T_1) but if 'fresh' blood flows into the slice, some inverted nuclear spins are replaced by new spins that have not been inverted, thus increasing the intensity of the signal detected at some later time. A second (control) measurement is then made in which the 180° pulse is non-selective, inverting nuclear spin populations throughout the sample and generating an image from the chosen slice that is unaffected by blood flow. The difference between the stimulus and control images highlights those regions of the brain where the blood flow has increased as a result of neural activity. The increased inflow of fresh, polarized nuclear spins partially cancels the effect of inverted spins in the voxels under investigation (§ 12.10). In favorable circumstances the change can be measured quantitatively in terms of millilitres of blood supplied to one gram of brain tissue per minute.

When brain imaging is performed one slice at a time, and if the pulse sequence induces some partial saturation, then increased local blood flow into the neurologically active regions of the slice causes an increase in NMR signal for those particular pixels. This mechanism would provide a neat (even glib) explanation for the 'lighting up' of the active areas of the brain, but in fact blood flow is only one factor in a far more complex story. This can be established by repeating these same measurements at a sufficiently low pulse repetition rate that complete spin–lattice relaxation occurs between consecutive excitations; this particular inflow effect is then excluded.

17.2 Blood oxygen

The level of blood oxygenation must also be considered. Whole blood contains about 40 % of red blood cells which contain the haemoglobin; white blood cells make up less than 1 % of the blood and can be neglected for these purposes. Arterial blood is oxygenated and has about the same magnetic susceptibility (§ 6.3) as the surrounding tissue. In this form it causes little or no distortion of the magnetic field at the boundaries between the blood vessels and brain tissue itself. This situation changes dramatically when the red blood cells give up oxygen.

Neural activity requires energy, which is generated by metabolizing glucose in a sequence of reactions that eventually yield carbon dioxide and lactate. The main glycolysis pathway involves oxidation, and this oxygen is derived from haemoglobin found in the red blood cells. Brain activity uses up oxygen and converts haemoglobin into deoxyhaemoglobin, which is a paramagnetic substance, that is to say, it concentrates the magnetic lines of force, thus generating a local non-uniform magnetic field within and around the blood vessels. This additional magnetic field in the vicinity of a particular capillary varies with distance from that blood vessel, causing local magnetic field *gradients* that are strong in proximity to the blood vessels carrying the deoxyhaemoglobin, but diminish with distance.

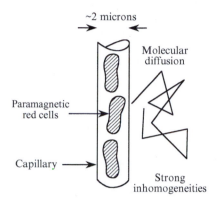

Diffusion of water molecules through these regions induces a random dephasing of the NMR signals, shortening the spin–spin relaxation time so that a spin echo refocused by a 180° pulse loses intensity irreversibly (§ 12.12). This is sometimes called 'dynamic averaging'. If a T_2-weighted image (§ 12.9) is recorded, it shows a decrease in NMR signal intensity in these regions.

But a decrease in signal intensity is *not* what is observed! The usual functional MRI response is positive. It turns out that neural activity also increases the cerebral blood flow and thus overcompensates for the consumption of oxygen, leading to a *lower* deoxyhaemoglobin concentration in the red blood cells. There is a natural mechanism that dilates the capillaries and thereby increases the flow of blood. So there is less induced paramagnetism, and the observed NMR signal *increases* with increased brain activity. The technique has been named BOLD (blood oxygen level dependent) contrast.

But this is not the whole story. Experiments conducted with high resolution in the time domain (using relatively large voxels to maintain acceptable sensitivity) indicate that the well-documented *positive* NMR response described above is in fact preceded by an earlier *negative* dip in the signal. So, after all, the rate of production of deoxyhaemoglobin does in fact rise soon after the stimulus, causing local magnetic field inhomogeneities and signal loss by dynamic averaging, but is soon swamped by a rush of blood that dilutes the deoxyhaemoglobin concentration again, leading to the strong positive magnetic resonance response reported in most functional MRI studies. Typically the deoxyhaemoglobin concentration peaks at about 3 seconds after the initial stimulus, and this delay seems quite reproducible. These observations confirm there are at least two main physical phenomena at play, conversion of haemoglobin to deoxyhaemoglobin and increased perfusion, operating in competition.

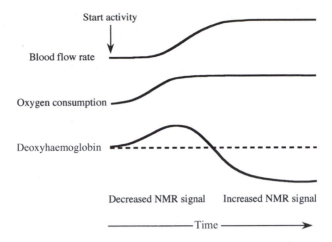

In a sense, the deoxygenated blood acts as a natural contrast agent that shortens T_2 but its effect is progressively negated as the natural control mechanism arranges for an increase in blood supply.

17.3 Pinpointing the response

It is claimed that the early negative fMRI signal is spatially more specific than the later positive response. This is important because it suggests that signal enhancement caused by the increased blood flow may have spread to regions of the brain beyond the initial site of the activation, thereby falsifying attempts to pin down the location of the neural event. One would then conclude that the early surge in oxygen consumption is more intimately related to neural activity than the later increase in blood flow. However, to date the majority functional MRI studies of the brain have concentrated on the main effect—the *increase* in signal intensity due to enhanced blood perfusion.

A BOLD investigation starts with the acquisition of a high-resolution anatomical MRI scan so that the later functional magnetic resonance images can be related to known anatomical 'landmarks' in the brain. Given the complexity of BOLD mechanism and the fact that the blood in question is moving, it is important to establish whether the spatial location of the observed magnetic resonance response does indeed correspond to the actual site of the neural activity. Macroscopic blood flow in venules or veins can give misleading fMRI results because of signal enhancement due to in-flow effects, combined with the more spatially extensive magnetic field distortions caused by larger blood vessels. These effects may highlight voxels at some distance from the true site of the neural activity. Note that spatial resolution of less than a millimetre can be achieved in fMRI maps, with a slice thickness of the order of 1 to 3 mm. To help minimize these unwanted complications from the veins and venules it is preferable to have the BOLD response dominated by changes in and around the capillaries, which are distributed in a rather uniform manner throughout the brain tissue. This should ensure that the fMRI response is in very good registration with the actual brain activity.

There is a way to achieve this important discrimination. For the larger blood vessels the variation in the magnetic field caused by deoxyhaemoglobin extends over larger distances where the (short-range) molecular diffusion has only a small effect. In these more distant regions the magnetic resonance signal is predominantly attenuated by the distortion of the magnetic field, which causes individual 'spin isochromats' to get out of phase with one another. The resulting loss of the macroscopic signal shows up best on T_2^*-weighted images obtained with the gradient-recalled echo sequence (§ 9.2). This effect is sometimes called 'static averaging' to distinguish it from the 'dynamic averaging' caused by haphazard molecular diffusion. With increasing blood vessel diameter there is a gradual progression from dynamic to static averaging. To be sure of good spatial specificity, we seek to emphasize the contribution from dynamic averaging at the expense of static averaging in order to minimize the influence of the larger blood vessels. This entails detecting the diffusion effect with T_2-weighted images obtained by the Carr–Purcell spin echo method (§ 9.3).

Unfortunately the functional MRI response of a T_2-weighted image is intrinsically rather weak, but it improves quadratically as the strength of the main magnetic field is increased. Consequently, a spin echo experiment with a relatively long delay (TE) before the echo, and carried out at 4 tesla or, better still, 7 tesla, does indeed emphasize the response arising from the capillaries, and largely excludes the influence of large blood vessels. In this manner we concentrate on the behaviour in brain tissue around the capillaries, arguing that this represents the actual site of the primary neural response.

When these precautions are taken, the transient magnetic resonance responses do indeed pinpoint the sites of increased neural activity. The voxel area within a slice can be as small as $0.5 \times 0.5\,mm$ and misregistration by flow effects can be neglected. Further progress may be anticipated when the spatial and temporal resolution of the technique are improved, but already functional MRI has provided some quite fascinating insights into the way the brain operates.

Of course the ability to focus attention on a very small activated region of the brain becomes useless if there is any physical displacement of the head during the measurement. Understandably, functional imaging is highly sensitive to head movement, and physical restraints may be required, backed up by a motion correction algorithm. The problem is mitigated when echo planar imaging (§ 12.7) is employed because a complete image can then be acquired in a time as short as 50 milliseconds, thus reducing the residual effects of head movement. This is particularly important for head scans of young children.

17.4 Time-scale

The 'snapshot' mode is important for the study of event-related fMRI, where the patient is presented with a task and the subsequent fMRI signal is detected. At low magnetic fields (1.5 tesla) the attainable signal-to-noise ratio is usually so poor that it is necessary to make several successive measurements and combine the results (§ 5.6). At higher magnetic fields (4 or 7 tesla) the sensitivity is high enough to permit the functional MRI response to be measured *in a single shot*, so that possible variations attributable to the subject (learning, mistakes, habituation) are not obscured by time averaging.

It is important to remember that functional MRI does not detect the brain activity directly; it is only a secondary indicator of neural events. One disappointing consequence is that the development of the fMRI response is quite slow, of the order of several seconds, whereas the time-scale on which neurons fire is much faster (milliseconds). In this aspect, fMRI compares unfavorably with the electroencephalograph (EEG) which can pinpoint neural events with a precision of a thousandth of a second. Fortunately, the time-lag between neural activation and the maximum change in blood flow is quite reproducible, varying by less than half a second. Furthermore, although the response is delayed, in some circumstances fMRI can detect the effects of an external stimulus lasting only as long as a tenth of a second.

To a certain extent the time-lag problem can be circumvented by devising a more sophisticated experiment. Suppose we have identified the location in a rat's brain that is activated during tactile stimulation of the left paw, and have also identified a different region that responds to stimulation of the right paw. If the left-paw stimulus is applied, and then, after a short delay τ, the right-paw stimulus, an interesting interference effect is observed. When we plot the second fMRI response as a function of the delay τ, we see a graph of the following general form:

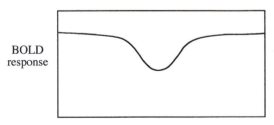

BOLD response

Delay τ (milliseconds)

Somehow, at a particular value of the delay, the effect of the first stimulus partially suppresses the response to the second. The dip in the BOLD response appears at a delay of about 50 milliseconds, which is interpreted as the time taken for information to travel between the two activated sites in the rat brain. This is clearly a function of the distance between the two sites. We might conclude that, for this type of activity at least, there is some advantage in possessing a physically small brain.

We should always bear in mind the fact that an fMRI response is the difference between two large quantities, the magnetic resonance signal elicited after some stimulus and that detected during the control scan. What is measured is only a small *change* in neural activity, something of the order of a few per cent of the total. This means that experiments to test perception or cognitive functions must be carefully designed so as to avoid any possible interference effects. Fortunately, results show that the method is reproducible and reliable when properly set up.

17.5 Degenerative brain disease

As life expectancy increases, we are forced to face up to the increasing problem of mental decline in the elderly. Alzheimer's disease, an age-related brain disorder, progresses gradually and inexorably; it leads to loss of memory, behavioural and personality changes, and a decline in the ability to think clearly. It presents a major health-care challenge which is increasing as the population ages, and it puts heavy psychological burdens on those who have to care for an elderly relative.

Although Alzheimer's disease has received a great deal of attention, there are other factors responsible for progressive mental impairment, such as stress, hormonal changes, or simply decreased blood supply to the brain. The problem is to distinguish these other cases of mental decline from those attributable to Alzheimer's disease; then the appropriate therapies can be used. The detection of certain brain metabolites by single-voxel MRS offers one possibility that has already been mentioned (§ 14.4). Another is the more conventional form of MRI, which can be used to measure the size of various structures in the brain and thus detect, for example, the shrinkage of the hippocampus that occurs in the early stages of Alzheimer's disease.

Functional MRI may also be able to make an important contribution. By monitoring the specific regions of the brain that are activated during cognitive functions such as learning, memorizing, recalling and reasoning, one might hope to identify the early changes in the brain that herald the onset of the disease. More importantly, if we could pinpoint one specific location in the brain where the first deterioration occurs, there might be a possibility of finding a treatment to slow the progression of this illness. There is evidence (unrelated to MRI) that the physical changes characteristic of Alzheimer's disease begin in the entorhinal cortex, spread to other parts of the hippocampus, and then progress to the temporal cortex, parietal cortex and frontal cortex.

In a study by Dr Scott A. Small[4] a group of non-demented elderly subjects with mild cognitive decline was examined by functional MRI. These subjects were compared with an age-related control group with a normal memory function. The results seemed to divide the experimental group into two different subsets, each with a distinctly different pattern of changes within the hippocampus. The first subset of patients had changes in the entorhinal cortex that appeared to be indistinguishable from those of patients with clinically diagnosed Alzheimer's disease. Patients in the other subset exhibited changes to the subiculum, a different region of the hippocampus, but had a normal entorhinal cortex. This appears to offer a new way to identify potential 'Alzheimer patients' at an early stage of cognitive decline. By tracking the progress of those with the dysfunction of the entorhinal cortex to see if they eventually develop Alzheimer's disease, the investigators hope to establish that functional MRI can indeed serve as an early indicator of susceptibility to the disease. The method relies heavily on the very fine spatial resolution that can be achieved by MRI.

17.6 How does the brain work?

The focus now switches to healthy subjects, with a view to studying 'normal' mental processes of all kinds. There have been many measurements designed to test the visual, auditory or motor functions of the brain, using flashing lights, various sounds, or tactile stimuli. More sophisticated experiments explore a cognitive task, for example a 'mental rotation test' involving two computer-generated images. These represent three-dimensional objects that are either identical or are related as mirror images, and one is rotated in space with respect to the other. The subject examines the two images, decides whether or not they are mirror images and then presses the YES or NO button. As expected, the subject's response time seems to depend on the relative rotation angle between the two images.

The opportunities to exploit functional imaging of the brain appear to be endless. One study gives an explanation for that long-standing conundrum. 'Why is it impossible to tickle oneself?' In a manner similar to the interference observed in the rat's paw experiment outlined above, the site in the brain involved in initiating the tickling stimulus appears to 'warn' a distinctly different site to expect the tickling sensation, and thereby negates the effect.

Just recently the world's press reported a study on aircrew that repeatedly fly long-haul east-west routes with only short rest periods between flights. One very disturbing finding, over and above the expected jet-lag, was an apparent reduction in size of their temporal lobes. In addition, a cognitive fMRI study established that these subjects performed poorly on a short-term visual memory test. One tongue-in-cheek newspaper headline read: 'This is the captain speaking. Er, where are we going?'

On a more serious level, magnetic resonance offers an unprecedented opportunity to probe the functioning of the human mind. Cognitive neuroscience employs fMRI simply as a tool, concentrating more on the design of the experimental protocol to extract new insights into how the brain works. For example, if it can be shown that a well-defined region of the brain responds specifically and selectively to a particular type of image (say the human face) then it can be argued that there is a special purpose mechanism for the perception of faces, rather than a general purpose algorithm for the processing of images. Kanwisher et al.[5] have carefully explored this idea, demonstrating that a specific region of the ventral occipito-temporal cortex called the *fusiform face area* is involved in the recognition of images of the human face. Functional magnetic resonance images of 6 mm near-coronal slices were obtained at a magnetic field of 3 tesla, using echo planar imaging (§ 12.7) and a bilateral surface coil (§ 14.3) to improve sensitivity for the chosen region of the brain. Averaged over all 'active' voxels, the strongest fMRI response represented 2 % of the 'resting' baseline signal, and was delayed by between 4 and 6 seconds after the stimulus. While this is a relatively small change in the total MRI signal, it could be reliably detected with adequate signal-to-noise ratio in a single shot, that is to say, without multiscan averaging.

The stimuli were grey-scale photographs or drawings representing head-only, full-body, and body-only images of humans and animals. A benchmark maximum response was elicited from full-face photographs, while pictures of inanimate objects acted as the minimum stimulus. The volunteer subjects were given two tasks—passive viewing of an image and a 'repeated image' test where they were asked to press a button whenever they saw two identical pictures in a row. Standard reordering and data analysis techniques were employed. The strongest responses (2 %) were to images of the human face, weaker responses were obtained from human heads (1.7 %), whole human bodies (1.5 %), and animal heads (1.3 %).

These researchers conclude that the fusiform face area of the brain responds selectively to faces, not merely to anything human or animate. The response to the back of the human head (with no face visible) was very low. Animal heads and whole animals produced a fairly strong response, supporting earlier findings of a strong response to cat faces, but this might be expected because human and animal faces have many features in common. Although the response to images of animals was slightly stronger than that to images of inanimate objects, this was no longer true when the animal faces were obscured. Faces are special. One could speculate about possible evolutionary reasons for this finding.

An even more exciting question arises when we consider mental imagery. Is there a functional magnetic resonance response when we conjure up an image 'in our mind's eye' and if so, is it as strong as the response from the actual image? O'Craven and Kanwisher[6] attacked this question by comparing fMRI responses from the fusiform face area to those from the ventromedial cortical region called the *parahippocampal place area* which responds strongly and selectively to images of scenes. This comparison study was designed to circumvent the difficulty in establishing a baseline level for mental imagery; it is hard to 'make your mind a blank'. To test perception, the subjects were shown photographs of the faces of famous people and familiar scenes from the campus of the Massachusetts Institute of Technology. To test mental imagery, they closed their eyes and heard the names of the people and places they had seen during the corresponding perception runs. Now it is known that individuals vary considerably in their ability to create a mental image, so it is not surprising that the results were not conclusive for all the subjects tested. Nevertheless, seven out of eight subjects exhibited activation from imagery of local scenes in the region of the brain that also 'lit up' during the perception test for these same scenes, and four of the eight subjects tested for mental imagery of faces showed activation in the region associated with direct perception of faces. One way to quantify these effects is to set a 'significance threshold' for the detected signal and count the number of voxels that show a response above this threshold. Most of the voxels activated during mental imagery fell within the region activated for direct perception (92 % for places; 84 % for faces).

One interesting finding from these experiments was that the magnitude of the magnetic resonance excitation was lower during the mental imagery tests than during the direct perception runs. This is consistent with the widely-held expectation that actual images provide a more vivid stimulus than imagination, although it might have been argued that forming a 'mind's eye' picture imposes heavier demands on the mental processing and should therefore yield a *stronger* response.

In his novel *Nineteen Eighty-Four*, George Orwell's hero maintained that 'Big Brother' would never be able to monitor what went on inside a person's skull, so absolute control by the state was not possible[7]. Kanwisher's findings appear to represent the first step along a path that may contradicts Orwell's comforting proposition. The magnetic resonance responses at 3 tesla had a sufficiently high signal-to-noise ratio in one measurement to detect a single mental 'event'. No repetition was required for multiscan averaging (§ 5.6), and there was no need to combine results from different subjects. Without any external stimulus, a pure act of will can create a mental image with a detectable fMRI response. At the very least this should alert us to the possibility of constructing a virtually fool-proof lie detector, and perhaps some future scheme for mind control, however alarming as this prospect may seem.

Permissions

I am grateful to the following for permission to reproduce diagrams:

Academic Press Inc. for Figure 11.2 from F. Del Rio-Portilla and R. Freeman, *J. Magn. Reson.* A. **108**, 124 (1994); Figure 11.4 from E. Kupče and R. Freeman, *J. Magn. Reson.* A. **105**, 234 (1993); Figure 11.8 from T. H. Mareci and R. Freeman, *J. Magn. Reson.* **48**, 158 (1982); Figure 11.9 from M. H. Levitt and R. Freeman, *J. Magn. Reson.* **34**, 675 (1979); Figure 11.10 from M. Woodley and R. Freeman, *J. Magn. Reson.* A. **109**, 103 (1994); Figure 11.11 from H. Barjat, G. A. Morris, S. Smart, A. G. Swanson and S. C. R. Williams *J. Magn. Reson.* B. **108**, 170 (1995); Figure 14.3 from S. Blüml, *J. Magn. Reson.* **136**, 219 (1999).

The American Chemical Society for Figure 15.1 adapted from J. K. Nicholson, et al., *Anal Chem.* **67**, 793 (1995).

Peter Barker for the unpublished images and spectra in Figures 12.6, 12.7, 12.8, 12.11, and 14.10.

General Electric Medical Systems for the photographs in Figures 2.2 and 3.3.

Laurie Hall for the image in Figure 12.12.

Toshiaki Nishida for the unpublished spectra in Figures 8.1, 8.2, 11.3, 11.5, and 11.7.

Pergamon Press for the spectra in Figure 15.3 from J. K. Nicholson and I. D. Wilson, *Progress in NMR Spectroscopy*, **21**, 449 (1989).

Brian Ross for the spectrum in Figure 14.1 and the scatter plot in Figure 14.2.

Taylor and Francis for the spectra in Figure 15.2 adapted from J. K. Nicholson, et al., *Xenobiotica*, **29**, 1181 (1999).

References

Chapter 1

1. E. M. Purcell, H. C. Torrey and R. V. Pound, *Phys. Rev.* **69**, 37 (1946).
2. F. Bloch, W. W. Hansen and M. E. Packard, *Phys. Rev.* **69**, 127 (1946).
3. W. G. Proctor, *Phys. Rev.* **77**, 717 (1950).
4. W. C. Dickenson. *Phys. Rev.* **77**, 736 (1950).
5. G. Lindstrom, *Phys. Rev.* **78**, 817 (1950).
6. H. A. Thomas, *Phys. Rev.* **80**, 901 (1950).
7. J. T. Arnold, S. S. Dharmatti and M. E. Packard, *J. Chem. Phys.* **19**, 507 (1951).
8. J. Larmor, *Philos. Mag.* **44**, 503 (1897).
9. H. S. Gutowsky and C. J. Hoffman, *Phys. Rev.* **80**, 110 (1950).

Chapter 2

1. F. A. Nelson and H. E. Weaver, *Science*, **146**, 3641 (1964).
2. F. Bloch, *Phys. Rev.* **102**, 104 (1956).
3. C. J. Bauer, R. Freeman, T. Frenkiel, J. Keeler and A. J. Shaka, *J. Magn. Reson.* **58**, 442 (1984).
4. H. Geen and R. Freeman, *J. Magn. Reson.* **93**, 93 (1991).
5. J. Baum, R. Tycko and A. Pines, *Phys. Rev. A.* **32**, 3435 (1985).
6. E. Kupče and R. Freeman, *J. Magn. Reson. A.* **115**, 273 (1995).

Chapter 3

1. N. V. Bloembergen and R. V. Pound, *Phys. Rev.* **95**, 8 (1954).
2. P. Styles, N. F. Soffe, C. A. Scott, D. A. Cragg, F. Row, D. J. White, and P. C. J. White, *J. Magn. Reson.* **60**, 397 (1984).
3. W. A. Anderson, W. W. Brey, A. L. Brooke, B. Cole, K. A. Delin, J. F. Fuks, H. D. W. Hill, M. E. Johanson, V. Y. Kotsubo, R. Nast, R. S. Withers, and W. H. Wong, *Bull. Magn. Reson.* **17**, 98 (1995).
4. C. E. Hayes, W. A. Edelstein, J. F. Schenck, O. M. Mueller and M. Eash, *J. Magn. Reson.* **63**, 622 (1985).
5. A. G. Redfield and R. K. Gupta, *Adv. Magn. Reson.* **5**, 81 (1971).
6. H. S. Black, *Modulation Theory*, Van Nostrand, Princeton, New Jersey (1953).
7. J. W. Cooley and J. W. Tukey, *Math. Comput.* **19**, 297 (1965).

Chapter 4

1. E. L. Hahn, *Phys. Rev.* **76**, 145 (1949).
2. R. L. Vold, J. S. Waugh, M. P. Klein and D. E. Phelps, *J. Chem. Phys.* **48**, 3831 (1968).
3. A. W. Overhauser, *Phys. Rev.* **92**, 411 (1953).
4. T. R. Carver and C. P. Slichter, *Phys. Rev.* **92**, 212 (1953).
5. R. Damadian, *Science* **171**, 1151 (1971).

Chapter 5

1. T. A. Barbara, *J. Magn. Reson. A.* **109**, 265 (1994).
2. D. L. Olson, T. L. Peck, A. G. Webb, R. L. Magin, and J. V. Sweedler, *Science*, **270**, 1967 (1995).
3. S. Sibisi, J. Skilling, R. G. Brereton, E. D. Laue, and J. Staunton, *Nature*, **311**, 466 (1984).
4. G. A. Morris, *J. Magn. Reson.* **80**, 547 (1988).
5. R. N. Bracewell, *The Fourier Transform and its Applications*, McGraw-Hill, New York (1986).
6. R. R. Ernst and W. A. Anderson, *Rev. Sci. Instr.* **37**, 93 (1966).
7. J. C. Leawoods, D. A. Yablonskiy, B. Saam, D. S. Gierada and M. S. Conradi, *Concept. Magnetic Reson.* **13**, 277 (2001).

Chapter 6

1. J. T. Arnold, S. S. Dharmatti, and M. E. Packard, *J. Chem. Phys.* **19**, 507 (1951).
2. J. T. Arnold, *Phys. Rev.* **102**, 136 (1956).
3. F. Bloch, *Phys. Rev.* **94**, 496 (1954).
4. L. Axel and L. Dougherty, *Radiology*, **171**, 841 (1989).

Chapter 7

1. N. F. Ramsey, *Phys. Rev.* **78**, 699 (1950).
2. R. Freeman, G. R. Murray and R. E. Richards, *Proc. Roy. Soc. A.* **242**, 455 (1957).
3. J. D. Roberts, *ABC's of FT NMR*, University Science Books, Sausalito, California (2000).
4. E. D. Becker, *High Resolution NMR: Theory and Chemical Applications*, Academic Press, New York (2000).
5. A. D. Buckingham, T. Schaefer and W. G. Schneider, *J. Chem. Phys.* **32**, 1227 (1960).
6. C. C. Hinkley, *J. Amer. Chem. Soc.* **91**, 5160 (1969).
7. J. K. M. Sanders and D. H. Williams, *Chem. Commun.* 422 (1970).
8. G. M. Whitesides and D. W. Lewis, *J. Amer. Chem. Soc.* **92**, 6979 (1970).
9. S. Forsén and R. A. Hoffman, *J. Chem. Phys.* **39**, 2892 (1963).

Chapter 8

1. M. Karplus, *J. Chem. Phys.* **30**, 11 (1959).
2. M. H. Levitt and R. Freeman, *J. Magn. Reson.* **33**, 473 (1979).
3. A. J. Shaka, J. Keeler and R. Freeman, *J. Magn. Reson.* **53**, 313 (1983).
4. M. H. Levitt, R. Freeman and T. Frenkiel, *J. Magn. Reson.* **47**, 328 (1982).
5. E. Kupče and R. Freeman, *J. Magn. Reson. A.* **115**, 273 (1995).

Chapter 9

1. E. L. Hahn, *Phys. Rev.* **80**, 580 (1950).
2. A. Abragam, *The Principles of Nuclear Magnetism*, Clarendon Press, Oxford (1961).
3. H. Y. Carr and E. M. Purcell, *Phys. Rev.* **94**, 630 (1954).
4. E. O. Stejskal and J. E. Tanner, *J. Chem. Phys.* **42**, 288 (1965).
5. E. L. Hahn and D. E. Maxwell, *Phys. Rev.* **88**, 1070 (1952).
6. S. Meiboom and D. Gill, *Rev. Sci. Instr.* **29**, 688 (1958).
7. M. H. Levitt and R. Freeman, *J. Magn. Reson.* **43**, 65 (1981).

Chapter 10

1. G. E. Pake, *J. Chem. Phys.* **16**, 327 (1948).
2. E. R. Andrew, A. Bradbury and R. G. Eades, *Nature* (London) **182**, 1659 (1958).
3. J. S. Waugh, L. M. Huber and U. Haeberlen, *Phys. Rev. Lett.* **20**, 180 (1968).
4. S. R. Hartmann and E. L. Hahn, *Phys. Rev.* **128**, 2042 (1962).
5. N. Tjandra and A. Bax, *Science* **278**, 1111, (1997).
6. G. Drobny, A. Pines, S. Sinton, D. P. Weitekamp and D. Wemmer, *Faraday Symp. Chem. Soc. (London)* **13**, 49 (1979).

Chapter 11

1. W. P. Aue, E. Bartholdi and R. R. Ernst, *J. Chem. Phys.* **64**, 2229 (1976).
2. J. Jeener, Ampère International Summer School, Basko Polje (1971) and published in *NMR and More: In Honour of Anatole Abragam*, eds. M. Goldman and M. Porneuf, Les Editions de Physique, Les Ulis, France, (1994).
3. J. Jeener, B. H. Meier, P. Bachmann and R. R. Ernst, *J. Chem. Phys.* **71**, 4546 (1979).
4. B. D. Ross, G. K. Radda, D. G. Gadian, G. Rocker, M. Esiri and J. Falconer-Smith, *New England Journal of Medicine*, **304**, 1338 (1981).
5. A. W. Overhauser, *Phys. Rev.* **92**, 411 (1953).
6. A. Bax and R. Freeman, *J. Magn. Reson.* **44**, 542 (1981).
7. F. Del-Rio Portilla and R. Freeman, *J. Magn. Reson. A.* **108**, 124 (1994).
8. S. R. Hartmann and E. L. Hahn, *Phys. Rev.* **128**, 2042 (1962).
9. L. Braunschweiler and R. R. Ernst, *J. Magn. Reson.* **53**, 521 (1983).
10. G. A. Morris and R. Freeman, *J. Amer. Chem. Soc.* **101**, 760 (1979).
11. T. H. Mareci and R. Freeman, *J. Magn. Reson.* **48**, 158 (1982).
12. M. H. Levitt and R. Freeman, *J. Magn. Reson.* **34**, 675 (1979).
13. M. Woodley and R. Freeman, *J. Magn. Reson. A.* **109**, 103 (1994).
14. C. S. Johnson Jr., *Prog. Nucl. Magn. Reson. Spectrosc.* **34**, 203 (1999).
15. E. O. Stejskal and J. E. Tanner, *J. Chem. Phys.* **42**, 288 (1965).
16. K. F. Morris, P. Stilbs and C. S. Johnson, *Anal. Chem.* **66**, 211 (1994).
17. S. J. Gibbs and C. S. Johnson, *J. Magn. Reson.* **93**, 393 (1991).
18. G. A. Morris, *J. Magn. Reson.* **80**, 547 (1988).
19. H. Barjat, G. A. Morris, S. Smart, A. G. Swanson and S. C. R. Williams, *J. Magn. Reson. B.* **108**, 170 (1995).

Chapter 12

1. P. C. Lauterbur, *Nature* (London) **242**, 190 (1973).
2. R. Damadian, *Science* **171**, 1151 (1971).
3. W. A. Edelstein, J. M. S. Hutchinson, G. Johnson and T. Redpath, *Phys. Med. Biol.* **25**, 751 (1980).
4. D. I. Hoult, *J. Magn. Reson.* **26**, 165 (1977).
5. A. Kumar, D. Welti and R. R. Ernst, *J. Magn. Reson.* **18**, 69 (1975).
6. A. N. Garroway, P. K. Grannell and P. Mansfield, *J. Phys. C.* **7**, L457 (1974).
7. P. Mansfield, *J. Phys. C.* **10**, L55 (1977).

8. M. Doyle, B. Chapman, R. Turner, R. J. Ordidge, M. Cawley, R. Coxon, P. Glover, R. E. Coupland, G. K. Morris, B. S. Worthington and P. Mansfield, *Lancet* **2**, 682 (1986).
9. R. Freeman and H. D. W. Hill, *J. Chem. Phys.* **54**, 3367 (1971).
10. P. T. Callaghan, 'Rheo-NMR: Nuclear Magnetic Resonance and the Rheology of Complex Fluids', *Rep. Prog. Phys.* **62**, 599 (1999).

Chapter 13

1. F. G. Shellock and J. V. Crues, *Radiology*, **167**, 809 (1986).
2. F. G. Shellock, B. Rothman and D. Sarti, *Am. J. Roentgenol.* **154**, 1229 (1990).
3. F. S. Prato, K. P. Ossenkopp, M. Kavaliers, et al., *Magn. Reson. Imaging*, **5**, 9 (1987).
4. N. Prasad, L. T. Kosnik and K. H. Taber, *Society of Magnetic Resonance in Medicine*, Book of Abstracts, Berkeley, California, **1**, 275 (1990).

Chapter 14

1. D. I. Hoult, S. J. W. Busby, D. G. Gadian, G. K. Radda, R. E. Richards and P. J. Seeley, *Nature* (London) **252**, 285 (1974).
2. J. J. H. Ackerman, T. H. Grove, G. G. Wong, D. G. Gadian and G. K. Radda, *Nature* (London) **283**, 167 (1980).
3. S. Blüml, *J. Magn. Reson.* **136**, 219 (1999).
4. R. J. Ordidge, A. Connelly and J. A. B. Lohman, *J. Magn. Reson.* **66**, 283 (1986).
5. P. A. Bottomley, *Ann. N. Y. Acad. Sci.* **508**, 333 (1987).
6. J. Frahm, K. D. Mehrboldt and W. Hanicke, *J. Magn. Reson.* **72**, 502 (1987).
7. T. R. Brown, B. M. Kincaid and K. Ugurbil, *Proc. Natl. Acad. Sci. USA* **79**, 3523 (1982).

Chapter 15

1. J. K. Nicholson, P. J. D. Foxall, M. Spraul, R. D. Farrant and J. C. Lindon, *Anal. Chem.* **67**, 793 (1995).
2. E. T. Fossel, J. M. Carr and J. McDonagh, *New Engl. J. Med.* **315**, 1369 (1986).
3. J. K. Nicholson, J. C. Lindon and E. Holmes, *Xenobiotica* **29**, 1181 (1999).
4. K. P. R. Gartland, S. M. Sanins, J. K. Nicholson, B. C. Sweatman, C. R. Beddell, and J. C. Lindon, *NMR in Biomed.* **3**, 166 (1990).
5. F. Y. K. Ghauri, J. K. Nicholson, B. C. Sweatman, C. R. Beddell, and J. C. Lindon, *NMR in Biomed.* **6**, 163 (1993).
6. J. P. Shockcor, S. E. Unger, I. D. Wilson, P. J. D. Foxall, J. K. Nicholson and J. C. Lindon, *Anal. Chem.* **68**, 4431 (1996).
7. J. R. Bales, P. J. Sadler, J. K. Nicholson and J. A. Timbrell, *Clin. Chem.* **30**, 1631 (1984).
8. J. R. Bales, J. K. Nicholson and P. J. Sadler, *Clin. Chem.* **31**, 757 (1985).

Chapter 16

1. P. A. Keifer, *Drug Future*, **23**, 301 (1998).
2. H. Sterlicht, G. L. Kenyon, E. L. Packer and J. Sinclair, *J. Am. Chem. Soc.* **93**, 199 (1971).
3. J. I. Crowley and H. Rapoport, *Acc. Chem. Res.* **9**, 135 (1976).

4. S. K. Sarkar, R. S. Garigipati, J. L. Adams and P. A. Keifer, *J. Am. Chem. Soc.* **118**, 2305 (1996).
5. P. A. Keifer, S. H. Smallcombe, E. H. Williams, K. A. Salomon, G. Mendez, J. L. Belletire and C. D. Moore, *J. Comb. Chem.* **2**, 151 (2000).
6. S. B. Shuker, P. J. Hajduk, R. P. Meadows and S. W. Fesik, *Science*, **274**, 1531 (1996).
7. J. Feeney, *Angewandte Chemie* (International Edition) **39**, 290 (2000).

Chapter 17

1. S. Ogawa, T-M. Lee, A. S. Nayak and P. Glynn, *Magn. Reson. Med.* **14**, 68 (1990).
2. S. Ogawa, D. W. Tank, R. Menon, et al. *P. Natl. Acad. Sci. USA*, **89**, 5951 (1992).
3. P. A. Bandinetti, E. C. Wong, R. S. Hinks, R. S. Tikofsky and J. S. Hyde, *Magn. Reson. Med.* **25**, 390 (1992).
4. Reported by K. DeMott, *Clin. Psychiat. News*, **27**, 5 (1999). Se also: S. A. Small, G. M. Perera, R. DeLaPaz, R. Mayeux, and Y. Stern, *Ann. Neurol.* **45**, 466 (1999); S. A. Small, E. X. Wu, D. Bartsch, G. M. Perera, C. O. Lacefield, R. DeLaPaz, R. Mayeux, Y. Stern and E. R. Kandel, *Neuron*, **28**, 653 (2000).
5. N. Kanwisher, D. Stanley and A. Harris, *NeuroReport*, **10**, 183 (1999).
6. K. M. O'Craven and N. Kanwisher, *J. Cogn. Neurosci.* **12**, 1013 (2000).
7. George Orwell, *Nineteen Eighty-Four*, Secker and Warburg, New York (1949).

Index

Page numbers in **bold** indicate main sections

Berkshire County
Metropolitan
Library

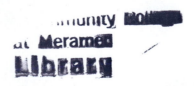
...munity Co...
at Meramec
Library